THE
ATHLETIC
WOMAN'S
SOURCEBOOK

THE
ATHLETIC
WOMAN'S
SOURCEBOOK

How to Stay Healthy and Competitive in Any Sport

JANIS GRAHAM

Foreword by Lisa R. Callahan, M.D.

AN AVON BOOK

With love and thanks to my brother John,
who inspired me to get to the starting line
and is always there to see me at the finish.

THE ATHLETIC WOMAN'S SOURCEBOOK is not intended as a substitute for medical advice from your physician. Always consult your doctor before beginning any new regimen that can impact your health. The author and publisher disclaim any liability arising directly or indirectly from the use of this book.

AVON BOOKS, INC.
1350 Avenue of the Americas
New York, New York 10019

Copyright © 1999 by Janis Graham
Cover illustration by Liz Kenyon
Inside back cover author photo by Lewis McClellan
Published by arrangement with the author
ISBN: 0-380-79667-8
Library of Congress Catalog Card Number: 99-94871
www.avonbooks.com/wholecare

First Wholecare Trade Printing: August 1999

WHOLECARE TRADEMARK REG. U.S. PAT. OFF. AND IN OTHER COUNTRIES, MARCA REGIS-
TRADA, HECHO EN U.S.A.

Printed in the U.S.A.

OPM   10   9   8   7   6   5   4   3   2   1

Contents

Foreword

Historically, the athletic field has belonged to men. Since the early years of the Olympics, when the mere *presence* of women at an athletic competition was discouraged, women have struggled for equal playing time. Today, however, the years in which women were forced to yield the ball, the field, the court to their male colleagues are all but gone. Wistful yearning on the sidelines has given way to an explosion of interest in women's sports, with record numbers of women participating in athletics, from the recreational athlete to the competitive one.

Sports participation bestows benefits upon girls and women of all ages. Studies show that girls who participate in sports are more likely to graduate from high school, have good self-esteem, and avoid teen pregnancy. As they age, girls and women who participate in regular exercise reap tremendous health rewards. Studies have long concluded that regular physical activity helps to decrease the risk of heart disease, which remains the number-one killer of women. Current research shows that many of the diseases with a high prevalence in women—osteoporosis, depression, breast cancer, diabetes, hypertension, and obesity—can be improved or possibly avoided altogether by exercise.

As a physician who specializes in the care of active and athletic women, I continue to be impressed that women who exercise display superior levels of energy and vitality, as well as better general health than women who are sedentary. We are at the dawning of a new understanding of women's health, wherein the best prescription your doctor may be able to give you is not for a pill, but for a soccer ball, pair of running shoes, or tennis racket!

But as women become more active, taking up a new (or old!) sport, there is a need for solid, up-to-date information to help maximize the benefits of exercise, while reducing the risk of illness or injury. That is why *The Athletic Woman's Sourcebook* is so valuable. It is filled with medically sound information and practical advice on a wide range of issues important to female athletes of all ages, in all sports. In both my personal experiences as an avid recreational athlete and my professional ones as a sports medicine specialist, I have seen women search, not always successfully, for the answers collected in this authoritative resource. Whether you read it cover to cover or use it as a reference book, you'll find it provides well-balanced insight and solutions to common problems that can help your next run be a little faster, your next throw a little more accurate, your next game a little more fun.

Play on, girls!

—Lisa R. Callahan, M.D.
Co-founder, Medical Director,
Women's Sports Medicine Center,
Hospital for Special Surgery,
New York

Introduction

This book is for any woman who loves being active and takes pleasure in engaging in her sport. You don't have to be an Olympic medalist, a national champion, or even feel all that comfortable about using the word *athlete* to describe yourself. But if you're dedicated to living an active life, this book is for you. It aims to provide answers to all those exercise-related health questions that crop up throughout a physically active woman's lifetime.

In Part One you'll find informed, practical advice from sports medicine experts in the fields of gynecology, dermatology, nutrition, obstetrics, psychology, podiatry, orthopedics, gerontology, and others. Throughout, news from the latest research and scientific studies has been carefully included.

There are solid solutions for minor exercise snafus, like gnarly black toenails, breast discomfort, and unintentional urine leaks, as well as information on how to overcome more major problems, like unusual fatigue or debilitating precompetition jitters. You'll find details on matching your diet to your activity level, exercising throughout your pregnancy, and staying active during menopause.

In Part Two there's a sport-by-sport resource that will guide you to new athletic challenges as it makes trying a new sport accessible and easy. You'll also hear the personal experiences of top athletes. There's the U.S. racquetball champion who finally found a remedy for her killer cramps; the first baseman on the 1996 gold-medal winning U.S. Olympic softball team who thinks the players' diet of plane food and candy bars compromised their performance; the Olympic gold-medal winning skier who battled a nervous breakdown to become competitive again; the U.S. women's bobsled team member who exercised harder throughout her pregnancy than most women who aren't expecting ever do; the winner of the prestigious Yachtsman of the Year award who would run off her boat to nurse her baby during breaks in competition; the Hall of Fame masters swimmer who has stayed strong and fast during menopause and beyond. These are just a few of the athletes who shared their stories with me.

Who am I? Besides my credentials as a health and medical journalist, I am a recreational runner and sometimes triathlete. I don't clock exceptional times and I will never wow the world with my sporting achievements. Still, I take my athletic pursuits seriously. I'm proud of the finisher medals (i.e., everybody who finishes the race gets one) I've earned in my marathon running and of the "best for my age group" trophies I've managed to win at local events.

My motivation for writing this book was personal. I've often sought advice on different exercise-related issues, but I haven't always found the information I needed. Before my first marathon, for example, I wanted to know what to expect if I got my period, I questioned whether I really needed to keep hydrated with sports drinks, and I wondered why, since I began training, my lips were suddenly chapped all the time. In the spirit of finding answers to all those questions as well as to the many others that female athletes of all caliber and from all sports have, this book was born.

May it help you stay out there, healthy and playing hard!
—Janis Graham

PART ONE

Your Active Health

I

YOUR MENSTRUAL CYCLE

Lisa Rainsberger of Colorado Springs, Colorado, age thirty-seven, winner of five major marathons, refused to be ambushed by her period. "I'll never forget it. I was set to defend my title at the 1989 Chicago Marathon—I had won the year before and there were a lot of competitors hungry to beat me. I got up the morning of the race to discover I had started my period. It was a blow, because my flow is always quite heavy the first few days."

Naturally, Rainsberger worried about how having her period might affect her ability to run 26.2 miles in top form. "But I had done all this training and I was really prepared and I just determined to not let it get in my way."

In fact, what most concerned Rainsberger was the color of her uniform. "I was being sponsored by New Balance, who had mandated I wear these pure white shorts. There's absolutely no time to stop and change a tampon when you're running hard to win. So all I could do was use a super tampon then pray 'please, please don't let me bleed all over the place during the race!'"

Rainsberger didn't leak, but she recalls "I did keep feeling wet, probably from sweating, and so whenever I would grab water off the water table, I would quickly glance down at my crotch to check. But even if I had started leaking, what could I have done? I know I would have run through it, then dealt with my embarrassment later."

In the end, Rainsberger's period didn't get in her way—

she won, bettering her time of the previous year by a minute (2 hours, 28 minutes, 15 seconds).

But for every athlete like Rainsberger who can overcome her symptoms of menstruation and go on to win (or simply get in a good workout) there's someone like twenty-seven-year-old Michelle Gould, the 1998 female World Champion in both professional and amateur racquetball. "I used to be completely useless when I had my period. My flow was really heavy and my cramps were so intense that I would have to take to my bed for at least two days. There was no way I could train during my period. Forget about competing!"

However, Gould eventually found a solution for her severe symptoms. She followed the advice of her doctor who recommended she try oral contraceptives. "If it hadn't been for the Pill, I seriously doubt I could have made it as far as I have in my sport. I simply would have been out of commission too much to be a top competitor," says Gould. "The Pill makes my periods much less intense, so that they are completely tolerable. Taking it also shortens the number of days in which I bleed and makes my flow lighter, which is absolutely fantastic."

The experiences of Gould and Rainsberger are as different as day and night, but together they make an important point: Whatever challenge your menstrual cycle presents you with, there's probably a strategy for dealing with it that doesn't compromise your athletic ambitions.

In this chapter, you'll find tactics for coping with a wide range of menstrual and gynecological concerns. Whether you're worried about heavy flow, severe PMS, bad bloating, urine leaks—or you're anxious because you've lost your periods—there are steps you can take to ease your problem and which don't require you to quit exercising or competing.

MONTHLY CRAMPS AND OTHER PAINS

Being active puts you one giant step ahead in the battle to reduce preperiod woes, according to most research. One study, from the University of British Columbia, Vancouver, found that six women who participated in a six-month running program of gradually increasing intensity experienced a significant decrease in overall premenstrual symptoms, especially breast tenderness and fluid retention, when compared to six inactive women.

Another larger study from the University of Arkansas, in which 968 members of the National Association of Girls and Women in Sport answered a questionnaire about their menstrual cycle, found that those who scored highest in activity—the "trained" group—also reported the least problems with pain, cramping, bloating, backaches, mood changes, breast tenderness, heavy flow, and headaches.

Still, the University of Arkansas study found that almost half of the "highly trained" women did experience some premenstrual symptoms, some of the time. In other words, exercise may help alleviate some symptoms, but it's not a cure-all, as any athlete who suffers from any of the monthly discomforts listed below knows.

Cramps. Why do we get them? As you get ready to bleed each month, the lining (called the endometrium) of your uterus produces prostaglandins, chemicals that encourage the uterine muscles to contract. These contracting muscles serve to close the blood vessels on the uterine wall, while simultaneously expelling menstrual blood out of the uterine cavity. It's believed that the higher your prostaglandin levels, the more prolonged and violent your uterine contractions and therefore the more painful your cramps. In addition, prostaglandins contribute to the gastrointestinal distress (nausea and diarrhea) and headaches that sometimes accompany cramps.

The trick, then, is to lower prostaglandin release. One way to do this is via a class of medicines called NSAIDs (nonsteroidal anti-inflammatory drugs). NSAIDs like ibuprofen (brand name Advil, Motrin, or Nuprin), naproxen sodium (brand name Aleve), and ketoprofen (brand name Actron, Orudis KT) actually block prostaglandin release from body tissues and thus prevent the cascade of events that cause menstrual cramps. These same drugs can also do wonders combating backaches and headaches; they are good at heading off the nausea and diarrhea that come with cramps too.

To get the best relief, however, you need to start taking these medicines before prostaglandin levels get high—i.e., the minute your period begins or you begin to feel the first hint of pain. Not only is it harder to curb cramps once they've begun, once prostaglandins get churned out they often trigger nausea and vomiting too, symptoms that can make it hard for you to keep medicines down.

NSAIDs can irritate your stomach so it's best to down your dose with a glass of milk or in conjunction with a meal. Road-test your tolerance, too: Take a dose, then do your normal work-out to make sure you don't suffer any adverse side effects—you don't want to run into unforeseen problems during a competition. It's also important to keep hydrated (drink a lot of liquids) when taking NSAIDs since that helps your kidneys me-tabolize the medicine. There's evidence that kidney function can be impaired by overexposure to NSAIDs. Signs of this impair-ment include swelling, a decreased output of urine, and a change in the color of your urine. In addition, anyone who has a chronic kidney condition, ulcers, or aspirin allergies should check with a doctor before using NSAIDs.

You might also want to try taking fish oil supplements, either in conjunction with NSAIDs or as an alternative. In a small study conducted at the Children's Hospital Medical Cen-ter in Cincinnati, Ohio, when forty-two adolescent girls who regularly experienced cramps began taking daily fish oil supple-ments (containing 1080 mg icosapentaenoic acid, 720 mg doco-sahexaenoic acid, and 1.5 mg Vitamin E), the majority reported feeling a "marked reduction" in cramps.

If all else fails, ask your doctor about the safety of upping the standard NSAID dose for two days during your cycle. If that doesn't work, ask about some of the stronger prescription drugs available. If your cramps are really terrible, you may need to consider taking the birth control pill too. Oral contra-ceptives (OCs) curtail the development of the endometrium, the uterine lining that produces prostaglandins. As a result, there are lower levels of prostaglandins and a decrease in cramps. Not all women, however, find that OCs completely erase

---

◓ Three Ways to Slow Your Menstrual Flow (So you don't leak during competition)

1. Take 800 mg of ibuprofen or other NSAIDs prior to the event
2. Try Instead or the Keeper—new diaphragmlike devices that can be worn twice as long as tampons.
3. Wear two tampons

cramps; some OC users may still need NSAIDs to manage their pain at times.

Heavy Flow. It's the day of an important competition and you're bleeding profusely—is there anything you can do, beyond just hoping you don't leak all over the place?

Some women are able to insert two tampons for extra assurance (others find it too uncomfortable); some rely on extra-absorbent sanitary napkins (others, like bikers and swimmers, find them impractical); and many athletes are testing out some new, innovative devices being marketed as alternatives to traditional tampons and pads.

One is a new diaphragmlike device called Instead, designed by a triathlete named Audrey Contente and produced by a company called Ultrafem, Inc. Basically it's a soft, nonlatex, disposable plastic cup that catches instead of absorbs menstrual flow. It can be worn twice as long as a tampon, for up to twelve hours (on a heavy flow day it would probably need to be changed within four to six hours). The cup sits below the cervix and is made of a heat-sensitive material that, once inserted, is supposed to conform to your internal shape to create a personal fit, thus preventing leakage. Lab studies performed by the company did not find that Instead promoted growth of the bacterium believed to cause most cases of the rare but potentially life-threatening disease, Toxic Shock Syndrome (TSS), but the product hasn't been used extensively enough to document the real TSS risk. Instead costs around $6 for a sixteen-pack, which means it costs about the same as tampons. (To get more information, call 800-INSTEAD).

Another new product, called The Keeper, is also worn internally. Unlike Instead, however, the Keeper, which is made of rubber, is reusable: when it's full, you use a tab that is attached to the bottom of the cup to remove it, dump its contents into the toilet, then wash it out with water before reinserting. The Keeper can hold an entire day's worth of fluids, although its manufacturers recommend you change it more often. It costs about $35, but can be reused for up to ten years. (For more information, call 800-500-0077).

In addition, anecdotal evidence suggests that ibuprofen and other NSAIDs can help reduce menstrual flow. "The dose that is most effective is 800 mgs, taken three times a day (2,400 mgs total). This dosage is frequently prescribed for women who are having problems with heavy flow, but since it is more than triple the standard recommended dosage, you should talk to your doctor about it first," advises Elizabeth Joy, M.D., assistant professor in the department of family and preventive medicine, University of Utah, Salt Lake City. Taking NSAIDs at this dose for one day is probably perfectly safe for most women and according to many doctors as well as women who have used NSAIDs, they can be quite effective at stanching your flow. However, taking this high dose for consecutive days could be risky to your kidneys and is a practice that should be avoided. So in addition to getting your doctor's okay, test your tolerance beforehand and be extra vigilant about staying hydrated to avoid straining and damaging your kidneys.

I know it sounds counterintuitive, but one of the best ways to fight bloating is to drink a lot of fluids.
—LISA R. CALLAHAN, M.D, MEDICAL DIRECTOR OF THE WOMEN'S SPORTS MEDICINE CENTER, NEW YORK

Bloating. In the University of Arkansas study, bloating was experienced by 85 percent of all the women, at least sometimes. Complaints about premenstrual bloating, in fact, seemed to cut across the issue of activity level, being almost equally common in the highly trained and inactive groups.

Preperiod bloating may be triggered by the high amounts of estrogen that circulate in the bloodstream in the week to ten days before the onset of menstruation. Estrogen binds salt and salt binds water, which could lead to water retention and swelling. Another theory is that the bloating is caused by the rise in progesterone that occurs premenstrually. Higher progesterone levels may blunt the action of hormones, such as aldosterone, which normally help the body rid itself of excess fluid.

But what can you do about bloating—that unpleasant sensation of abdominal fullness? Drink more water for starters, advises Lisa R. Callahan, M.D., a former competitive runner and medical director of the Women's Sports Medicine Center at the Hospital for Special Surgery, New York. "I know it sounds counterintuitive, but drinking fluids helps your kidneys flush excess salt from the body, plus stimulates them to process body fluids more efficiently." The standard advice to drink about eight 8-ounce glasses of water daily is a good place to start, although it may not be enough for active athletes, who lose a lot of fluids through sweating. If you're already drinking that much, try increasing your fluid intake even further to see if it helps.

In addition, some women find that cutting down on their intake of salt and limiting salty foods for at least a week before their periods is a good way to put the brakes on water retention. Studies haven't shown this is effective, though. In fact, there's some evidence to the contrary. A small study published in the *Annals of Internal Medicine*, in which thirteen women cut their sodium intake by 30 percent for two months, found that breast tenderness and bloating was not helped by sodium restriction.

Another tactic is to concentrate on eating more foods high in fiber, to promote the speedy passage of wastes from your digestive system: That helps counteract the tendency many women have in the days before their periods toward slower bowel activity, which can lead your abdomen to feel congested and "overstuffed." Things like artificial sweeteners (especially sorbitol), chewing gum, and drinking liquids through a straw are all notorious promoters of gastrointestinal gas and thus can aggravate your bloating, so it makes sense to avoid these things as much as possible too.

What about using diuretics, medicines that encourage your body to eliminate surplus water? Most doctors don't recommend them for women who are active. "Diuretics are, for the most part, a no-no in my opinion—they can make you feel less bloated, yes, but they can also dehydrate you and make you feel tired, washed out, and fatigued," says Dr. Callahan.

Dr. Joy voices a similar opinion: "Diuretics can cause an athletic woman to excrete too much potassium and put her at a higher risk for dehydration and electrolyte imbalances. That's why, as a general rule, I'm reluctant to prescribe them. Still, to every rule there are exceptions and I can think of circumstances in which diuretics might make sense. I know of one endurance athlete who has pretty significant bloating around her periods. She also happens to be a nurse who is very knowledgeable about medications. She uses half of a prescription diuretic tablet for about five days of her cycle, a dose that is quite safe, and she clearly derives a great benefit from it."

If you are considering using a diuretic, it's important to consult with your doctor to review the risks versus the rewards.

Your doctor can also make sure your bloating is caused by normal hormonal ups and downs, since bloating can also be caused by digestive problems, like lactose intolerance or irritable bowel syndrome.

Breast Tenderness. In the two weeks before your period, estrogen activates receptors in the glands of your breast, triggering growth and making your breasts feel heavy, achy, and sore. Your best defense against this is to wear a comfortable, supportive bra (see How to Choose a Sports Bra, page 119). In addition, try the tactics for combating bloating, described above, since they can help fight edema or swelling of your breasts.

Solutions for Combating Premenstrual Mood Swings
- Avoid excessive caffeine and alcohol.
- Get adequate calcium, magnesium, and zinc.
- Try herbal remedies (St. John's wort or evening primrose oil).
- Schedule a strenuous workout (to boost your endorphin levels).

Mood Swings. It's believed that mood swings are caused by changes in the brain's chemistry that occur in response to the monthly hormonal shifts of estrogen and progesterone. For instance, your levels of serotonin—a brain chemical linked to depression, fatigue, anxiety, and sleep disturbances—may become abnormally low premenstrually. In addition, your changing hormonal tides may also have an impact on your levels of endorphins—mood-lifting chemical compounds that are also released during exercise.

It's no wonder a common recommendation for combating premenstrual moodiness is to exercise. For women who already work out regularly, the best defense may be to push yourself just a little harder or further—that will ensure your endorphin levels get elevated, plus you'll get a psychological boost from knowing you went that extra little bit.

Other steps to keep your emotions on an even keel? Avoid excessive caffeine and alcohol intake since they can heighten feelings of jumpiness and can contribute to sleep problems. Studies have linked adequate consumption of calcium, magnesium, and zinc to fewer mood swings too. If you take a supplement, make sure it includes these minerals at dosages equal to (but not more than) 100 percent of the RDA (Recommended Daily Allowance). You won't get a benefit from taking more than the RDA, and you might even be harmed, since zinc, in particular, can be toxic in high doses.

Some preliminary studies suggest that St. John's wort, an herbal remedy available at health food stores, may help relieve mild to moderate premenstrual moodiness. A common dosage is 300 mgs taken three times a day, although no research has really established how much is enough or too much. So far, St. John's wort is not associated with any serious side effects.

Another popular, but unproven, herbal remedy is evening primrose oil, often sold in capsule form. It contains essential fatty acids that are purported to help regulate hormones and moderate prostaglandin output. A common dose is 1,000 mgs a day.

Another remedy, sold over the counter at pharmacies and supermarkets is the dietary supplement called PMS Escape—it's a flavored powder you mix with water to make a drink that contains dextrose (a sugar), various vitamins and minerals, and 47 g of carbohydrate. Developed by Judith Wurtman, Ph.D., a research scientist, the drink is based on studies that have suggested that carbohydrates can boost your mood by increasing serotonin and tryptophan levels in the brain. PMS Escape can be convenient, but many nutritionists doubt that it really offers a significant advantage over simply eating a carb-dense snack.

What about vitamin B_6, which has long been touted as a reliever of premenstrual depression and fatigue? The studies have not been consistent and you need to be wary of high doses, since B_6 can cause nerve damage if you take too much. However, Dr. Joy says that if nausea is also part of your constellation of symptoms you might get some relief from taking 25 mg of B_6 twice a day. "Since it has been proven to help with pregnancy-related morning sickness, it's likely to help with other hormone-related nausea. And at that dose, it's very safe."

Finally, if you are facing an important event, keep in mind that your irritability or moodiness may not be totally caused by your cycle. "I get very edgy, uptight, and sensitive before competition. If I also happen to be premenstrual, it is easy to blame my moods on my cycle when it is more of a problem of prerace jitters," says Lisa Rainsberger. She adds, "My husband says I get PMS, but it's not premenstrual syndrome, it's pre*marathon* syndrome."

Food Cravings. So why do you feel as if you can't live without chocolate—or that you'll die if you don't get some salty chips during the days before your period? Premenstrual rises in hormones (researchers aren't sure whether estrogen or progesterone is the main culprit) probably create bona fide cravings for sugar and other carbohydrates. In addition, your munchies may be related to an increase in your metabolic rate—in other words, your body may need more calories because its resting metabolic rate goes up before your period.

On the one hand, it's okay to indulge yourself a little. If you know a cookie will lift your mood right now, experts advise "don't deny yourself." If you do, it could backfire and lead you into an all-out binge. Obviously, bingeing is best to avoid for many reasons. First, your spirits aren't going to be much lifted if you start putting on pounds. Second, if you binge on salty items, it might exacerbate your bloating.

A better alternative is to make a conscious effort to eat smaller, healthier, more frequent meals. That way your hunger won't build and become uncontrollable. Also, some women find they benefit by eating a lot of low-fat carbohydrates like pasta, potatoes, and whole-grain breads. Several studies have linked carbohydrate consumption to an increase in the level of serotonin in the brain, and some researchers believe that premenstrual cravings for sweet, starchy foods are the body's attempt to combat moodiness and irritability by increasing serotonin levels.

COPING WITH SEVERE PMS SYMPTOMS

Given that some of the chemical changes that occur in the brain during premenstrual syndrome are nearly identical to those that occur during depression, it should come as no surprise that severe PMS is frequently treated with antidepressant medications. For example, in a 1997 study of two hundred women with extremely severe premenstrual symptoms (severe enough to disrupt job performance and personal relationships), 62 percent of the women treated with Zoloft showed "marked or much improvement" in symptoms, compared with 34 percent of patients who took a placebo, according to findings published in the *Journal of the American Medical Association* (*JAMA*).

Many women who experience depressed mood, anxiety, and mood swings premenstrually can derive benefits from using antidepressants such as Prozac or Zoloft for two weeks before every period. However, says Dr. Joy, "studies indicate that you would probably be helped more if you took the medication continuously for the entire month. Still, some women resist taking antidepressants daily because it makes them feel as if they have been diagnosed with depression when they are more comfortable with the diagnosis of PMS."

In addition, oral contraceptives (OCs) help about a third of the women who suffer from severe PMS (about a third find they feel worse, while the other third don't notice any change). In general, the best choice for PMS sufferers are OCs that are monophasic—ones that deliver the same amounts of estrogen and progesterone every single day (except for the days when you have your period). With monophasic OCs, your hormone levels are steady, which means your moods are more likely to be too.

DOES YOUR PERIOD AFFECT YOUR PERFORMANCE?

Coping is one thing, but what about successfully competing at "that time of month?" Are you stronger or weaker, faster or slower, depending on where you are in your menstrual cycle (for a refresher course on what happens during your cycle, see The Four Phases of Your Menstrual Cycle, page 38).

Medical researchers have long suspected the answer is yes—that changes in hormone levels over the course of a month might affect energy metabolism, muscle fiber strength, and oxygen utilization during exercise. For example, researchers have speculated that when a woman's estrogen levels are at their highest, she may have the potential to reach her peak in terms of endurance, because studies have demonstrated that estrogen has a positive effect on the storage and utilization of glycogen—the chief energy source for muscles during exercise.

But when you sift through the archives of studies, the ones that have found links between the menstrual cycle and athletic prowess have been less than definitive. In fact, the bulk of the research has found no significant differences in performance at different times of the cycle.

—〰〰〰—

You can't be a winning athlete if you take a week off every month because you're having a rough time with your period.
—LISA RAINSBERGER, WINNER OF FIVE MAJOR MARATHONS

—〰〰〰—

One of the more recent—and thorough—studies, for example, from the Department of Sport, Leisure, and Exercise Science at the University of Connecticut, in Storrs, involved sixteen women, ages eighteen to thirty-seven, who were running a minimum of thirty-five miles a week for at least a year. Half of the women had regular periods (they were *eumenorrheic*) at intervals of twenty-three to thirty-three days and half of the women hadn't menstruated for three or more months (they were *amenorrheic*).

The women with normal cycles gave urine samples regularly so that their hormone levels could be checked and their menstrual phase status accurately documented. Then, in the early follicular phase and the midluteal phase of their cycles, the women performed a series of exercise tests (and also had a series of blood samples drawn both before and after exercise). Some of the measures of endurance and performance that were tracked included VO_2max, the body's maximal capacity to take in, transport, and utilize oxygen; levels of plasma lactate—a measure of the capacity of the muscle to utilize oxygen; and how high the athletes themselves rated their perceived exertion.

Here's what the researchers found: First, there were no differences in exercise performance between the eumenorrheic and amenorrheic runners. In other words, the women who didn't get their periods did not gain any advantage from being free of normal hormonal fluctuations when compared to the runners who were menstruating regularly.

Second, there were no differences in aerobic capacity, heart rate, and other metabolic measures of performance during the different phases of their menstrual cycles within the group of women who were menstruating.

Similar findings came from a Canadian study. That study, conducted at the Allan McGavin Sports Medicine Centre at the University of British Columbia, Vancouver, looked at aerobic capacity, endurance performance, high-intensity running performance, and strength during the early follicular phase and the midluteal phase in sixteen regularly menstruating women, ages eighteen to forty.

As in the American study, the Canadian researchers found no cycle-related differences in endurance, intensity, or strength performance. However, the Canadian researchers did find that the athletes had slightly lower VO_2 max or aerobic capacity during the luteal phase of their cycle. Theoretically, this change in aerobic capacity could have meaningful implications for the athlete who competes at the elite level, where the difference between first and second place is often measured in fractions of seconds.

But the finding that aerobic capacity may be lowered during the luteal phase is still tentative. In fact, the researchers aren't sure if their finding is meaningful. As they explained, "given the limitations of the statistical analysis, and the ranges of equipment error in measurement, this change in aerobic capacity is of borderline statistical significance."

Of course, it's always possible that the performance of some women is more susceptible to the effects of hormonal ups and downs. Or that future research will uncover minor menstrual cycle–related differences in physiological responses to exercise. The big surprise is that many experts think that even if differences are found it doesn't necessarily follow that performance will be affected.

"There is a lot more to performance than just physiology," says Dr. Callahan. "One of the biggest variables in how well you perform is your mental attitude. As a lot of professional athletes will tell you, the only thing that sometimes makes the difference between them and the competitor in the next lane is mental attitude. In other words, if you think you are going to do great, you may do better than you physiologically should really expect to." (For more on the mind's impact on performance, see Chapter 4.)

In the same vein, if you don't think you can do well, chances are you won't. Which brings us to the crux of what many experts feel is the crucial link between menstrual status and performance: "Many women have been mentally conditioned to believe they can't do well when they're menstruating," says Dr. Callahan. "Remember when you were encouraged to get exempted from gym in high school simply because you had your period? The belief that you can't perform well during your period is often planted very early in a young girl's life."

Or, because you don't *feel* your best around period time, you may assume you can't *do* your best, thus setting up a self-fulfilling prophecy. No one ever said you would necessarily feel great while you performed well. Most of the research to date simply implies that if you wanted to put forth maximal effort— i.e., if you really wanted to overlook and override the fact that your breasts are achy and your belly bloated—physiologically there is probably no reason why you can't. Even though you may not feel tiptop, you may still be capable of doing great things athletically if you decide to make an all-out effort.

The experience of ski racer Hilary Lindh, twenty-nine, of Park City, Utah, the 1997 World downhill ski champion and 1992 Olympic medalist is telling. "It's funny, if I'm not busy, if it's a slow time for training and competition, it seems my period has more of an effect on me. I'll really notice being achy and I'll be a lot more bothered by my symptoms," she says. "But if it's an important time and I don't have the luxury to give in to my symptoms, I just don't. I hardly even notice them. I started my period the day of the World Championship in 1997 and it was my best performance ever. I don't think having my period has ever lowered my ability to compete well."

In fact, the most persuasive proof that there isn't one time of the month when most women are necessarily weakest or strongest is women like Lindh, who have set records and won competitions at all phases of their cycles—before, during, and after their periods.

If you think there's a chance you are prey to the myth that menstruation is incompatible with a great workout, the best way to learn if you are just as strong before or during your period is to try training at all times of the month. After all, competitive, menstruating athletes who don't take oral contraceptives (OCs) must learn to cope with hormonal ups and downs.

"You can't be a winning athlete if you take a week off every month because you're having a rough time with your period," notes Rainsberger. "You also can't control when events are scheduled—you need to be prepared to perform whether you have your period or not." Clearly, the more you train through every stage of your cycle, the more reassurance you'll feel that being premenstrual or having your period is not something that is going to make or break your performance.

◆ Five Reasons Athletes Like Oral Contraceptives (OCs)
1. You can plan when to have (and not have) your period.
2. You bleed less heavily, for fewer days.
3. You usually have less pain and cramping.
4. Your risk of anemia is reduced.
5. It's 99 percent effective as a form of birth control.

WHY THE PILL MAKES SENSE FOR SOME ATHLETES

"I used to have spotting and a period every two weeks. I never knew when I was going to begin to bleed and it was really frustrating," recalls thirty-year-old Diann Roffe-Steinrotter, winner of a 1994 Olympic Gold Medal and one of the top ski racers in the history of the sport. "Although I had heard lots of negative things about how oral contraceptives can make you gain weight and impair your performance, I decided to try them anyway because I was so uncomfortable with all the bleeding and cramps I was experiencing. I was desperate to regulate my cycle."

Getting their menstrual cycle to be normal and regular is just one of the reasons some athletes opt for oral contraceptives. Other reasons are these:

1. OCs are 99 percent effective as a form of birth control when used correctly. The peace of mind you get from using such an effective form of birth control is considerable: It means that doubts about whether your contraceptive worked don't get piled on top of anxieties you may be experiencing about an upcoming athletic event.

2. On OCs you bleed less, for fewer days, and have less pain and cramping. That's because OCs work by stopping ovulation; when you don't ovulate, there is less buildup of the uterine lining and less tissue that must be shed during menstruation. So you don't have to worry about heavy flow and leaking

as much during races or meets. The chance that you'll be incapacitated by cramps diminishes too.

3. OC use reduces your risk of iron-deficiency anemia (a decrease in the blood's oxygen-carrying red blood cells). Many endurance athletes, in particular, have a hard time keeping their iron stores up and use the Pill to help prevent problems with anemia.

4. When you take the Pill, you can plan not to have your period during important competitions. You can either stop taking your Pill about seven days early to prompt your period or extend the time you take hormones to delay its onset. However, experts recommend you only manipulate your periods for events of special importance. Although the practice doesn't appear to be harmful, constantly adjusting your Pill schedule might have an adverse effect on its contraceptive effectiveness.

In addition, the Pill also offers some nonathletic benefits. Recent medical research has shown that taking the Pill can reduce a woman's risk of ovarian cancer (a particularly deadly cancer) as well as protect her against cancer of the endometrium, the uterine lining (probably because there is less buildup of it each month). The Pill also cuts the risk of pelvic inflammatory disease, a sexually transmitted disease that is a major cause of infertility (since the Pill causes a thickening of cervical mucus, which makes it harder for infections to reach pelvic organs).

Scares about a long-term link between the Pill and breast cancer seem to have been largely laid to rest by a 1996 study published in the medical journal *Contraception*: For this study, a group of two hundred researchers brought together virtually all the studies ever done on the subject, representing 153,536 women from twenty-five countries, and found that there is no increased chance of being diagnosed with breast cancer ten to twenty years after stopping use of the Pill.

But the Pill does carry some serious health risks. Namely, women on the Pill are more likely to form blood clots in the deep veins of their legs. These clots can break off and travel to other organs, causing stroke, lung embolism, or even blindness if they travel to the eye. The risk of this happening is small for most healthy, nonsmoking women; the risk goes up for women over thirty-five who smoke, which is why the Pill should not be used by them.

Another potential health hazard of the Pill is that it may encourage the development of cervical cancer, a highly treatable form of cancer when detected early. The jury is still out about whether the Pill really is a factor in cervical cancer, but in the meantime, it is important that any woman who uses the Pill have yearly Pap tests.

Finally, a question that isn't completely settled is whether the Pill has an impact on athletic performance. Although most studies have found the Pill has no impact, one study, by Constance Lebrun, M.D., a sports medicine researcher at the University of Western Ontario, found a slight lowering of VO_2 max (your body's maximum oxygen consumption) in Pill users. But even Dr. Lebrun is reluctant to make sweeping conclusions from this research, given how small the study was and how wide the variety of different combinations of hormones and choices of OCs is. Still, there does remain the remote possibility that certain types of OCs may have a slightly negative effect on aerobic capacity in elite-level athletes.

Of course, for every athlete who finds the Pill is the answer to her menstrual difficulties and/or her contraception needs, there is one who finds it doesn't agree with her. "I tried all different kinds, of the most minimum dosages possible, but while I was on them I just cried all the time; they made me very depressed," recalls professional triathlete Sue Latshaw, thirty-six, of Boulder, Colorado, winner of the 1997 Ironman Germany and a three-time top finisher at the Hawaii Ironman World Championships. "I also tried using oral contraceptives to interrupt my menstrual cycle so it wouldn't interfere with an event and I ended up not doing well at that event. I don't know if it was because I screwed around with my hormones or if I just wasn't fated to do well that day. But I've found that I just don't like the way the Pill takes away my natural cycle. I like to be able to feel what is happening in my body."

Besides depression, other side effects sometimes associated with OC use include breast tenderness, more frequent headaches, and water retention, especially in the fingers and ankles. Some Pill users also experience nausea or light spotting and staining between periods, although these symptoms usually diminish after a few months. The pill also has a (undeserved) reputation for promoting weight gain, but the most weight you would add from today's low-dose pills is probably three pounds from water retention.

If you're considering taking the Pill, you may want to ask your doctor about taking a monophasic pill, which delivers the same amount of progesterone and estrogen in each daily pill, rather than a triphasic pill, in which hormone levels delivered by the each pill vary over the course of the month. "If an athlete ever intends to manipulate her period using the Pill, then a monophasic pill is preferable," notes Dr. Joy. "Also, if you are taking the Pill as a way to even out menstrual cycle–related moodiness or bloating, you may find you do better on a monophasic pill."

BEYOND THE PILL

"Although taking the Pill was an improvement, I still had a lot of problems because of how often I had to travel across different time zones. Especially when I was zigzagging back and forth to Europe, losing or gaining six hours each day I flew, I found it very hard to figure out when to take a pill. And because I was having such a hard time keeping on schedule, I still experienced some spotting," recalls Roffe-Steinrotter.

Interestingly, the solution that finally worked for her is one many experts wouldn't recommend: injections of the contraceptive Depo-Provera. Says Dr. Joy, "I don't like to prescribe it because it's often associated with significant weight gain—up to fifteen pounds—which can be completely intolerable for an athlete."

Says Roffe-Steinrotter: "Depo-Provera has been the perfect solution to my problems with my period. I haven't had any bad side effects, no weight gain or bloating, maybe because I am so active. I am absolutely content with it."

The bottom line, as Roffe-Steinrotter's story illustrates, is that there is no one right contraceptive choice for every athlete. Here, then, is a quick look at some birth control options other than the pill and how they might have an impact on your athletic endeavors. (For details on the full spectrum of benefits, drawbacks, risks, and side effects of the various methods, a good source is *The Birth Control Book* by Samuel A. Pasquale, M.D., and Jennifer Cadoff, (Ballantine Books, 1996). A helpful feature of this book is that it explains and highlights why someone is—and isn't—a good candidate for each method.

Diaphragms/Cervical Caps

How They Work: a soft, natural latex rubber device inserted into the vagina blocks sperm from entering the uterus and tubes, while spermicide held in the bowl of the device provides additional protection by killing sperm around the cervix.

Effectiveness: 82 to 96 percent

Pros: There is no tampering with your body's chemistry, which is important to some athletes who feel strongly about keeping in touch and in tune with their body's natural rhythms. Since no hormones are involved, there is no potential for side effects like bloating, headaches, or weight gain.

Cons: The diaphragm must be kept in for six hours after intercourse and the cervical cap for eight hours, so if you have intercourse in the morning you'll need to train with the device in place. Since spermicides sometimes seep out, you may also have to wear a panty liner. However, there is no evidence to indicate that being physically active with the diaphragm or cervical cap in place compromises the effectiveness of either device. Both the diaphragm and cervical cap may increase the risk of urinary tract infection because they exert pressure against the urethra.

Female Condom

How It Works: it lines the vagina, creating a physical barrier so that sperm cannot enter the reproductive tract.

Effectiveness: about 85 percent

Pros: It does not interfere with your menstrual cycle or your hormones and involves no use of chemical agents, so it is completely natural. It should be removed immediately after intercourse—a plus since it means you never have to contend with it in place during training or competition.

Protects against sexually transmitted diseases (STDs), including HIV, the virus that causes AIDS (the only protection that is more effective is avoiding sex altogether). This disease-blocking protection can provide tremendous peace of mind and shouldn't be undervalued—after all, how could you possibly perform your best if you were worried about having placed yourself at risk for AIDS?

Cons: Some women experience irritation on the outside of their vagina from the outer ring of the condom. This can make it uncomfortable to wear snug workout clothes (such as biking shorts, running tights, or close-fitting bathing suit) after using the device.

Male Condom

How It Works: A thin, latex sheath made to be worn over the penis, it captures ejaculated sperm, thus preventing it from entering the vagina.

Effectiveness: up to 90 percent if used with a spermicide; 70 percent if used without a spermicide

Pros: It doesn't effect hormone levels or the menstrual cycle. Like the female version, it protects against STDs, including HIV. Since the condom is worn by the man, there isn't any device left inside you that you must contend with during training.

Cons: Almost none, in terms of your exercise goals.

Intrauterine Device (IUD)

How It works: It is not known exactly how pregnancy is prevented by an IUD, a small T-shaped device approximately 1 inch wide that is inserted into your uterus by a physician. It may work by interfering with the sperm's ability to move freely and gain access to the egg and/or it may trigger an inflammatory response in your uterine lining, which prevents a fertilized egg from implanting.

Effectiveness: 98 percent

Pros: It's convenient—once inserted, you don't need to remember to use it—you can forget about it until it's time for your physician to remove it. The type of IUD most widely used by women in the United States can be left in place for up to ten years.

Cons: It can increase your menstrual bleeding, spotting, and cramping as well as increase the chances you'll become anemic, all of which can interfere with your training. Also, young, childless athletes are not candidates for an IUD since it may increase the risk of pelvic inflammatory disease (PID), which can cause infertility. IUDs are designed primarily for women in monogomous relationships who have already had children.

Norplant

How It Works: Six toothpick-size rods containing the pregnancy-preventing hormone progestin are inserted under the skin on the inside of your upper arm. Once in place, the rods slowly and steadily release progestin for five years.

Effectiveness: up to 99 percent

Pros: You don't need to take pills, which can be challenging to schedule if you travel across time zones frequently. Your periods may be less painful and lighter.

Cons: In athletic women with low body fat and good upper body muscle tone, the rods may be quite visible. Breakthrough and irregular bleeding are common, which can be a nuisance. Many women stop having periods altogether when using this hormone-based method, which could be positive, in terms of sheer convenience. It could also turn out to be negative, since amenorrhea may be linked to a decrease in bone density, which could increase your risk of broken bones currently and osteoporosis, brittle-bone disease, later in life. At this point, it isn't known if Norplant use leads to lower bone density.

Depo-Provera

How It Works: Works like Norplant, except the progestin is delivered via injection and lasts only three months.

Effectiveness: 97 percent

Pros: Same as Norplant, with the additional benefit that there is no device visible (in other words, no one needs to know about it). It's more easily reversible too, since you can just stop going in for your shots (instead of having to go to a doctor's office to have the rods removed) if you decide you don't like the effect it is having on your body.

Cons: Irregular bleeding is common; some women stop bleeding altogether, which as noted with Norplant, could be a health risk. Headaches, nausea, and acne and skin problems are reported up to 20 percent of the time. Also, weight gain seems to be a bigger issue with Depo-Provera than with Norplant or oral contraceptives. According to the package insert, over half of all women gain five pounds during the first year on Depo-Provera and then continue to gain a little in subsequent years of use. And since the gain appears to be in fat (as opposed to water or muscle), these added pounds can be hard to shake even after you stop receiving injections.

The Emergency Morning-After Pill

How It Works: Within seventy-two hours of unprotected sex, a woman takes a first dose of oral contraceptives and then another dose twelve hours later. The number of pills you take each time varies according to the brand. The pills appear to prevent pregnancy by affecting the lining of the uterus, making it a hostile environment for a fertilized egg to implant in or the pills may delay ovulation.

Effectiveness: 75 percent

Pros: Less expensive, as well as less emotionally, philosophically, and physically complicated than abortion, the combined pill regimen is a wonderful thing to fall back on when you're worried that unprotected sex may have led to pregnancy. Some women can continue with their training during treatment, although others will be put out of the action for a few days.

Cons: The combined pill regimen often causes two days of nausea and sometimes vomiting. Ask your doctor about taking an antinausea medicine at the same time. Another common side effect is breast tenderness. Also, you may find your cycles are irregular for up to two months afterward. Finally, the method should be used only rarely, for emergencies. Using high doses of hormones regularly is not considered a safe or effective means of daily birth control.

Tubal Ligation

How It Works: Surgery is performed (via laparoscope—a thin, small instrument that is usually inserted through a tiny incision in your belly button) to separate a woman's fallopian tubes from her uterus so that sperm can no longer reach the egg.

Effectiveness: 99 percent

Pros: It's immediately effective and permanent. You then have natural menstrual cycles but no need to worry about birth control or accidental pregnancy.

Cons: Even though it's same-day surgery, many women find it really takes a few weeks to get back to normal, so it's important to schedule the operation during a time when you don't need to do a lot of training. For reasons unknown, some women's periods become heavier and more irregular after the surgery. Finally, the surgery should be considered irreversible, so any woman who isn't completely sure about whether she is finished with childbearing isn't a candidate.

Fertility Awareness Methods

How They Work: Also known as natural family planning, most of the approaches include charting the days of the menstrual cycle, keeping track of changes in the quality of cervical mucus (a barometer of when ovulation occurs), and avoiding intercourse during fertile days.

Effectiveness: possibly up to 80 percent

Pros: It's completely natural—it involves no drugs or devices inside your body. It expands your awareness of your body and the changes it undergoes over the course of a menstrual cycle; this training in "listening to your body" could possibly help you become more sensitive to your body's athletic capabilities and limitations.

Cons: It is a very hard method to use reliably if your periods are irregular. Because the risk of an unplanned pregnancy is higher with this method than with almost any other method, you may also have to contend with a lot of worries about whether or not you are pregnant each month, anxieties that can interfere with focused training and competition.

Skipping or losing your period can have serious consequences. It may be convenient, but you pay a high price in terms of your health.
—AURELIA NATTIV, M.D., TEAM PHYSICIAN AT UCLA

WHEN YOU SKIP PERIODS OR THEY STOP ALTOGETHER

In some sports, as many as 50 percent of the athletes who are competitive may suffer from what's known as exercise-induced or athletic amenorrhea (in which you stop having periods altogether) or oligomenorrhea (cycles lasting longer than forty days, leading to fewer than ten menstrual periods per year). In comparison, the prevalence of these problems is only 5 percent in the general population.

These menstrual disturbances are often viewed by athletes as a welcome relief from the hassle of dealing with their periods every month. For some, losing their period is even an emblem of "athletic success," notes Aurelia Nattiv, M.D., assistant clinical professor in the department of family medicine and department of orthopedic surgery at the UCLA School of Medicine and team physician at UCLA. "But what these women don't realize is that skipping or losing your period can have serious consequences. It may be convenient, but you pay a high price in terms of your health."

Why Your Period Is Important

Over the past ten years or so, research has shown that when a woman doesn't menstruate regularly, she loses bone density.

When you have regular cycles, you produce adequate levels of estrogen, a hormone that helps keep calcium in your bones and thus helps keep bones strong. In contrast, when you don't menstruate regularly, it's a sign that your estrogen levels are low—without adequate estrogen, calcium is lost and your bones become thinner, weaker, and more brittle. An immediate consequence of this is that you become more prone to stress fractures—cracks in your bones, especially in your feet and legs. For example, a study of fifty-three competitive track-and-field

athletes aged seventeen to twenty-six found that those with irregular periods were six times as likely as the others to have
had a stress fracture, according to researchers at La Trobe University in Victoria, Australia. In addition, you become more
prone to osteoporosis—a disease in which your bones become
quite brittle and easily broken—later in life.

What's not known at this point is how "regainable" lost
bone is. Although most studies indicate that once a woman
resumes having normal periods, she stops losing bone, it's still
unclear to what extent it is possible to catch up and retrieve
what has been lost.

The Exercise Link

But what is it about exercise that can lead you to miss
periods? Interestingly, exercise, in and of itself, is probably not
the culprit, which may explain why some athletes never lose
their periods, while others do. Instead, amenorrhea in athletes
appears to be triggered by an "energy drain," an imbalance
between the energy you put out and the energy you take in.

Dr. Nattiv explains: "Although the theory about what
causes athletic amenorrhea is still evolving, right now the pre-
vailing belief is that when an athletic woman takes in too few
calories to support her energy expenditure—that is, when she
burns more calories every day than she eats—her body shuts
down reproductive function as a way to conserve the little energy that is available."

Stress, which appears to affect how the brain releases and
secretes hormones, may play a role too. "Although people respond very differently to stress, in some it appears that the
psychological stress of competition can interfere with normal
hormonal secretion patterns," notes Melinda M. Manore, Ph.D.,
R.D., professor of nutrition at Arizona State University,
Tempe, Arizona.

In other words, inadequate nutrition and possibly stress—
not strenuous training per se—may be the keys to why you
skip or lose your periods.

Correcting the Problem

Some athletes lose their periods for pretty obvious reasons:
They are obsessed with their appearance and with being thin;
they believe the thinner they are, the better they'll perform, and
so they intentionally—and drastically—limit their food intake.

These athletes have unhealthy—and often unrealistic—body weight goals. At the root of their amenorrhea is usually an eating disorder (for a complete discussion of the diagnosis and treatment of eating disorders, see Chapter 2).

But not every athlete who loses her periods has a psychologically based eating disorder. "A lot of these amenorrheic women have great diets. They don't have eating disorders and they are not necessarily restricting their eating for their sport," says Dr. Manore. "But their training schedule really interferes with mealtimes. When they choose not to eat at certain times it has nothing to do with denying their hunger, it just isn't convenient or practical to begin a workout right after a big meal. As a result, they just don't get enough calories."

Eating more, for example, turned out to be the simple solution for swimmer Melanie M. Valerio, age twenty-eight, a Gold Medalist at the 1996 Atlanta Olympic Games in the 400-meter free relay event. "I had taken a year off of training and I was trying to get back into competitive condition. I decided I would improve my diet and eat healthy food. I wasn't trying to lose weight—I've always been tall and skinny—I just thought I might be even healthier and stronger if I stopped eating so much ice cream, candy, potato chips, and fast food," she remembers. "So I started eating lots of vegetables, fruits, lean poultry and fish, rice, pasta, and that sort of thing. I was eating a lot of food—just no junk. But it sort of backfired. I began to lose weight, stopped getting my periods, and felt really tired. The doctors couldn't find anything wrong. Finally, I stopped trying to stick so closely to my so-called healthy diet. I began to let myself have things like ice cream and hamburgers when I wanted them and before long I got my period back, my weight went back up, and I had the energy I needed to perform well. It seems pretty clear to me now that I just wasn't getting enough fat and calories to properly fuel my metabolism."

For other women, the problem isn't that they need to eat more. Instead, they simply need to eat *more often* throughout the day. "When you eat only one big meal a day, your metabolic rate goes down as a way to conserve energy for the long stretches in which there is no food intake. Consequently, if an athlete begins to eat more frequent meals throughout the day, she may find her periods resume," says Dr. Nattiv.

The good news, then, is that you may be able to get your menstrual cycle back on track by simply improving your diet.

You may not have to reduce your training. Here are the general guidelines many experts use when treating amenorrhea or oligomenorrhea in athletes:

1. First, check for medical causes of amenorrhea. Pregnancy, low thyroid, and polycystic ovarian disease commonly cause missed periods and so should be ruled out.

2. Start increasing your calcium intake right away to help halt further bone erosion. If your periods have stopped altogether, you need to take 1,500 mg a day; if you just skip periods now and again, you need 1,200 mg daily. Most women find that the easiest way to get enough calcium is by drinking or eating calcium-dense dairy products (milk, yogurt, cottage cheese) and taking a supplement too.

3. If you have had irregular periods for less than six months, a three-month trial in which you improve your diet makes sense. You'll probably need to put on a few pounds (usually 2 to 5) in addition to learning what and when to eat. (A nutritionist can help you design the right diet.) If you know already that you couldn't bear the prospect of putting on any weight, you should probably forgo this trial and proceed directly to hormonal treatment (see number 5). You may also want to think about whether or not you might be suffering from an eating disorder (see page 73).

4. Some, but not all, women may also need to consider moderating their training schedule. In some cases, that may mean taking one day off each week or trading two days of endurance work (like long-distance running or biking) for weight training. If the idea of cutting back makes you nervous, it's important to remember that many athletes find that their performances actually improve when they build more rest and repair time into their training schedules.

5. For women who have not had a period for six months and/or are unable to resume their periods through lifestyle and diet changes, the best course of action may be to take hormones, although there is some controversy about how much estrogen and progesterone are needed to protect bones in female athletes. Some experts recommend birth control pills, since the hormones they contain may help protect bones, and they provide contraception. But others worry that oral contraceptives will further prevent the body from jump-starting its own cycle and so they prescribe lower, noncontraceptive doses of estrogen and progesterone. If you are sexually active (and don't want to get pregnant), it probably makes sense to opt for birth control pills, since you then reap the contraceptive benefits. But if you are uncomfortable with the idea of taking hormones in general, the lower-dose option may be better. If you don't experience a period even when taking oral hormones, additional hormone therapy, in the form of a vaginal gel called Crinone 4 percent, which you insert every other day for about twelve days, appears to be quite effective in bringing on a cycle almost immediately.

Whatever course of treatment you choose, it's important to remember treatment is crucial—even if you feel young, strong, and immortal, if you don't take action now, there is a high risk you won't be able to "stay in the game" later in life.

THE HIDDEN MENSTRUAL CYCLE CHANGE

Strenuous exercise may also trigger the onset of a subtle menstrual disturbance called a luteal phase defect or luteal suppression. It's when you don't secrete enough progesterone in the days after ovulation (called your luteal phase) to support a pregnancy. In addition, your luteal phase is shortened—lasting ten days or less instead of the usual fourteen. Some evidence indicates that almost half of all female athletes experience this temporary, reversible condition.

Like the more serious problem of amenorrhea, a luteal phase defect appears to be a menstrual cycle alteration that occurs when an exercising woman expends more calories than she takes in. But unlike amenorrhea, most athletic women who have a luteal phase defect have no idea whatsoever that they have the problem. That's because their periods stay perfectly regular and their entire cycle length may be more or less normal.

So is there something to be worried about?

"If you are getting normal periods, you have no reason to worry about whether you are experiencing luteal suppression or not: The research now indicates very clearly that women with subtle menstrual disturbances like luteal phase defects do not have the risk of losing bone mass that women who skip or lose their periods do," says one of the chief researchers in the field, Mary Jane De Souza, Ph.D., at the Center for Fertility and Reproductive Endocrinology at New Britain General Hospital in Connecticut.

Still, if you want to get pregnant, a short luteal phase could be a concern, since these defects may prevent the fertilized embryo from successfully implanting in the uterus. But don't panic or jump to conclusions. Just because you are an athlete doesn't mean you'll necessarily have a short luteal phase or that you'll have trouble getting pregnant because of one. First of all, every woman appears to have a different threshold: For example, one woman may be able to run 60 miles a week and have her cycle be unaffected whereas another woman may experience luteal suppression when she runs 20 miles a week.

So before becoming overly anxious about whether you might have trouble conceiving because of a luteal phase defect, give yourself some time to try to get pregnant. Most experts recommend you give yourself a year to get pregnant—if you are under age thirty. If you're older, the risk of there being a problem with your ability to conceive increases, so it makes sense to seek medical advice sooner. There are age-specific guidelines: women between age thirty and thirty-five should see a doctor after six to nine months of unprotected intercourse; women between thirty-five and forty after six months; and women over forty should see their doctor if they haven't gotten pregnant in three months.

Then, if you're concerned about a luteal phase defect, ask your doctor about being tested for it. If your luteal phase turns out to be a problem, you might consider trying to resolve it yourself first (rather than rushing to resolve it via hormone therapy) by increasing your caloric intake and/or reducing your training volume for a few cycles.

OTHER GYNECOLOGICAL WOES

Besides throwing a big monkey wrench into your training schedule, problems like an itchy vaginal yeast infection or uncontrollable urine leakage can actually be worsened by certain workout practices. Here, then, is a rundown of ways to get quick relief, plus some pointers on how best to prevent and treat the most common female irritations:

Stress Incontinence

It's the problem no one wants to talk about: leaking urine when you don't intend to. Yet, approximately 40 to 60 percent of young women under age forty experience mild, occasional urine leakage. "Leaking a little urine, every once in a while, is an extremely common occurrence. In my opinion, it's not abnormal—it's simply a natural consequence of how a woman's urogenital tract is designed. With enough vigorous activity, practically anyone would lose drops of urine," says Ingrid Nygaard, M.D., associate professor of obstetrics and gynecology at the University of Iowa College of Medicine in Iowa City.

Another 5 to 10 percent of young women experience more severe leakage, which is considered leaking urine at least once a week.

There is no evidence that high-impact sports, such as basketball, volleyball, running, or aerobics, cause the problem, but these activities can certainly provoke incontinence. Luckily, remedying the problem rarely requires surgery in young women; in fact, some very simple self-help measures are usually all you need to keep dry.

But to correct the problem, it helps to understand what causes it. In young women, the problem is sometimes related to a weakness in the tissues and muscles that support the pelvic organs (the bladder, uterus, and vagina). If these muscles, which

---

○ Four Ways to Stop Urine Leakage During Workouts

1. Strengthen your pelvic floor muscles by doing Kegel exercises twice a day.
2. Wear a tampon—it puts pressure on your urethra, thus preventing urine from dribbling out.
3. Insert your diaphragm—it elevates the angle of the neck of the bladder, supports the urethra, and stops leakages.
4. Train your bladder to hold urine better. Follow a timetable to store and release urine every hour. Then, using fifteen-minute increments, gradually extend the time you can last. Aim to be able to go two to three hours without urinating.

are called the pelvic floor muscles, are slack, your bladder will often leak small amounts of urine whenever you cough, laugh, lift heavy objects, sneeze, or exercise.

But these muscles can be strengthened by specific exercises called Kegels (named after the physician who invented them). In a study led by Dr. Nygaard of seventy-one women of all ages with various types of incontinence, one-third of the participants who learned how to do these simple, no-risk, no-cost exercises reported excellent improvement and desired no further treatment. In the study, the women only did the exercises twice a day, for five minutes each time. Here's how to do them: First, to make sure you know which muscles you are supposed to be working, sit on the toilet and stop the flow of urine midstream and/or squeeze the muscles you would use if you were trying to prevent yourself from passing gas. These are the muscles you need to exercise to prevent urine leakage. You can also lie down, place a clean finger in your vagina, and squeeze—you should feel a tightness on your finger if you are squeezing the right muscles.

While exercising, be sure to squeeze only the pelvic floor muscles—don't tighten your stomach, legs, or other muscles and don't hold your breath. Then, simply pull in your pelvic floor muscles for a count of three, then release for a count of three. Repeat for a total of five minutes, changing your position, so that you sit, stand, and lie down during those five minutes. Using these three positions helps exercise all the different muscles. With time, you should try to lengthen the time of your contractions so that you increasingly hold the muscles for longer counts. It may take from three to six weeks for you to notice an improvement in your leakage problem—as an added benefit, you may find sex becomes more enjoyable as your muscle tone improves.

Other ways to deal with leakage:

• Wear a tampon during workouts. Insert it a little lower in your vagina than usual (although it should still feel comfortable). The tampon puts pressure on your urethra, thus preventing urine from dribbling out.

• Wear a diaphragm during exercise: It elevates the angle of the neck of bladder, supports the urethra, and stops leakages.

• Urinate on schedule: You can train your bladder to hold urine better. Follow a timetable to store and release urine every hour, then, using fifteen-minute increments, gradually extend the time you can last. Aim to be able to go two to three hours without urinating.

• Consider biofeedback training. A vaginal probe equipped with a sensor is painlessly inserted into your vagina, then as you contract your muscles you can see how well you're doing on a TV screen. "I've been really impressed with the results of this—women get a lot of positive feedback when they use the device—and so I refer a lot of women for this training," notes Dr. Joy.

• Consider diet changes. Drinks like coffee, colas, tea, and alcohol can make bladder control harder.

For young women, a combination of the above do-it-yourself techniques is usually enough to keep dry. But even if your problem is more severe, there are still lots of treatments available.

The newest nonsurgical option for keeping urine in your bladder is called FemAssist (manufactured by Insight Medical, Bolton, Massachusetts, 800-232-4344). It's a small, soft silicone cap that fits over the urethra and is held in place by a slight vacuum. Each cap, which can be used for a week, costs about $10.

Other anti-incontinence prescription devices currently available include Introl, a reusable soft, silicone, U-shaped device that holds the neck of the bladder in its proper position and Reliance, a disposable tamponlike device that employs an inflatable balloon to block the bladder neck and prevent leakage. Collagen injections to add bulk to the tissue around your urethra and keep your sphincter muscles tightly closed are also an option. For more information, a good place to contact is the National Association for Continence (800-252-3337); for a list of urogynecologists in your state, send a self-addressed, stamped envelope to the American Urogynecologic Society, 401 North Michigan Avenue, Chicago, Il 60611-4267, 312-644-6610.

Urinary Tract Infections (UTIs)

About 25 to 35 percent of women between the ages of twenty and forty have had at least one UTI, according to the American Medical Association. UTIs are bacterial infections that need to be diagnosed by a doctor and treated with antibiotics.

The two unmistakable symptoms of the most common UTI, the bladder infection cystitis, are a stinging, searing pain when you urinate and feelings of pressure in your abdomen that lead you to believe you absolutely must urinate—only to be frustrated to find you can pass only a few burning drops.

The good news for competitive athletes who can't afford to be put out of the action or distracted by a bout of cystitis: The medication Uristat, which numbs the bladder, relieving pain and discomfort until an antibiotic can kick in and cure the problem, is now available in drugstores over the counter. Uristat is a great way to get instant relief, but it's important to remember that it doesn't treat the infection itself. An untreated bladder infection can progress to pyelonephritis, a serious kidney infection that often needs to be treated in a hospital with intravenous antibiotics.

But why are young women so cystitis-prone? Anatomy is partly to blame. In women, the short distance between the rectum and the entrance of the urethra (the narrow canal that funnels urine from the bladder to the outside of the body) is only 1 to 2 inches long, which means that bacteria can easily travel from one to the other. Especially during sex, bacteria from the vaginal/rectal area may be pushed into the urethra. From there, they travel upward, where they irritate the bladder lining.

In addition, diaphragm users and women who use spermicide-coated condoms are at increased risk for cystitis. By pressing on the bladder neck, a diaphragm may partially obstruct the flow of urine, thus allowing bacteria to pool and grow. And spermicides change the vagina's bacterial balance, allowing invaders to flourish.

To diagnose a UTI, a doctor does a simple dipstick urinalysis. Or there's a new over-the-counter test kit, available in drugstores for less than $10, called UTI, which lets you confirm whether symptoms should be treated with antibiotics. Almost all first-time cases of UTI clear up surprisingly quickly—all it takes is as little as one to three days of antibiotic treatment.

However, anyone who has experienced one UTI should consider herself at risk for another, since statistics show that 80 percent of women who have had one occurrence will have another within about eighteen months. To keep UTIs to a minimum, here are nine easy-to-implement prevention strategies:

1. Down plenty of liquids—advice most athletes need to follow anyway. Drinking at least eight 8-ounce glasses of water a day helps keep your urine diluted (it should be pale to clear yellow in color) and ensures bacteria get flushed from the bladder regularly.

2. Drink 10 ounces of cranberry juice cocktail a day. A group of Israeli researchers found that cranberry juice contains a protein that prevents bacteria from attaching to the inner lining of the bladder (the protein was also found in blueberry juice, which is harder to find in grocery stores). In a study of 153 elderly women conducted by researchers at Harvard Medical School, only 15 percent of those who drank cranberry juice for six months had urinary tract infections, compared to 28 percent of the women in the placebo group. A second study is now underway to determine whether cranberry juice is as helpful for younger women with histories of frequent urinary tract infections.

3. Urinate frequently over the course of the day—healthy urine is sterile and cleanses the surrounding tissues and carries bacteria away from the urethra and vagina.

4. Urinate before and after sexual intercourse. Drinking a full glass of water before you make love helps ensure you'll have a good stream of urine to flush away bacteria from the bladder afterward. Try to urinate as soon after intercourse as possible.

5. Wash your genitals (and have your partner wash his) before intercourse to minimize the chance that bacteria from the anus and vagina will be introduced into the urethra during sex.

6. Wipe properly—from front to back—when you go to the bathroom. This keeps bacteria from the bowel away from the urethral entrance.

7. Don't use feminine hygiene products, such as douches, sprays, and deodorants, since the chemicals in them may irritate the urethra. For the same reason, most experts say women who experience frequent UTIs should avoid bubble baths, perfumed toilet paper, and heavily scented soap or powders in the vaginal area.

8. Avoid wearing tight exercise pants or shorts for long stretches of time since they can encourage bacterial growth as well as irritate the urethra. Same goes for hanging around in a wet swimsuit. Tight jeans can be trouble too. If you are prone to recurrent UTIs (or yeast infections, which are described next), you might save your sleek, tight exercise wear for competition use and limit wearing it during training to see if the change helps.

9. Change pads or tampons frequently during your period.

Yeast Infections

When there is an overgrowth of *Candida albicans,* a fungus that normally resides in the vagina (as well as rectum and oral cavity), you have what's known as a yeast or *Monilia* infection. The symptoms are a white, curdy discharge that resembles cottage cheese, a yeasty odor, and itching as well as painful swelling and sensitivity in the vagina.

Any woman who must take antibiotics is at increased risk for a yeast infection, since these medicines kill the "good" bacteria (*lactobacillus*) that help keep yeast growth in check.

Most yeast infections can be self-treated, with over-the-counter, single dose or three-day vaginal cream treatments. The trick, however, is to be sure you know what you're treating. Vaginal discharge can also be caused by sexually transmitted diseases as well as bacterial infections. Yeast treatments won't help these problems and can even cause them to worsen, by causing you to delay seeing a doctor. So if this is your first yeast infection, if you doubt your diagnosis, or if your symptoms don't resolve as promised by a yeast cure, it's best to get checked out by a doctor.

To prevent future yeast infections: Choose loose, breathable, natural-fiber workout gear whenever possible. If you must wear tight running or biking shorts, for example, make sure they

SPECIAL FOCUS

◖ The Four Phases of Your Menstrual Cycle

The cycle of a healthy, regularly menstruating woman has four phases, each with its own distinct mix of hormones. A twenty-eight-day cycle would be divided like this:

1. It starts on the first day of menstrual bleeding (Day One) and lasts for about five days. It's characterized by low levels of both estrogen and progesterone. At this time, your pituitary gland starts releasing pulses of FSH (follicle-stimulating hormone); the FSH stimulates the follicles in your ovaries to grow, which, in turn, stimulates several of your stored eggs to mature.

2. Called the follicular phase, from days six to thirteen the presence of FSH increasingly causes the follicles to grow, which triggers the production of estrogen within them. As your level of estrogen rises, the preparation of the uterine lining—the endometrium—starts. It begins to get thick and spongy with a wealth of new blood vessels so as to be able to receive and nourish an embryo.

3. On approximately Day Fourteen, the most dominant follicle releases an egg, a process called ovulation. Your estrogen levels are at their peak; the hormone progesterone, which controls the final maturation of the uterine lining, begins to be produced in higher amounts too.

4. If you haven't become pregnant, during the luteal phase—Days Fifteen to Twenty-eight—your levels of estrogen and progesterone stay elevated for about seven days, then begin to fall rapidly, reaching their lowest point at the end of the monthly cycle. As this is happening, the lining of your uterus bgins to break up, leading once again to menstruation.

have a roomy cotton crotch and change out of them as soon as possible. Change and shower after swimming in chlorinated pools. Whenever you must take antibiotics, make it a daily habit to eat 8 ounces of yogurt with live cultures of *Acidophilus lactobacilli*—these bacteria replace the ones killed by antibiotics and help keep yeast growth in balance. Finally, avoid douching, since it washes out the bacteria that keep yeast controlled.

Herpes Flare-up

The possibility of a herpes outbreak right before an important competition is, unfortunately, a real risk since the virus is reactivated and stirred up by high levels of stress and anxiety. But you may not have to wait until you feel the first signs of an impending outbreak to begin treatment. Instead, discuss suppressive therapy, sometimes called prophylactic therapy, with your doctor. This involves taking a regimen of medication to suppress the activation of the virus; in other words, you begin to take medicine before any sign of active disease surfaces. In this way, if you tailor your medication schedule to fit your competition schedule, you are more likely to head off an outbreak entirely so you don't have to deal with the tingling, itching, or burning of lesions at the same time you are trying to perform your athletic best.

2

YOUR DIET

Sheila Cornell Douty, age thirty-five, first baseman on the 1996 Gold-Medal-winning U.S. Olympic softball team, feels the team could have played even better—if it had eaten better.

"Before the Olympics, we went on a two-and-one-half-month twenty-city tour. We were traveling constantly during this time. So, for starters, we had to eat a lot of plane food. While at the stadiums, it was candy bars. Then it was a lot of fast food, barbecue, and banquet-type meals, since we often had to eat late at night, after playing a doubleheader, and we didn't have the time or facilities to cook fresh foods.

"Our diets were horrendous! In fact, I know that the team was in much worse shape by the time the tour ended and the Olympics rolled around, since we had only a short interval of three weeks in which to get back on a decent diet after those months of unhealthy meals. Personally, I really felt the effects of constantly eating the wrong kinds of foods. It made me feel more tired and sluggish. Plus, I gained about five pounds over the course of all the traveling, which doesn't make much sense given how much I was playing softball. If I had had access to the foods I wanted, I'm sure my weight would have been stable."

Yet, if diet is so important, how does Douty explain that the team consistently won? "It's true that we played well. On the whole, you can't be disappointed with our performance. But even so, I definitely believe we would have been even more powerful if we had been able to eat right. I can't prove it, but

I feel sure that there wasn't a single athlete on the team who wouldn't have benefited greatly from better food."

Like Douty, most athletes feel there is room for improvement in their diets. In addition, most of us are intrigued by the concept of "peak performance eating"—after all, wouldn't it be wonderful if by simply eating better, you could perform better? In fact, it's the rare athlete who doesn't aspire to—or at least think about—eating a so-called healthier diet.

Yet, according to many top experts, there is no such thing as a perfect diet formula.

"No eating plan prescription fits everyone. The right diet for a one-hundred-fifty-pound ultra-marathoner is not the same as the one for an eighty-five-pound gymnast," says Ann C. Grandjean, director of the International Center for Sports Nutrition, Omaha, Nebraska, and a consultant for over twenty years to the U.S. Olympic Committee. "Not only do different sports dictate different nutritional needs, there are a slew of other factors, such as your food preferences, your body size, your training regimen, and your age, that have an impact on what your particular nutrient requirements are. In fact, even two one-hundred-fifty-pound ultra-marathoners of the same age might not thrive on the same food choices."

So how do you find the diet best for you and your athletic pursuits? "It's surprisingly simple," says Grandjean. "Just follow some general commonsense guidelines, then listen to your body."

That's what many elite athletes do. Highly tuned to the subtleties of their bodies, they pay attention to how they feel after eating meals. They ask themselves: Did that make me feel good? Did it give me more energy? Has it affected my mood or performance?

"As long as you know the basics of good nutrition, using yourself and your body's reactions as a guide to what foods to choose is far more likely to lead to high performance than any preprinted, superimposed diet plan," says Grandjean.

In fact, the best thing an athlete can do is to *not* overly obsess about exact calorie counts or strict diet regimes, says Debra M. Vinci, Ph.D., R.D., director of the health education department at Hall Health Primary Care Center at the University of Washington, Seattle. "Just because you're an athlete doesn't mean you have to start calculating grams, percentages, and calories of everything you put in your mouth," Dr. Vinci notes. "There really isn't all that much that has to be different in the diet of an athlete compared to the diet of any other healthy person. You don't have to be compulsive about food; you should still be able to enjoy food."

With this perspective in mind, here are seven basic principles of smart *everyday* eating. Then you'll find details on what to eat before, during, and after competition; the pros and cons of various sports supplements; and how to lose (or gain) weight safely. The point of the chapter is not to tell you exactly what to eat, but to arm you with information you can use to evaluate, and if necessary, redesign, your diet.

◑ Seven Rules of Healthy Eating for Female Athletes
   1. If it works (i.e., you feel great and perform well), don't fix it!
   2. Know your carbohydrates—they are the body's chief energy source.
   3. Don't neglect protein.
   4. Beware of fat phobia.
   5. Get enough iron.
   6. Make calcium intake a priority.
   7. Hydrate, hydrate, hydrate!

AN ATHLETE'S GUIDE TO EVERYDAY EATING— SEVEN RULES

If It Works, Don't Fix It

Those are the words from many nutritionists. If you feel good, your body weight is stable, and you are happy with the way you are performing in your sport, there is no reason to start tinkering with your diet, even if your eating habits go against the grain of what other athletes are doing.

Recalls Grandjean: "I had a conversation with a cyclist who was worried because she didn't eat like the rest of the competitors. The other cyclists constantly gave her a hard time, always 'ragged' on her because she ate a lot of eggs and dairy products. When I asked this woman how she felt, she said 'Great'; when I asked her what her ranking was, she replied, 'I am the number one female cyclist in my country.' Well, to me that said it all.

I simply told her, 'Don't screw with it—your diet is obviously working for you!' "

Know Your Carbohydrates

Carbohydrates are the backbone of most athletes' diets because they are the body's chief energy source. When you eat carbohydrates, your body quickly transforms them into glucose, the predominant fuel for every cell in your system. Glucose that is not needed is stored in the form of glycogen in your muscles and liver—these glycogen stores are what your body taps into to fuel muscle fiber contraction and energy output during exercise. Without good muscle glycogen storage, you simply won't go as far or as fast as you might be able.

Carbohydrates come in two forms: The simple carbohydrates are the sugars—from white, refined sugar to maple sugar to the sugars that naturally appear in some fruits and dairy products. The complex carbohydrates are primarily starches, which are found in bread, cereal, rice, oatmeal, and pasta as well as vegetables such as corn, beans, peas, lentils, and potatoes.

The key to healthy eating is to *not* treat all carbohydrates alike. Instead of emphasizing simple ones (like a doughnut for breakfast), the focus should be on complex ones (like a bowl of Cheerios or Wheaties or Shredded Wheat instead) since these carbohydrates come naturally packaged with a lot of vitamins, minerals, and fiber in addition to being topnotch energy sources.

A commonly accepted rule is that carbohydrate-containing foods should comprise at least half of what you eat every day. A general recommendation for a balanced diet breaks down like this:

Carbohydrates—50 to 60 percent of total calories
    10 to 20 percent simple (fruits, juices, special treats)
    40 to 50 percent complex (whole grains, legumes, vegetables)
Proteins—15 to 20 percent
    animal (fish, poultry, meats, eggs, dairy)
    vegetable (nuts, seeds, legumes)
Fats—25 to 30 percent
    10 percent saturated (meats, eggs, butter, dairy products, coconut and palm oils)

10 percent polyunsaturated (corn, safflower, sesame oils)

10 percent monounsaturated (nuts, seeds, avocado, olive, canola, peanut oils)

However, if you regularly work out for more than an hour a day, you may find you need to shift this balance a little more toward carbohydrates, although most nutritionists don't recommend you go beyond getting 65 percent of your calories from them.

Don't Neglect Protein

Why is protein so important? It's what our body's tissues are composed of. Muscles, internal organs, some hormones, and enzymes are all largely made up of protein. The protein in these tissues is constantly being used and then replaced, and that's where the protein from your diet comes in. Without enough of it, your organs can't replenish the protein lost during normal functioning. One of the key warning signs of insufficient protein is slow recovery after exercise. That is, you may begin to feel unusually tired after long workouts, and your muscles will stay sore for longer periods afterward. You simply can't rebound as well when you are running short on protein.

Yet, many female athletes embrace diets that are so extremely high-carbohydrate and low-fat that they become protein deficient. "They've taken the message that 'carbs are good' to an extreme, even becoming a bit phobic about eating any protein and fat because they are afraid it will cause them to gain weight. They view meats and dairy products as completely off limits," says Page Love Johnson, M.S., R.D., a nutritionist for the U.S. Tennis Association National Sport Science Committee and for the Atlanta Track Club and Atlanta Marathoner's Group. "But without good protein balance, your performance eventually begins to suffer."

Other athletes go to the opposite extreme and follow high-protein diets, such as that popularized in *Enter the Zone* by Barry Sears, Ph.D., or *Protein Power* by Michael and Mary Eades. These diets usually recommend eating only 40 percent of your daily calories from carbohydrates, 30 percent from protein, and 30 from fat; these diets are also based on the assertion that a high-carbohydrate diet tips the body's hormonal balance, making it "insulin resistant," a phrase that implies that the body can't process the sugar in carbohydrates. As a result, this reasoning goes, the sugar is stored as fat, which leads to weight gain as well as chronic diseases like high blood pressure and Type II diabetes.

To date, the concept that a high-carbohydrate diet promotes a state of insulin resistance hasn't been well documented. What's more, compared to the mountains of research that shows a diet high in complex carbohydrates is best for replenishing an athlete's muscle glycogen stores, there are almost no studies that show that athletes, in particular, do better on a high-protein regimen.

Still, many people claim to feel remarkably better on these high-protein regimens. "I think one of the reasons these diets initially seem so effective, leading to a sense of well-being, is that so many people weren't eating enough protein and fat to begin with," notes Vinci. "Plus, many people were overeating things like oversized bagels and fat-free SnackWell cookies. They lose weight when they go on one of these high-protein diets because they eat fewer calories."

◗ Protein Calculator

Here's how to figure your requirements:

1. *If you aren't active . . .*
   ____ (your weight) ÷ by 2.2 = ____ × .8 = number of grams of protein you need daily
2. *If you exercise aerobically at least three times a week . . .*
   ____ (your weight) ÷ 2.2 = ____ × 1.2 = number of grams of protein you need daily
3. *If you are an endurance athlete in training . . .*
   ____ (your weight) ÷ by 2.2 = ____ × 1.5 = number of grams of protein you need daily

---

Okay, so how much protein is enough, but not too much? Don't look to the standard RDAs (Recommended Daily Allowances) since research suggests that athletes have increased protein requirements compared to the general population. The recommended daily requirement for sedentary women is about 0.8 grams of protein per kilogram (2.2 pounds) of body weight; active women who exercise regularly probably need about 1.2 grams per kilogram of body weight, with endurance athletes needing even more, up to 1.5 grams per kilogram of body weight. Most of the evidence suggests that getting more than 2 grams of protein per kilogram of body weight does no good and could be harmful to your health—besides causing your body to lose needed calcium and to become dehydrated, it can strain your kidneys, which must work overtime to flush the by-product of excess protein, nitrogen, out of your system.

To estimate your own requirements: Divide your weight by 2.2, then multiply that amount by .8 (if you aren't active right now) or 1.2 (if you exercise aerobically several times a week) or 1.5 (if you are an endurance athlete—a marathoner, for example—actively training). The amount you come up with equals the number of grams of protein you need to eat each day.

Meat, fish, and poultry are excellent sources of protein, containing about 30 grams per 4-ounce serving. (Keep in mind that a 4-ounce serving is pretty small, roughly equivalent to a deck of cards or the palm of your hand.) There's plenty of protein in other foods too: kidney beans, lentils, chickpeas, and other legumes contain about 7 grams of protein per ½ cup serving; one large egg contains 6 grams; a 1 cup serving of many breakfast cereals contains 10 to 12 grams; 2 slices of bread, a bagel, English muffin, or pita contains about 6 grams; 1 cup of milk contains 8 grams, and 1 cup of cottage cheese contains 25 grams of protein.

As evidenced by this list, there are plenty of good nonmeat protein sources that athletes who are vegetarians can rely on. In fact, if you eat eggs, milk, and cheese, a vegetarian diet can easily include enough protein. (If your diet doesn't include dairy products and eggs, you'll have to work a little harder to meet your protein needs. See The Vegetarian Athlete, page 56.)

Beware of Fat Phobia

You can't live without a little body fat—or some fat in your diet. Body fat is necessary to provide a protective padding around internal organs; it serves to help insulate your body—a layer of fat under your skin helps your body maintain its proper core temperature; it also serves as a source of stored energy; especially at moderate levels of exercise intensity, fat can be utilized as a fuel for muscles, thus helping to spare their stored glycogen stores.

Fats from food transport the fat-soluble vitamins (A, D, E, and K) through your bloodstream; supply essential fatty acids, which are the building blocks for several hormones; help maintain healthy skin; and also give you a feeling of satiety after a meal, possibly because they slow the transit of food from the stomach.

Yet many women attempt to steer clear of any form of fat, for fear it will make them fat. What are the dangers of an active athlete eating a diet that is too low in fat (below 10 to 15 percent)? You have no energy source to fall back on when your limited glycogen stores are depleted. Simply put, you'll become exhausted more quickly and take a lot longer to recover. A diet too low in fat can also lead you into problems with nutrient deficiencies, can make you very susceptible to feeling chilly, can make your skin unusually dry and crepe-papery, plus lead your nails to become brittle.

Of course, the infamous downside of too much fat in the diet is that it is linked to obesity, heart disease, and an array of different cancers.

The trick, then, is to get just enough fat, but not too much.

The American Heart Association and USDA's Dietary Guidelines for Americans recommend that you get between 25 and 30 percent of your calories from fat. However, there's evidence that certain types of athletes may actually perform better if they eat a diet slightly higher in fat. In a study conducted at the State University of New York in Buffalo, runners who trained at least 40 miles a week and increased their fat intake from 15 percent to as much as 42 percent increased their endurance time by 40 percent—yet their body weight, cardiovascular risk, and immune function were not adversely affected.

"We know that many elite endurance athletes—triathletes and road cyclists, for example—eat a lot more fat than is usually recommended. This higher percentage may be necessary sometimes to meet their high calorie needs, which can range from four thousand to six thousand calories a day," says Grandjean.

But for anyone who is not an elite endurance athlete, getting more than 30 percent of your calories makes little sense. Not only will it increase your disease risk and possibility of weight gain, according to Johnson, "Eating too much fat tends to decrease carbohydrate intake and carbohydrate stored as glycogen, which is really the preferred fuel for your muscles during high-intensity exercise."

To calculate how many grams of fat a day you need to keep to the 30 percent limit, you first need to estimate how many calories you eat a day. For example, if you maintain your weight on approximately 1,800 calories a day, no more than 30 percent, or 540, of those calories should come from fat. Since there are 9 calories to each gram of fat, that means you would consume about 60 grams of fat each day.

A tablespoon of just about any type of oil has 13 gs of fat; 1 ounce of chocolate has approximately 9 gs of fat; 1 ounce of tortilla chips has about 8 gs; 1 ounce of cheese generally has between 7 and 13 gs of fat, depending on the type; 3 ounces of lean meat has between 6 and 8 gs; fatty meats like spareribs can have as much as 25 gs of fat per 3 ounce-serving. On food labels, it helps to refer to "fat grams per serving," since that will give you a number you can easily apply to your daily total.

In addition, your fat grams should be—at the very least—evenly distributed among the three different kind of fats. Here's why:

- Saturated fats are solid at room temperature and come primarily from animal foods—meat, dairy products, butter—although palm and coconut oils are also saturated. Saturated fats are believed to clog your arteries and raise your blood cholesterol, thus raising your risk of heart disease. That's why you don't want to get more than 10 percent of your daily fat calories from foods that are high in this kind of fat. (Note: Since all foods contain a mixture of saturated and unsaturated fats, they tend to be characterized by the fat they contain the most of. For example, butter is referred to as saturated fat because it is 67 percent saturated fat and 33 percent monounsaturated; olive oil is just the opposite—it's considered a monounsaturated fat because it contains 71 percent monounsaturated fat, 14 percent saturated and 7 percent polyunsaturated).

- Polyunsaturated fats are predominant in corn, safflower, sesame, and soybean oils. The health story on these oils is not clear: For example, some studies indicate they may have a protective effect when it comes to heart disease, but other studies hint that they may increase the risk of breast cancer slightly. Limit them to 10 percent.

- Monounsaturated oils. Olive oil is the richest source, followed by canola, peanut, and sunflower oils. There's a wealth of evidence linking olive oil, in particular, to heart disease prevention and lower breast cancer risk. That's why it's a good idea to substitute olive oil for other oils (especially shortening and stick margarine, which contain trans fats, a type of fat linked to a higher risk of heart disease) whenever possible. In addition, you may want to get more than 10 percent of your calories from monounsaturated fats as long as you don't increase your total fat intake.

Get Enough Iron

It's estimated that around 15 percent of women under age forty-five suffer from some degree of iron deficiency. In addition, a recent study of sixty-two young women athletes conducted at Purdue University in West Lafayette, Indiana, found that long-term moderate exercise was associated with a decrease in iron status.

Even if you eat a balanced, healthy diet, it's easy to experience an iron shortfall—particularly if you bleed heavily each month during menstruation (since this blood loss leads to iron loss), if you are vegetarian (since the iron found in plant food tends to be less available to your body than the iron derived from meat sources), and/or you are an endurance athlete (the reasons for this aren't well understood, but it may be that you excrete more iron during prolonged exercise).

Iron is a very important mineral for athletes to get enough of because it plays a crucial role in carrying oxygen to your muscles as well as getting the oxygen to circulate within the muscles. In fact, training and performance suffer almost immediately, resulting in shortness of breath, weakness, and loss of strength when you experience anemia caused by iron deficiency (anemia can also be caused by other deficiencies, such as B_{12} or folic acid, as well as other diseases). But even when your iron stores are just low (you are not quite anemic) your ability to utilize oxygen becomes impaired and your performance potential declines, according to studies conducted by researchers at the Division of Nutritional Sciences at Cornell University in Ithaca.

"When I was training for the Olympic marathon trials in 1987, I began to have horrible, horrible workouts where I felt like I couldn't breathe and where I would experience diarrhea during runs. And that had never happened to me. I knew something was wrong," recalls professional triathlete Karen Smyers, age thirty-seven, female winner of the 1995 Gatorade Ironman

Triathlon World Championships in Hawaii (an event comprising a 2-mile swim, 115-mile bike race, and a 26. 2-mile run). But my doctor just said, 'Why do you run so much? Stop running.' He also said, 'You're getting older.' I was only twenty-six years old and he was telling me I was finished! When I asked him point blank if I might be anemic, he said, 'No.' Although my hemoglobin tested low, it was still in the normal range. I left thinking my problem was mental."

Eventually Smyers mentioned her problem to a coach she knew, who urged her to get a test of her level of serum ferritin, an indicator of the body's iron stores. Today, more doctors are aware of the importance of not just testing hemoglobin (the amount of iron circulating in red blood cells) but also testing levels of serum ferritin (your iron reserves, which your body taps into when iron requirements aren't met by the diet). "There's no question that testing both hemoglobin and serum ferritin values is the best way to screen for anemia risk," notes Ruth D. Verhegge, R.D., clinical dietitian at East Tennessee State University's Eastman Center for Nutrition Research in Johnson City.

◑ If Your Iron Stores Are Low, Your Performance May Suffer

Best sources of iron:
- beef, lamb, pork, and dark meat poultry
- fortified breakfast cereals
- a multivitamin that contains the RDA for iron

Eat vitamin C–rich foods to boost your body's ability to absorb iron.

As it turns out, Smyers' ferritin values were way below normal; once she began to take an iron supplement, her strength returned. "It was such a relief to know that something was the matter—that the problem wasn't all in my head and that I wasn't over the hill. Since then, I've found that I need to take iron supplements regularly—even though I eat red meat at least once a week, whenever I stop taking supplements, I start feeling weaker." Smyers has also never had a problem with diarrhea during runs since taking iron supplements, which are known to be binding (even constipating) in some women.

The best way to prevent the problem of iron deficiency is simply to pay attention to your intake, and possibly have your hemoglobin and serum ferritin levels checked once a year. The RDA for iron for women aged eleven through fifty is 15 mg daily. Animal foods are the best sources of iron because they contain heme iron, a form of iron that is more highly absorbed than nonheme iron, which is found in plant foods. Beef is a particularly good source of iron, containing 3 mg per 4-ounce serving; dark meat poultry contains about 2 mg per 4-ounce serving; 1 egg or 3 ounces of tuna contain 1 mg.

A good nonmeat source of iron is fortified breakfast cereals—1 cup of Total or Raisin Bran contains 18 mg—all the iron you need for a day.

If you eat a vitamin C–rich food, especially citrus fruit, along with your iron source, you'll boost your body's ability to absorb iron. Likewise, if you take an iron-containing supplement, taking it with a glass of orange juice is a good idea.

But should you take a supplement? "If you are an athlete, it probably wouldn't hurt to take a multivitamin that contains the RDA for iron—and it could very well help prevent you from running into problems," says Verhegge. However, she adds, "If you haven't been diagnosed as needing a therapeutic dose of iron, there is absolutely no good reason to self-prescribe iron at levels higher than the RDA. Large doses of iron can damage your liver, pancreas, and heart."

If you find an iron supplement doesn't agree with you and provokes nausea or constipation, Verhegge's advice is to take it at bedtime, just before you go to sleep. Or you may find it helps to split up your dose and take half in the morning, half in the evening. Finally, some women find children's chewable multivitamin multimineral tablets to be the easiest to digest.

Make Calcium Intake a Priority

The importance of getting enough calcium when you are young in order to prevent the brittle bones disorder, osteoporosis, when you're older has been making medical headlines for years. Yet, just because you've probably heard about the importance of calcium doesn't necessarily mean you're doing anything about it. The most recent USDA Nationwide Food Consumption Survey data, for example, shows that fewer than 30 percent of women between the ages of nineteen and fifty get enough calcium on any given day.

The simple truth is that many of us can't get very worked up about a disease that might not strike for another forty or fifty years. Athletes, in particular, often feel that they're out of danger when it comes to osteoporosis because they engage in regular weight-bearing exercise (which has been shown to increase bone-mineral density and strength).

But here's news that might jolt you to drink more milk: "Calcium is required for transmission of nerve impulses and we suspect that inadequate calcium consumption may be the culprit in leg muscle cramping; the calcium connection may explain why some athletes have more of a problem with cramping than others," says Verhegge.

In addition, a 1990 study of nineteen female athletes with lower extremity stress fractures, published in the *Annals of Internal Medicine*, found that these injured athletes had significantly lower calcium intakes and intakes of dairy products than their uninjured competitors. "We think that you increase your risk of stress fractures if your diet is deficient in calcium," says Verhegge. "All the evidence indicates that a lot of the hairline fractures we see in young female athletes is the first sign of a weakening of the bones."

In other words, you don't have to wait until you are old to reap the benefits of getting enough calcium, there are plenty of potential payoffs—i.e., fewer muscle cramps and stress fractures—right now.

The National Institutes of Health recommends women under the age of twenty (but over age ten) get 1,200 mgs of calcium a day, while women between the ages of twenty and fifty get 1,000 mgs of calcium a day. However, "most of us think athletes, in particular, who are over the age of twenty also need more, from twelve hundred to fifteen hundred milligrams a day," notes Verhegge.

What is the best way to meet your calcium needs? Eat more dairy products and calcium-fortified foods. Dairy products are a particularly important source of calcium because your body absorbs the calcium in them very well, plus they often come packaged with vitamin D, which is essential for optimal calcium utilization.

Milk, yogurt, buttermilk (whether whole, low-fat, or skim), products formulated for lactose-intolerance, and calcium-fortified juices (orange and apple are available in many markets) provide about 300 mg of high-quality, highly absorbable calcium per 1 cup serving. Of course, other foods contain calcium, but few really make sense to depend on as daily sources. For example, how likely are you to consume 4 ounces of canned salmon, 2½ cups of broccoli or 2 cups of cottage cheese, each of which provides about 300 mg of calcium? Think of these foods as bonus sources of calcium. (Other good sources of extra calcium include kale, collards, and bok choy. However, green leafy vegetables such as spinach are not good choices because they contain oxalic acid, which binds calcium and makes it unabsorbable.)

As far as supplements go, most nutritionists feel that food sources are superior to pills. "First and foremost, you should try to get as much calcium as you can by eating a healthy diet," says Terri Karl, R.D., sports nutritionist at the Women's Sports Medicine Center at the Hospital for Special Surgery, New York. "When you get your calcium from foods, you get an array of other important vitamins, minerals, and food compounds that help fight disease and promote overall health at the same time."

But what if you know that despite your best efforts you run a calcium shortfall in your diet? "If you can't seem to eat enough to meet your calcium requirements, then it definitely makes sense to supplement," says Karl.

To determine how many milligrams of calcium you need to take daily in the form of a supplement, use this formula:

1. Multiply by 300 the number of cups of milk, yogurt, or calcium-fortified orange juice you consume on a typical day.

2. Subtract this number from 1,200 (the minimum number of calcium milligrams most experts think athletes of all ages need daily).

3. The resulting figure represents your calcium deficit and the number of milligrams you need to get from a supplement.

The good news is that the calcium in many supplements is "highly bioavailable," according to Karl. Bioavailability refers to how well your body absorbs and utilizes the calcium from a particular source. What's more, the supplement options are pretty easy to narrow down if you are young and healthy (versus elderly, when the issue of which supplement to choose is often complicated by the number of other medications being taken). Tums, Os-Cal, and Caltrate are three brand-name choices that not only contain easily absorbable calcium (in the form of calcium carbonate), but also require you to take only one or two tablets daily. In contrast, supplements that contain calcium citrate may require you to take four to six pills a day. Two calcium sources that you often find in health food stores, bonemeal and dolomite, should be avoided, since they may contain unhealthy levels of lead.

If you want to make sure the supplement you choose dissolves properly in your stomach and thus is more likely to be well-absorbed, you can do this simple test: Put the tablet in a glass of vinegar (which mimics stomach acids), then stir every five minutes for a half hour. If the pill disintegrates completely, the calcium it contains will probably be well absorbed by your body.

Probably one of the most unknown things about dehydration is that women are far more prone to it than men.
—FELICIA BUSCH, RD, AMERICAN DIETETIC ASSOCIATION

Hydrate, Hydrate, Hydrate!

Fluids play a vital role in keeping you healthy: they regulate your body temperature, keep your blood volume up, carry nutrients and oxygen to your cells, help flush wastes from your system, provide cushioning for your joints and protect organs and tissues.

When you don't drink enough liquids every day, you run the risk of becoming chronically dehydrated, symptoms of which include feeling uncharacteristically fatigued, less motivated to work out and less energetic in general.

Women in particular need to pay attention to keeping properly hydrated all day, every day. "Probably one of the least known things about dehydration is that women are far more prone to it than men," says Felicia Busch, R.D., spokesperson for the American Dietetic Association and nutrition consultant in St. Paul, Minnesota. "Because water is stored primarily in muscle tissue, men, who have greater muscle mass, are able to stockpile more water than women. This means women have less available water to lose during strenuous workouts or hot weather conditions."

How much liquid do you need each day? The American Dietetic Association makes this recommendation: Your need for water increases with body weight and level of activity. So a good rule of thumb is to start with 8 cups a day and drink an additional 1 to 3 cups per hour as you increase your intensity and length of activity. For example,

• If you weigh 110 pounds and bike for an hour, you should drink 8 cups of water plus 1 additional cup, for a total of 9 cups of water for that day.

• If you weigh 125 pounds and participate in a 1-hour aerobics class, you should drink 8 cups of water plus 2 additional cups for a total of 10 cups of water for that day.

• If you weight 150 pounds and run for 1 hour you should drink 8 cups of water plus 3½ additional cups for a total of 11½ cups of water for that day.

Other experts recommend that if you exercise for more than 60 to 90 minutes, you drink 8 ounces of fluid for every 15 to 20 minutes you are exercising.

A good gauge of whether you are drinking enough every day is the frequency, color, volume, and odor of your urine— if you're voiding often and your urine is plentiful, light in color, and odorless, you're probably taking in enough. In contrast, if you don't urinate frequently, and your urine is darkly colored, has a strong smell, and is not abundant in volume, it's a clear sign you need to take in more fluids.

Thirst is not a good indicator of how much fluid you need ("by the time you are thirsty, you are already dehydrated," says Busch). For this reason, most experts advise you to schedule your fluid intake—for example, you might make it a habit to drink a full glass of water before and after meals, to drink a bottle of water during your morning and evening commute, to have a glass of water on your desk to sip on as you work, to have a water bottle (or two) on hand during workouts, and so on.

When it comes to what liquids to drink, water should be your first choice because it has no calories, caffeine, or alcohol.

Other good choices include juice, milk, herbal tea, and clear broth. To be avoided in excess: Caffeinated and alcoholic beverages (coffee, colas, black teas, beer, wine, and so forth), since these act as diuretics, causing you to excrete water.

For a full discussion about sports drinks and where they fit into the hydration picture, see page 63.

Applying the Rules

Truth be told, these seven rules for healthy everyday eating (and drinking) don't have special powers to increase your speed, coordination, endurance, or weight loss suddenly. But then, no diet has ever been proven to offer all that. Eating along these guidelines, however, ensures you'll enter competition in a well-nourished, nutritionally solid state.

What if you find your diet falls short when measured against the seven rules? Start small. Make changes gradually and one at a time. Instead of swearing never to eat fast food hamburgers again in your life, for example, just aim to cut back to one or two a week at first. That way you won't feel deprived of your beloved burgers—and you won't be as tempted to throw all attempts at reform out the window. In the same way, instead of vowing suddenly to drink two liters of liquid during workouts, up your intake in increments, since taking in a lot of fluids can be uncomfortable, leading to stomach upset, if you're not accustomed to the practice. The idea is to tweak your diet gradually so that healthy changes become a natural part of your life.

THE VEGETARIAN ATHLETE

You don't need to eat meat in order to compete well, but you do need to pay more attention to your diet, for the following reasons.

• Meeting your protein needs can be a challenge, especially if you stick to a vegan diet (i.e., one that includes no dairy products or eggs). "Typically, vegan diets are 11 to 12 percent protein," notes Virginia Messina, M.P.D., R.D., and Mark Messina, Ph.D., in *The Vegetarian Way* (Crown, 1996).

But if you train regularly and aerobically, your diet needs to be at least 15 to 20 percent protein for you to perform at your best. So vegan athletes may need to make a conscious, concerted effort to get adequate protein, by including meat analogues (vegetable burgers, vegetarian meatloaf, and other foods packed with plant protein) and soy products (such as tofu, soy milk, and tempeh).

In contrast, vegetarian athletes who consume dairy products, cheese, and eggs should have no trouble meeting their protein needs if their vegetarian diet is reasonably healthy and well balanced.

• Vitamin B_{12}, which is crucial for the formation of red blood cells and which athletes require in greater amounts than nonathletes, is found only in animal products. Athletes who consume dairy, eggs, and cheese can easily meet their RDA, but vegans need to take care either to supplement or choose B_{12}-fortified foods.

• Iron and zinc status may be hard to maintain on a plant-based diet since the predominant sources of these minerals are meats such as beef, lamb, pork, veal, and poultry. According to Susan M. Kleiner, Ph.D., R.D., in a review article on "The Role of Meat in an Athlete's Diet," "Iron and zinc are the two nutrients most often deficient in vegetarian or modified-vegetarian diets. Also, iron and zinc are the most cited nutrients that may be deficient in the diet of athletes."

In fact, regularly eating moderate portions of red meat is the easiest way for a woman who regularly engages in high-intensity exercise to avoid anemia and zinc deficiency. But vegetarian athletes can get enough of these minerals, according to Kleiner, if they "learn that it is not sufficient to merely cut meats out of the diet; these foods contain essential nutrients that must be carefully replaced by adding other foods to the diet." In addition, vegetarian athletes should have their iron and zinc levels monitored periodically (at least once a year) and should consider taking a multivitamin fortified with 100 percent of the RDA for iron and zinc daily.

• Finally, when you are both an athlete and a vegetarian, you are at particularly high risk for menstrual irregularity and amenorrhea—conditions that put you at greater risk of stress fractures, painful muscle cramps, and, later in life, osteoporosis.

First, female athletes in general (meat eaters and non–meat eaters alike) have a higher frequency of menstrual irregularities than sedentary women. (It is estimated that up to 44 to 70 percent of gymnasts, rowers, and runners have amenorrhea compared to about 5 percent of sedentary women, for example).

Second, female vegetarians as a group (exercisers and non-exercisers alike) experience more menstrual dysfunction. In a study of forty-one meat eaters and thirty-four vegetarians, for example, conducted at the Pennsylvania State University College of Medicine, the incidence of menstrual irregularity was 26.5 percent among the vegetarian women compared to 4.9 percent among the nonvegetarians. The researchers speculated that the reason for this difference is that vegetarians eat less fat and more fiber—dietary factors that appear to have an impact on a woman's estrogen levels.

So, it's likely that when you put the two things together—being an athlete and being a vegetarian—your risk of menstrual irregularity is probably pretty high. The way to avoid this problem is to eat enough calories and to meet protein and fat needs—all of which are possible on a vegetarian diet but may take some extra effort, especially if you are an endurance athlete or an athlete training on an elite or professional level. Another good source of information, beside *The Vegetarian Way*, is *Nancy Clark's Sports Nutrition Guidebook* (Human Kinetics, 1997); it also includes a large section addressing the nutrient needs of the vegetarian athlete and includes a lot of meal-planning tips and recipes.

WHAT TO EAT AND DRINK BEFORE AND DURING COMPETITION

Whether it's a swim meet, big basketball game, important soccer match, or road race, your pregame eating strategy needs to fill these three requirements:

1. It needs to provide adequate fuel for your muscles so they're loaded with energy and ready for action.
2. It needs to be easily tolerated—you don't want any foods or liquids you ingest to "talk back" in the form of constipation, diarrhea, or nausea.

3. It needs to prevent the performance-lowering (not to mention potentially life-threatening) ill effects of dehydration.

The Weeks Before

The rule for all athletes who participate in events that last over ninety minutes (this includes athletes, such as basketball, volleyball, or soccer players, who engage in a lot of high-intensity, aerobic, stop-start competition) is this: Eat a high-carbohydrate diet (about 60 percent) in the weeks and months that comprise your playing and/or training season. If you are preparing for one big competitive event, such as a marathon or triathlon, about two to three weeks in advance of the big event, you should also taper your training. In other words, you stick to the same diet but exercise less. As a result, you burn fewer carbohydrates and thus build up your glycogen stores. In a Canadian study of eleven triathletes preparing for the Ironman, for example, the athletes who tapered their training for two weeks prior to the event experienced a 16 percent improvement in their running scores.

The golden rule is to eat foods you like and tolerate well prior to a competition. If you eat something unfamiliar you risk getting gastrointestinal distress like diarrhea.
—ANN C. GRANDJEAN, NUTRITION CONSULTANT FOR OVER TWENTY YEARS TO THE US OLYMPIC COMMITTE

The Day Before

This may surprise you, but the growing consensus among top sports nutritionists is that the best foods to eat on the day before an important event are exactly the same foods you eat every day. "The golden rule for athletes prior to a competition is to eat familiar foods you both like and tolerate well," says Grandjean. "If you eat something unfamiliar you risk getting gastrointestinal distress like diarrhea."

In addition, you should eat the same amount of food you normally eat. The ritual among endurance athletes of stuffing themselves with large amounts of carbohydrate-rich food the night before competition in order to help stave off exhaustion the next day is not thought to be beneficial. A 1995 study published in the *International Journal of Sports Nutrition* found that your muscles get no better fueled when you take in excess carbohydrates the day or night before a competition than they do when you consume your normal amounts. Yet, as many athletes have discovered, the chances that an overly hefty pre-competition dinner will throw a monkey wrench in your performance are pretty high. Why? Overeating can throw your digestion process off its normal schedule, leading you to become constipated or to experience diarrhea, and/or leaving you with an uncomfortable, bloated feeling the next day.

Other considerations for the day before: If you've had problems with diarrhea during events, you might also make a point to eat a little less fruit and high-fiber grains (and drink less fruit juice and more water) the day before competition. Some women find that cutting back on these things for twenty-four hours can prevent the problem of frequent or diarrheal bowel movements the next day (see page 68).

Also, during the twenty-four hours prior to your event, it's extremely important to drink a lot of fluids. Be aggressive about it—keep a water bottle at your side at all times and drain it and refill it as frequently as possible since the benefits of entering a competition well-hydrated are firmly established. For example, in a study conducted at the Ball State University, Human Performance Laboratory, Muncie, Illinois, when runners were well-hydrated prior to a 10,000-meter track race, they consistently finished two minutes faster then when they ran the same distance in a dehydrated state.

The Day of the Event

As a general rule, most athletes—from figure skaters to distance cyclists—find that a meal high in carbohydrates and relatively low in fat (such as a banana, bagel, English muffin, or cereal bar) goes down most easily the morning of a big competition. Many athletes avoid milk on competition day because they find it hard to digest as well as linked to diarrhea. However, others find yogurt, in particular, goes down well on race day morning.

Of course, the timing of your last precompetition meal depends on several things. First, it depends on when you are scheduled to compete. If your meet is first thing in the morning and is likely to last over an hour, you should try to eat something light beforehand to prevent your energy from flagging and/or hunger from setting in mid-event. If your tournament is not until midafternoon, you may want to eat a normal-size breakfast, then a light snack for lunch. Or just eat a brunch midmorning. There's really no prescription that is right for every athlete, since some find they need two hours between a meal and competition, others need more time and yet others can scarf down a huge amount of food right before the start gun goes off.

The trick is to road-test your strategy as often as possible in training. Start by scheduling your training sessions at the same time you expect your event to begin. If the race starts at 10:50, make sure several of your training runs begin at that time, for example, or, if the big tennis match is at 3 P.M., make sure you practice at that hour. Then, see how different eating patterns work when coordinated with those training sessions. Do you feel better if your last meal is two hours prior to the session—or do you need more or less time? Did you experience hunger pangs? How did the food you chose sit—did you notice any problems with gas or stomach distention? And so on— finding the precompetition meal and the right timing of it ultimately takes some trial and error on your part, since it is such a highly individual matter.

Of course, there's always the chance that come the day of the big competition you find your stomach gets fluttery and your appetite completely flags. Or the stress and anticipation rev up your appetite, making you more hungry than usual. In either event, your aim should be to not veer too far from your norm. In other words, even though you're not really hungry try to snack on foods you know you can easily digest. Or, even though you are ravenous, hold yourself back to a level that is normal for you. The risk of letting yourself go hog wild before-hand, when you are not used to doing so, is that you'll suffer stomach cramps or other gastrointestinal ills once the event gets going.

What about drinking fluids the day of the big event? First, it's wise to know why fluids are so important. Muscles heat up during heavy exertion. Liquids are needed to maintain your blood volume so that the circulating fluid can penetrate the muscles and carry the heat away from the skin. The evaporation of sweat is the body's primary means of releasing heat during exercise. So, if you don't take in enough fluids, your body's internal cooling mechanism gets thrown out of whack and your core body temperature begins to rise. The first symptoms of this are fatigue and a reduction in your muscular work capacity; you may also begin to feel dizzy and experience muscle cramping.

To prevent this, the American College of Sports Medicine (ACSM) recommends you start by drinking "about 16 ounces of fluid about two hours before exercise to promote adequate hydration and allow time for excretion of excess ingested water." This recommendation is based on research that has found that athletes who drink fluids in the two hours before exercise have lower core temperatures and heart rates than those who don't ingest fluids.

Then, during exercise, the ASCM says "athletes should start drinking early and at regular intervals in an attempt to consume fluids at a rate sufficient to replace all the water lost through sweating, or consume the maximal amount that can be tolerated." In other words, you need to drink as much as you can without making yourself sick. Many experts suggest taking in about 8 ounces of fluid for every fifteen to twenty minutes of vigorous exercise. The way to do this is via practice: The more you get used to ingesting fluids during practice, the better able you'll be to tolerate large volumes of fluid during events.

It's important to remember, too, that fluids are crucial in all seasons. Most athletes know that when the weather is hot and humid, the risk of dehydration is especially high since it is accompanied by three attendant ills: (1) heat cramps, which are characterized by muscle pains and twitches, usually in the legs and abdomen. Nausea and vomiting during and after competition may also be caused by this. (2) Heat exhaustion, the symptoms of which tend to include chills, headache, weakness, fatigue, extreme thirst, confusion, and lack of coordination. And (3) heat stroke, the most serious of the heat-related ailments, which can cause dizziness, unconsciousness, extreme disorientation, rapid breathing, and elevated pulse. Heat stroke can be fatal.

But the problem of dehydration does not end just because you are not competing during the summer or in a hot climate. Studies indicate that winter athletes, especially skiers and snowboarders are also at high risk. Why? First, these athletes often stay on the slope for hours on end, only breaking to drink some fluids at lunch. Cold air also tends to be dry, which means you lose some water with each breath. Finally, if you heat up in warm clothes, you can lose a lot of fluid from sweating. Although the risk of the most serious heat-related illnesses are less, there is still the risk of your performance suffering and fatigue setting in if you fail to take in enough liquid. In other words, just about all women who participate in prolonged (over an hour) athletic events, including swimmers and athletes participating in events that take place indoors, need to focus on fluid replacement during their event.

Sports Drinks

By now, you're probably wondering: Where do sports drinks fit into this picture? The answer, it turns out, depends on how long you exercise.

If you exercise continuously for less than an hour, it isn't completely clear yet whether sports drinks offer any advantages—in terms of helping you keep hydrated or improving your performance—over plain water. Several small studies suggest ingesting sports drinks during bouts of exercise shorter than an hour might improve endurance capacity to a greater extent than water alone. However, the American College of Sports Medicine, in its position on Exercise and Fluid Replacement, says, "It would be premature to recommend drinking something other than water during exercise lasting less than one hour at this time."

To maintain blood glucose levels during continuous moderate-to-high-intensity exercise, carbohydrates should be ingested throughout exercise at a rate of thirty to sixty grams per hour.
—AMERICAN COLLEGE OF SPORTS MEDICINE

If you do exercise continuously and intensely for more than an hour, drinking sports drinks can have some well-established benefits over water. The carbohydrates contained in them help maintain blood glucose concentration and thus delay the onset of fatigue. Studies show that sports beverages containing 6 to 10 percent carbohydrate in the form of glucose or sucrose are most easily and quickly absorbed. Drinks in which fructose is the predominant carb, however, should be avoided since fructose is not readily converted to blood glucose, plus it is more likely to result in adverse gastrointestinal reactions.

Most drinks also contain electrolytes—salts—which are supposed to help replace the salts you lose through perspiration, thus helping you retain liquids and maintain adequate blood volume. However, this benefit has never been proven; the electrolytes contained in sports drinks have not been demonstrated—in a physiologic sense—to promote better water absorption or a more normal blood profile directly. But electrolyte-loaded solutions may offer some indirect benefits. First, they help make most sports drinks more tasty and palatable, which makes you want to drink more of them. Second, the salts they contain make you feel more thirsty, which triggers you to drink more.

The ASCM makes this recommendation: "To maintain blood glucose levels during continuous moderate-to-high-intensity exercise, carbohydrates should be ingested throughout exercise at a rate of 30 to 60 grams per hour." The preferred strategy is to meet carbohydrate and fluid needs at the same time. To do this means you would need to drink between 16 and 32 ounces of sports drink every hour (since most contain 28 to 38 g of carbohydrate per 16 ounces).

But never, never try a sports drink for the first time during a competition. You should test your tolerance during training, since some athletes find they can't stomach large doses of these drinks (they either feel nauseated or experience diarrhea). Diluting them 50 percent with water is often a solution that works (during road races, for example, many runners grab both water and sports drinks at the water stations. They then drink the entire glass of water, but throw away half of the sports drink).

Energy Gels and Bars

As a whole, this category of products aim to provide quick and convenient "energy replacement." As for their effectiveness, in terms of whether ingesting them actually leads to improvements in performance, the jury is still out since most haven't been rigorously tested (or tested at all!). In addition, the issue of whether it's better to get your carbohydrates in the form of liquids (sports drinks), goos (the gels), or solids (bars) hasn't been carefully studied. So far, however, all forms seem to be digested equally quickly as long as you take them with a lot of water. In fact, like so many things in sports nutrition, it probably comes down to personal preference—i.e., what you find works best for you.

Here, then, is a quick rundown of how you might experiment with using these energy aids:

Gels. Designed to be speedily absorbed into your bloodstream, easily carried and quickly slurped down (they come packaged in single-serve 1- to 2-ounce easy-to-open foil pouches or toothpastelike tubes with a flip-top cap), gels consist primarily of simple sugars and carbohydrates. Most have no fat or protein; some contain a dash of caffeine, electrolytes (salts such as potassium), ginseng (a natural stimulant), or other (sometimes exotic) ingredients as well.

Compared to sports drinks, gels are a more concentrated form of carbohydrate. On the plus side, that means you get good glucose replenishment—from 20 to 28 grams of carbohydrate—when you suck down a packet of gel. The downside is that some athletes have a hard time digesting carbohydrates that are so concentrated.

The general recommendation for using gels is to pop a pouchful every half hour during vigorous exercise, making sure to wash it down with a generous dose of liquids (water is crucial for a gel's proper digestion and absorption). Gels come in a wide variety of flavors, such as strawberry creme, chocolate espresso, and peach, and some are sweeter, syrupier, and/or gooier than others. Your best bet is to experiment with the different choices to see which one best suits your tastes—and to see how well you tolerate energy gels while working out. Make sure to road-test your gel of choice several times before using it in competition. Double this advice if you choose a gel that contains caffeine. Why? Besides giving you a bolt of energy, you may find the caffeine causes an unwanted side effect of stimulating your bowels.

Bars. Unlike sports drinks and gels, which don't tend to vary dramatically from each other in nutritional make-up, energy bars can vary widely in what they contain. Some are high-carb; some are high-protein; some are fat-free while others contain as much as 8 grams of fat per bar. So the first rule of thumb is to read labels so you know what you're buying. (In other words, if you're looking to maximize your carb intake during a marathon, make sure you don't buy a high-fat or high-protein bar.)

During long events, some athletes find taking bites on a bar more to their liking than slurping down a gooey pouch of gel. Others find the bars harder to digest and more bulky to carry than gels. It is strictly a matter of what works best for you, which means you'll probably have to do a fair amount of trial-and-error tasting and testing.

Sports bars can be wonderfully convenient pick-me-ups to eat during breaks of a long soccer match, tennis tournament, softball game, etc.—they are generally healthier and more easily digested than candy bars, too. Some athletes find that munching on a bar is an easy way to refuel after an event, since they are compact to pack, unlikely to trigger stomach distress, and pleasantly chewy and sweet.

WHAT TO DRINK AND EAT AFTER COMPETITION

To rehydrate after an event that lasts under an hour, plain water is the best beverage. To rehydrate after longer events, sports drinks may be better than plain water, according to some research. When the beverage you imbibe is loaded with electrolytes (salts), your body retains fluids, your palate craves more liquids, and you urinate less. That's why some experts feel a sports drinks (instead of water) is a better after-exercise choice for endurance athletes.

You should start sipping your sports drink as soon as you cross the finish line or the game ends. If you exercised continuously and intensely for more than sixty to ninety minutes, be sure to take in at least 3 cups of liquid during the first post-exercise hour. Then, match every hour that you exercised with an hour of good post-exercise hydration. For example, if you played soccer nonstop for two hours, drink 3 cups of fluid every hour for at least two hours after you finish playing; if you

---

⚙ **Postcompetition Fluid Replacement Rules**
1. Sports drinks may be preferable to water if you have exercised for over an hour.
2. Start sipping as soon as the race or game ends.
3. Take in 3 cups of fluids every hour post-exercise. Match every hour that you exercised with an hour of good post-exercise hydration.

completed a triathlon in four hours, drink 3 cups of fluids every hour for at least four hours after finishing and so on.

Most sports drinks are designed to be easily digested *during* exercise; in and of themselves, they are probably too diluted to supply you with enough replacement potassium and sodium *after* exercise.

This is where food comes in. Eating solid food—especially potassium/sodium-laden foods often found at the finish line, like bananas and bagels, as well as drinking right after exercise further helps you retain fluids, according to research conducted by Ronald J. Maughan, Ph.D., a professor and researcher at the University Medical School at Aberdeen, Scotland (who was once dubbed "the world's leading authority on fluid replacement" by *Runner's World* magazine).

As it turns out, eating immediately after prolonged (over an hour) exercise is also crucial when it comes to replenishing muscle glycogen stores. In a study conducted at the University of Texas at Austin, the cyclists who ate within fifteen minutes of completing their workout, had significantly greater muscle glycogen storage four hours later than those who waited two hours. Evidence from this same study also suggests that you should eat about .5 g of carbohydrate per pound of body weight every two hours, for about eight hours. So if you weigh 120 pounds, you would need to eat about 60 g of carbohydrate every two hours. Getting this much shouldn't be too hard when you consider the tallies of a just a few classic recovery foods:

1 cup of Gatorade: 14 g
1 banana: 25 g
1 PowerBar: 42 g
1 small bagel: 31 g
1 cup fruit yogurt: 50 g

Finally, a good way to promote rehydration and muscle glycogen replenishment after a prolonged event is to take some time off to rest. The more intense your event, the more rest you probably need. Marathoners, for instance, are often advised to take an entire week off before running again. Of course, if you are involved in a series—a basketball player with successive games lined up—rest may not be an option. In those circumstances, it is especially important you eat and drink properly after games so that you are refueled and ready to keep competing.

HOW TO PREVENT EXERCISE-INDUCED DIARRHEA

It's a surprisingly common problem. According to one researcher, Randall A. Swain, M.D., a family and sports medicine specialist at West Virginia University, Charleston, at least one in ten runners have either stomach cramps, a feeling of a need to defecate, a need to actually defecate, and/or diarrhea during exercise. In fact, among runners, the problem of diarrhea is so common it has been given a name, "runner's trots."

Some experts theorize that diarrhea is particularly a problem in sports that require bouncing, such as running, aerobics, or basketball, and less of a problem in sports like swimming or cycling. A proposed theory for what causes the problem is that exercise decreases the blood flow to the colon, which triggers it to spasm temporarily. Elevation of hormones during exercise may also be a culprit, since most hormones also effect the motility of intestines to some extent.

For anyone who has experienced diarrhea during training or competition, here are some tactics to help you avoid future bouts:

• Establish a ritual of having a bowel movement at the same time every day.

• Avoid too much caffeine, since it can lead you to have the trots. This said, some athletes find one cup of coffee in the morning is precisely what they need to trigger a bowel movement. The idea is to not overdo it when it comes to caffeine.

• Stay well hydrated—diarrhea can be a symptom of dehydration.

• Review your medicine use. One recent study published in *Medicine and Science in Sports and Exercise* found a link between aspirin intake in runners and increased gastrointestinal permeability, an alteration that could potentially lead to diarrhea and other complaints.

• Keep your diet lower in fiber than usual—avoid excessive fruit, bean, and whole-grain intake, especially the day before an important competition.

• Watch out for hidden causes of diarrhea and gas in your diet, such as colas, sorbitol-containing chewing gum or candies, and/or an excess of dried fruits and nuts.

• Try avoiding dairy products the day before a race—some athletes, even if they are not lactose intolerant, find dairy foods harder to digest when they are feeling a lot of stress and anticipation.

• As a last resort, you might consider taking an over-the-counter antidiarrheal agent containing loperamide (Imodium or Imodium A-D) at the strength recommended on the package a half hour before a big event. This is a controversial solution because loperamide may cause abdominal gas, dizziness, or nausea, and it increases your risk of dehydration. In other words, the side effects may be worse or as bad as the problem of diarrhea you are trying to avoid.

If these measures don't offer you relief and/or your urgency is continual and extreme (for example, if you find you actually soil yourself during an event), consult your doctor, who can rule out other causes, such as a parasitic infection, for your diarrhea.

◖ Stop the Trots: Four Preventive Steps

1. Avoid too much coffee, cola, or other caffeine-containing beverages before exercise.
2. Keep away from fruits and beans the day before a big competition.
3. Skip dairy products prior to workouts.
4. Keep hydrated—diarrhea can be a symptom of dehydration.

YOUR MORNING CUP OF COFFEE AND OTHER ERGOGENIC AIDS

Some athletes worry about the safety of drinking coffee, but studies haven't substantiated any strong connections between caffeine and adverse health effects such as infertility, osteoporosis, breast cancer, miscarriage, and heart disease. So on that count you can rest easy when you have your morning brew.

But there's another caffeine-related question that interests many athletes. Namely, can caffeine boost performance?

It might. A large number of studies have linked relatively moderate doses of caffeine—as little as two cups of coffee—to increased speed and improved endurance performance in cross-country skiers, sprinters, swimmers, runners, and cyclists. For example, in one 1995 study of well-trained distance runners conducted at the School of Human Biology, University of Gueph, Ontario, endurance performance was improved by 20 percent for those who ingested caffeine versus the group who had a placebo.

Experts don't understand why caffeine has seemingly "ergogenic" (i.e., performance-improving) effects. One theory holds that caffeine may work simply because it revs up your metabolism, but other theories suggest it may give you an advantage because it has a direct impact on your hormonal balance, your nervous system, or even on your muscles.

The International Olympic Committee has long considered caffeine a "controlled or restricted drug"—an athlete who is found to have more than 12 mcgs of caffeine per milliliter of urine can be banned from competition. But that's a lot of joe—a 150-pound person could drink six regular size cups of drip-percolated coffee one hour before competition and still produce a urine sample that would only approach the urinary caffeine limit, according to a review article on caffeine and exercise performance by Terry E. Graham, Ph.D., and Lawrence L. Spriet, Ph.D., professors in the department of Human Biology and Nutritional Sciences at the University of Guelph. "A caffeine level of about 12 ug/ml suggests that an individual has deliberately taken caffeine in the form of tablets or suppositories in an attempt to improve performance," note Drs. Graham and Spriet.

But even though lesser doses are legal, it doesn't mean coffee drinking makes sense for all athletes. Many people just can't stomach the stuff: it makes them jittery, nauseated, unsteady, anxious, and/or headachy. Caffeine also stimulates your intestines—which is fine if you are in the habit of having a cup of coffee then going to the bathroom every morning. But it's not so fine if you overdo it, since overstimulation of your intestines can lead to gas, abdominal pain, and diarrhea.

The other catch to caffeine is that its impact hasn't been as well studied in women as in men. Researchers like Drs. Graham and Spriet, for example, suspect that the effect in female athletes may be dependent on where they are in their menstrual cycle, since estrogen may influence how long caffeine circulates in your system. Also, if you're already a habitual coffee drinker, you may have built up a tolerance to caffeine that cancels out any performance benefits.

When it comes to caffeine in your diet, then, the key is to keep close tabs on how it makes you feel: Do you feel more alert (or more jumpy), do you actually clock faster times (or does the time just seem to go by faster?), do you recover as well the next day (or do you find you can't sleep that night?), and so on.

Know your doses too. Doses of caffeine as low as 200 mg have been shown to increase performance while doses higher than 400 mg start to be associated with side effects like dizziness, gastrointestinal distress, and insomnia. Here are the amounts of caffeine found in some common sources:

Drip brewed coffee (6 ounce cup) 100 mg
Instant coffee (6 ounce) 65 mg
1 Midol tablet 32 mg
1 Exedrin tablet 65 mg.
Cola (12 ounce) 35 mg
Mountain Dew (12 ounce) 55 mg
Tea (6 ounces) 35 mg
No-Doz (1 tablet) 200 mg
Espresso (1 ounce) 50 mg

What About Other Exercise Elixirs?

Walk into any health food store and you'll find an array of nutritional supplements that promise fat loss, muscle building, increased speed, better endurance, and so forth. There's creatine, an amino acid purported to decrease muscle fatigue, chromium picolinate, a trace mineral that is supposed to help reduce body fat and build muscle mass, there's ginseng, an ancient Chinese root herb that is believed to boost energy and speed recovery. Some of these substances may eventually be found to be effective (since some small studies support the claims made for them) while others may be proven to be pure hype (since some studies refute the claims made for them).

What do you do in the meantime? First, it's important to

realize that dietary supplements are treated under law differently from prescription drugs and over-the counter medicines; they are considered "food" and so manufacturers of the supplements don't have to prove they are safe or effective. Safety is a real issue. For example, creatine may have played a role in the deaths of three college wrestlers and in serious seizures suffered by two others; the Food and Drug Administration (FDA) is investigating this link. The FDA has also issued a warning urging consumers to consult a doctor before using creatine.

Dose is an important issue too. Right now, most of the supplements popular among athletes are sold in all kinds of different strengths. But little is known about how much is safe, how much is needed to get a performance boost (if indeed a substance is shown in the future to be helpful), and how much might be risky to an athlete's health.

Experts have concerns about the purity of the various products sold (purity doesn't have to be guaranteed with nutritional supplements) and worry that long-term use of nutritional supplements may reveal unforeseen health consequences and risk.

The easiest answer to the question of whether you should dabble in nutritional supplements is provided by the National Collegiate Athletic Association, which states in its guidelines, "There are no shortcuts to sound nutrition, and the use of suspected or advertised ergogenic aids may be detrimental and will, in most instances, provide no competitive advantage."

Still, if you're worried that competitors who use nutritional aids may be getting an unfair advantage you'll be tempted to try the various supplements. Before you jump on any bandwagon, consult your team physician, coach, or a health professional. Also, educate yourself as much as possible. A good place to start is *The Ergogenics Edge: Pushing the Limits of Sports Perfor-*

◔ The Female Athlete Triad

- Disordered eating
- Amenorrhea
- Osteoporosis

These three interrelated problems are so common in female athletes that researchers gave the syndrome a name: "The female athlete triad."

mance by Melvin H. Williams, Ph.D. (Human Kinetics, 1998). This book not only rates a wide array of supplements, it gives you the tools and know-how you'll need to evaluate any new elixir that hits the market.

IS YOUR EATING DISORDERED?

"The first time I made myself vomit I did it because my track coach in my senior year at Harvard made some vague remark about me needing to lose some weight. I desperately wanted to please him," recalls Ellen Hart Pena, age forty, a former top-ranked long-distance runner (in 1983, she posted the best 20k race time in the world).

"Of course, I thought vomiting was disgusting and I vowed it would be the only time I ever did it," continues Pena, who is now a mother of three and a spokesperson for the Harvard Eating Disorders Center Advisory Board. As it turned out, Pena was just at the beginning of a ten year struggle with bulimia—an eating disorder characterized by overeating, then purging.

"As I prepared for the first women's Olympic marathon trials in 1984, I remember thinking 'If I could just get a handle on this eating problem for six months, I'm sure I could make the team. Then I said, 'If I can just stop bingeing and purging for three months beforehand . . .' Finally, I thought, 'If I can only stop for three weeks before the trials . . .' But I couldn't. And when I finished eleventh instead of first, second, or third, I knew I had thrown away my chance to make the Olympic team."

How did Pena finally overcome her problem? "When I got pregnant with my first child, I thought I could quit vomiting, but I couldn't. It wasn't until I started to have premature contractions, and I thought I would lose the baby that I got scared enough to stop. But I'm sure I would have gone right back to bingeing and purging after my baby's birth if I hadn't been working closely with a therapist, who helped me understand some of the issues that were underneath my behavior."

No one knows exactly how many women suffer from disordered eating patterns—a broad array of unhealthy behaviors that range from mildly restrictive eating to life-threatening self-starvation. One of the reasons it's difficult to obtain accurate statistics is that women suffering from disordered eating patterns often keep them a secret and avoid professional help.

But research does indicate that the prevalence of disordered eating is very high in female athletes competing in sports where leanness and/or a specific weight is considered important for either performance or appearance, such as long-distance running, gymnastics, figure skating, tennis, and ballet. In a Norwegian study of 603 elite female athletes for example, 117 athletes or almost 20 percent were found to be at risk for eating disorders.

The Disorders Defined

The two disorders that get the most "press" probably because they are so serious and dramatic, are bulimia and anorexia nervosa. Bulimia is characterized by bingeing—eating huge amounts of food (such as a dozen donuts in one sitting), then purging with vomiting, laxatives, or some other drastic method (such as enemas or even excessive exercise) to lose weight. Anorexia nervosa, which appears to be rarer, is marked by a constant shunning of food and a compulsive drive to become thin—even as the woman becomes increasingly emaciated, she still believes she looks too fat.

Anorexia nervosa can be fatal; the dangers of bulimia include cardiac arrhythmias, dehydration, erosion of tooth enamel, swollen glands, gastrointestinal complications, decrease in metabolic rate, amenorrhea, an increased risk of stress fractures, and osteoporosis.

But the problem that many experts believe is most common among women, especially athletes, is less well known. Dubbed a "subclinical eating disorder" or SCED, it's characterized by chronic calorie restriction. In other words, you don't throw up after meals or shun food altogether, but you do consistently and intentionally deny yourself sufficient calories in an effort to keep unnaturally thin.

An SCED is different than simply "watching your weight," which is something virtually every woman does. It's perfectly normal, for instance, to forgo a rich dessert because you want to keep your weight in check. And it's fine, too, to be more attentive to your eating and weight during competition season. In fact, in our weight-obsessed culture, it can be hard to know when a woman crosses the line from "normal" to having an SCED, but common warning signs include:

- You frequently feel guilty or remorseful after meals.
- You're fat-phobic—i.e., you try to eliminate all fat from your diet.
- You almost obsessively try to avoid favorite foods, such as tortilla chips, cookies, or french fries, even in small amounts, because they are "bad."
- You skip meals to compensate for overeating—you may even very occasionally use a laxative or vomit as a way to compensate.
- You eat a monotonous diet of the same low-fat, low-calorie foods (such as an unbuttered bagel for breakfast, salad with fat-free dressing and plain rice cakes at lunch, and pasta with no-fat tomato sauce for dinner).
- Your moods depend on how successful you've been in restricting your eating—that is, you feel better and stronger on days when you've managed to eat less.
- You think a lot about food and feel persistent anxiety about getting fat.

But is a subclinical eating disorder all that serious? Yes, especially when it is accompanied by amenorrhea and osteoporosis. In fact, this trio of disorders is so common it has a name—"the female athlete triad."

"The athlete with poor nutritional habits may go for months, even years, with skipping or losing periods, which can be the result of very low estrogen levels. This, in turn may lead to premature bone thinning or osteoporosis," notes Aurelia Nattiv, M.D., assistant clinical professor in the department of family medicine and department of orthopedic surgery at the UCLA School of Medicine and team physician at UCLA. "Untreated, the female athlete triad can result in a woman of age twenty having the bone density of a woman over age fifty. And with this decrease in bone density comes an increase in her risk for all sorts of stress fractures as well as other abnormal fractures."

Another, quite ironic, risk of an SCED is this: Although women restrict their eating because they believe being thinner makes them better athletes, the reality is that it undermines their ability to perform their best. A chronic calorie deficit can lead to a reduction in aerobic capacity, decrease in immune function, low energy and fatigue, poor muscle glycogen replacement, decreased muscle mass and strength, slow injury recovery rate, mental dullness, an inability to concentrate, and a decreased heart rate.

In short, there is every reason to believe that an SCED leads to slow times, poor workouts, and weak performances.

In addition, the longer you restrict your eating, the more likely it is your metabolism will adapt in a way that makes it harder for you to lose weight. "It is well established that dieting leads to a drop in your resting metabolic rate—the rate at which your body burns calories," explains Melinda M. Manore, Ph.D., R.D., professor of nutrition at Arizona State University in Tempe. In other words, when your body senses a calorie deficit, it responds by burning less in an attempt to prevent starvation. That's why women on low-calorie diets often stop losing weight—their metabolism is trying to combat the effects of a reduced energy supply.

The Road to Recovery

Fortunately, all available evidence indicates that once you begin taking in adequate calories, not only do many of the adverse effects of an eating disorder reverse, but your performance may skyrocket too. In a study conducted at Arizona State University, for example, a nineteen-year-old amenorrheic runner set more personal records, broke two school records, and qualified for Nationals after engaging in a fifteen-week diet program in which she added 360 calories a day (in the form of one 11-ounce serving of GatorPro sport nutrition beverage) and adding one day of complete rest from training per week.

Of course, this runner was lucky—according to the researchers, she had no history of disordered eating and no negative or unhealthy attitudes regarding food. She just wasn't eating enough, and once she realized she needed to eat more, she did.

In fact, athletes with less severe problems often can overcome their disordered eating patterns by simply working with a nutritionist who is experienced in SCEDs. In conjunction with advice from a nutritionist, an athlete can sometimes help herself, by slowly giving herself permission to eat a little bit more and to weigh just a few more pounds. "The fact that an athlete's performance often gets much better when she begins eating and resting more can provide tremendous positive reinforcement for the changes," says Page Love Johnson.

But many women with SCED, bulimia, or anorexia have a serious mental block when it comes to heeding the advice to

SPECIAL FOCUS:

○ Eating Disorders Resource Guide

Women with disordered eating habits have a broad spectrum of resources to turn to for help. The list below is just a beginning; all of the organizations listed provide links to additional resources).

On-line Resources
www.eating-disorder.com
Not designed to compete with other sites, but to bring all of them together through links, E-mail, and references. Provides comprehensive, informative, detailed information about anorexia, bulimia, and compulsive overeating.
www.anred.com
A nonprofit organization that provides free and low-cost information about anorexia nervosa, bulimia nervosa, binge eating disorder, and other less well known food and weight disturbances. There's a special section on athletes and eating disorders. Material includes details about recovery and prevention.

Books
Gurze Books
P.O. Box 2238
Carlsbad, CA 92018
Phone: 800-756-7533
or 760-434-7533
Fax: 760-434-5476
E-mail: gzcatl@aol.com
Website: www.gurze.com
Publishes the Eating Disorders Bookshelf Catalogue containing over one hundred selected books and tapes; it also includes lists of nonprofit associations and advertisements for treatment facilities. It is circulated free.

National Resource Centers
American Anorexia/Bulimia Association (AABA)
293 Central Park West, Suite 1R
New York, NY 10024
212-575-6200

A source of public information, support groups, referrals, speakers, educational programs, professional training, and a quarterly newsletter.

National Association of Anorexia Nervosa & Associated Disorders (ANAD)
P.O. Box 7
Highland Park, IL 60035
847-831-3438
Distributes a listing of therapists, hospitals, and informative materials; sponsors support groups, conferences, advocacy campaigns, research, and a crisis hotline.

Anorexia Nervosa and Related Eating Disorders, Inc. (ANRED)
P.O. Box 5102
Eugene, OR 97405
541-344-1144
Provides free and low-cost information on eating disorders and compulsive exercise. Booklets, brochures, fact sheets, and a monthly newsletter.

"eat more." As Pena recalls, "I feared that if I ate normally, I would instantly balloon out. I thought that if I didn't restrict, I would lose control and just gain and gain weight." Fortunately, acknowledging that you have a problem puts you firmly on the road to recovery. Once you do that, you can start to seek out the appropriate help.

Right now, something called cognitive-behavioral therapy (CBT) is generally considered to be the treatment of choice, for women with an SCED who haven't been able to conquer their problem with the help of a nutritionist as well as for women with bulimia or anorexia. Psychologists, clinical social workers, and psychiatrists are the health professionals who offer CBT, which focuses on the eating problem itself; it does not delve into early childhood problems. CBT teaches women to be more flexible about eating: It encourages women to abandon notions of banned food and stresses eating regular meals and snacks in addition to developing healthy exercise habits and realistic expectations about body weight and shape.

Generally, CBT lasts about twenty weeks. As an adjunct to

CBT, antidepressants are often used; they can help to lift an initial veil of depression so that a woman can begin to feel emotionally strong and clearheaded enough to embark on a path of change. Although CBT in conjunction with antidepressants appears to be more effective than other forms of psychotherapy, it's not magic—it doesn't work overnight, it doesn't provide foolproof protection against relapse, and it doesn't work for everyone. Luckily, other therapies, such as body image work, interpersonal therapy, even dance/movement therapies can sometimes be helpful. The trick is to keep searching for something that works for you—and not despairing if recovery seems to be taking too long.

3

YOUR SKIN, HAIR, FEET . . .

"Competing in my sport undoubtedly took its toll on my skin. I probably could be a lot more beautiful if I hadn't been a cyclist," jokes Linda L. Brenneman, age thirty-four, a member of the 1996 U.S. Olympic cycling team who has recently retired from competitive cycling.

Brenneman found that participating in her sport created some special challenges when it came to caring for her skin properly. "There were many times I simply couldn't take care of it the way I knew I should," says Brenneman. "Although I always wore sunscreen with high protection factors, you are supposed to reapply most of these products after an hour or two. Yet when I was racing I would be out biking nonstop for four to five hours. My sweat would often cause the sunscreen to drip down my face. But I couldn't lose time and stop in the middle of a race to reapply sunscreen. As a result, I often ended up getting a lot more sun exposure than I know was healthy."

As Brenneman learned firsthand, your skin can really take a beating when you're an athlete. Depending on your sport, it may be regularly exposed to outdoor assaults ranging from the sun, chlorine, salt, and whipping winds to violent subzero temperatures. Even if you work out exclusively indoors, your skin stills tends to get subjected to heavy sweating and multiple washings many times a week.

Your skin suffers, too, when there's any kind of problem with the use, size, or design of your gear. For example, if the chin cup on your hockey helmet rubs you the wrong way, the result can be an eruption of unsightly blemishes. Or, if your athletic shoes don't fit quite right, you can end up with gnarly-looking black toenails or tender blisters. And these sports-related skin insults not only wreak havoc with your looks, they can be painful enough to get in the way of a good performance.

The good news is that many problems can be avoided entirely, while there are some pretty simple solutions for others. You don't have to sacrifice the health and appearance of your skin for your sport. The (literally) head-to-toe guide ahead will provide you with specifics on how to spot, remedy, and prevent most sports-related skin problems, from the common (such as athlete's foot and dry skin) to the more off-beat (such as exercise-induced hives). In addition to the "skin-deep" debriefing, you'll find a guide on how to prevent the most common sport injuries, information on how to choose a sports bra and what the best fabrics to wear for your sport are.

FIXING OVEREXERCISED HAIR

Probably the biggest mistake most athletes make when it comes to everyday is that they overwash their hair with strong shampoos, according to Ida Orengo, M.D., associate professor of dermatology at Baylor College of Medicine, Houston.

Although a coat of perspiration can leave your hair limp, grimy, and lifeless, washing it away only requires a very mild shampooing. In fact, using heavy-duty shampoos can have a rebound effect, actually leading your hair to become more greasy: strong shampoo strips your hair of all its protective oils, which causes your scalp to "perceive" an oil deficit, leading it to go into overdrive and step up oil production. Unfortunately, most of us respond to this increase in hair oiliness by using even stronger shampoos, thus creating a vicious cycle. The solution: choose shampoos that bill themselves as "gentle and mild"; shampoos formulated for dry hair also tend to be less harsh.

Two other "bad hair-care" tendencies among athletes: First, the overuse of conditioners. In excess, hair moisturizers can leave your hair feeling gooey and looking flat. "So if you wash your hair more than once a day you shouldn't moisturize each time. Once a day is enough," says Dr. Orengo. The other mistake: excessive blow-drying, which makes hair brittle and causes split ends to get worse (the more bone-dry the hair, the more likely it is the split will just keep traveling up the shaft). If you can't avoid blow-drying completely, first towel-dry your hair well, then blow-dry at low speed, at medium to low heat, and stop before your hair becomes thoroughly dried.

Other hair dangers:

• *Green hair.* Contrary to common belief, it's not the chlorine in swimming pools that allows natural or tinted blond, gray, or white hair to take on a greenish tinge. Instead it's that your hair shaft absorbs the metal copper. "These copper ions may be present either as naturally occurring elements in the water source or released from copper pipes used in the construction of some of the older swimming pools," according to a recent *Dermatology Nursing* article on skin injuries in women athletes. In addition, some algae-killing chemicals used in pools may contain copper.

Indirectly, chlorine may also contribute to the problem: Acting as a bleach, it lightens your hair, and the lighter the tint of your hair, the more vulnerable it is to the greening effects of copper (which tend to be most prominent and noticeable when your hair is wet).

Prevention, luckily, is a no-brainer: Wear a snug-fitting bathing cap. This acts as a physical barrier between the copper ions, the chlorine, and your hair. If you hate caps, you can sometimes prevent the problem by combing a hair-treatment oil into your hair before swimming—the oil repels water and thus creates a barrier to the chemicals.

Treating the problem isn't very difficult either. Applying 2 to 3 percent hydrogen peroxide and leaving it in your hair for 30 minutes will remove the color. (At that strength, hydrogen peroxide does not bleach the hair.) Alternately, you can use a shampoo, such as Ultraswim or Metolex, that is specially designed for pool swimmers and is formulated to remove copper from the hair shaft.

*Probably the biggest mistake most athletes
make when it comes to everyday hair care
is that they wash too frequently with strong shampoos.*
—IDA ORENGO, M.D., ASSOCIATE PROFESSOR OF DERMATOLOGY
AT BAYLOR COLLEGE OF MEDICINE, HOUSTON

- *Sunburn.* The thinner your hair and the fairer your skin, the more susceptible your scalp is to burns. Your hair can also suffer from sun overexposure, although it doesn't actually burn. Instead, the hair shafts tend to become dried out, less flexible, and more prone to breakage. In addition, the sun tends to fade colored hair (wash-in colors are especially vulnerable to the sun's effects) and further lighten naturally fair hair. To protect your scalp from burning as well as your hair from drying and discoloring, wear a hat with a wide (3 inches or more) brim or apply sunscreen, preferably in the form of a nongreasy, spray mist like the product Ombrelle, directly to your scalp and hair.

- *Ponytail breakage.* Any hairstyle that puts traction on your hair roots, such as the classic ponytail, can lead to hair loss. It can also encourage hair breakage, especially if you factor in a lot of vigorous movement.

  The trick to keeping medium-length to long hair healthy— yet out of your face during workouts—is to support the weight of your ponytail or braid so that it doesn't tug at your roots and doesn't pull at the point where it is secured with a coated rubber band or Scrunchie (never use regular rubber bands since they always rip hair out when removed). One way to do this is simply to double your ponytail or braid back up, then secure it to the back of your head with a large barrette. There are a lot of different ways to twist your hair into a snug, close-to-your-head bun, too. The goal, basically, is to avoid having your ponytail whip around as you exercise. The less tension placed on hair roots and the less friction placed on the hair tie, the less hair loss and breakage you'll experience.

FACE AND BODY SKIN TROUBLES

Here's a rundown of the skin troubles that commonly afflict athletes. You'll find a lot of information to help you identify any problems you already have, plus tips on avoiding ailments for which you might be at risk.

- *Acne mechanica.* Unlike *Acne vulgaris,* a type of acne that often strikes during the teenage years and may be triggered by hormonal fluctuations, *Acne mechanica* is sparked by direct physical or "mechanical" stresses, such as: the pressure of a hot and sweaty baseball cap on your forehead; the friction of a tight, clammy leotard on your shoulders or thighs; the pressure of a warm chin cup on your chin; and/or the heat and rubbing of a plastic-covered weight bench on your midback.

What happens is this: The excess heat, friction, and pressure of athletic gear causes moisture, oil, and dead skin to get plugged up in the skin's pores. This causes a buildup of debris under the surface of the skin, which, in turn, creates an ideal breeding ground for bacteria. As the bacteria multiply, the pore stretches, distends, and becomes inflamed. The result is a whitehead, blackhead, or pimple.

The first step to taming these eruptions is to change whatever factor is contributing to them. When wearing a baseball cap, for example, try to wear it a little more loosely, and switch hats whenever the one you have on becomes sweat-drenched. Similarly, if you work out on a plastic-covered weight bench, wear a clean, absorbent, soft cotton tee-shirt and/or place a dry towel over the bench first.

To keep an acne flare-up from getting worse (and to encourage its disappearance), it makes sense to clean the affected area before and after workouts with an antibacterial soap. That helps keep the total bacterial count down. Scrub gently, though, because overly vigorous and abrasive scrubbing can aggravate the problem.

After washing, apply one of the over-the-counter acne products containing benzoyl peroxide and keep the area dry. If your case of *Acne mechanica* is mild, this regime (in concert with eliminating the original source of friction/pressure/irritation) should clear the problem within two months. If the problem persists, or it's more severe, it's time to see a dermatologist and to resort to prescription medications.

In general, the most effective course of action is to combine a prescription topical agent with oral antibiotics (tetracycline is usually the first choice, then minocycline or doxycycline). Some experts recommend following this program for at least five months.

In severe cases that resist these remedies, the oral drug isotretinoin can be very effective in clearing the skin completely. "Isotretinoin is a wonderful medicine, but like a sharp knife—must be used carefully," warn dermatologists Ronald C. Savin, M.D. and Lisa M. Donofrio, M.D., in an article titled "Aggressive Acne Treatment," published in *The Physician and Sportsmedicine*.

A big risk for athletes is that isotretinoin, which should be taken for twenty weeks, can cause joint and muscle pain as well as make you feel lethargic and lacking in energy. For that reason alone, many athletes may want to avoid it—or, at the very least, postpone using it until their competitive season is over. The other very serious risk of isotretinoin is that it produces birth defects. So if you take the drug you need to stick to a super-strict pregnancy prevention regime.

• *Bikini bottom.* This bacterial infection on the skin of your buttocks is characterized by deep, inflamed red patches; it's caused by sitting for hours on end in the same tight-fitting, damp swimsuit. The reaction, however, may be delayed, with the rash only appearing three to five days *after* you've spent a full day at a beach, pool, or lake.

"Untreated, this malady can run a protracted and frustrating course, making sitting in one position for any length of time quite unpleasant," according to a *Dermatology Nursing* article.

Treatment involves taking a course of oral antibiotics to kill the bacteria and not wearing swim gear for at least ten days. Topical antibiotics may also be prescribed. Then, to prevent future flare-ups, you simply need to get in the habit of getting out of your swimsuit whenever possible when it's damp and/or removing it for several hours (and donning a pair of loose shorts or a dress, for example) if you are spending the entire day at water's side. You might also want to apply an absorbent powder after drying yourself off, to further reduce the risk of a recurrence.

◔ Dried-Out Gym Skin: Three Ways to Fight It

1. Avoid long, hot showers after workouts (they strip your skin of hydrating natural oils).
2. Only soap your groin and underarms.
3. Apply a light moisturizer after your shower, while your skin is still damp.

• *Chafing.* When two of your body parts repeatedly rub together or an article of clothing continuously rubs against your skin during exercise, the result is chafed skin, which tends to be irritated, reddened, and inflamed as well as sensitive to the touch. The area that tends to be most vulnerable in women is the upper thighs, although the inside of your upper arms may become chafed if they continually rub against the rough seams of a jog bra, for example.

The treatment for chafing is to use a lubricant, such as petrolatum (Vaseline) or other similarly greasy ointment to reduce friction and create "slide." Wearing the right gear can help tremendously too. A *Dermatology Nursing* article recommends: "Garments such as 'bun huggers' for volleyball players and tights for runners are an excellent option for those afflicted, as are sport shorts with longer legs made of low-resistance fabric." Finally, you might want to try using a sports powder, such as Zeasorb, to further reduce the risk of uncomfortable chafing.

• *Chapped lips.* "Lip skin is thinner than other facial skin. It doesn't have a lot of layers or lubricating glands, so it's very vulnerable to the harsh, drying effects of the sun, wind, salt, and cold," says Dr. Orengo. "Athletes also have a tendency to lick their lips—if you're in the middle of a workout and your lips feel dry, the natural inclination is to lick them. But this sets up a vicious cycle, since each time you lick your lips, you cause them to dry out more."

Clearly, getting out of the habit of licking your lips is the first step to repairing damaged lips. Step two is to use a thick, waxy, or petrolatum-based balm to seal in moisture and help heal cracks. If your lips are actually burned (from sun exposure) or bleeding (from being exposed to cold temperatures), try a lip ointment that contains analgesics for soothing. You might want to take an over-the-counter NSAID, such as ibuprofen, too, suggests Dr. Orengo, to reduce the inflammation.

To prevent future lip troubles, always wear lip balm to seal in moisture and prevent the harmful effects of the elements. Stay away, too, from the new "long-lasting," "stay-on," "rub-off proof" lipsticks since these tend to dry out lips.

Most important, whenever outdoors, make sure the lip balm you wear contains a sunblock with an SPF of at least 15 and be sure to apply it repeatedly over the course of the day. "Lips are extremely prone to developing skin cancer, and unfortunately the cancers that grow on the lip usually act more aggressively than other skin cancers," notes Dr. Orengo. Protecting your kisser with sunblock also helps prevent the development of vertical lip wrinkles, brown spots, and premature thinning of lip skin.

• *Dry skin.* In the winter, practically everyone's skin is more prone to dryness because the air indoors tends to be hot and dry, while outdoors it's cold, dry, and windy. But athletes, in particular, often have dry-skin problems all year round primarily because they tend to bathe so frequently, often more than once a day; take long, hot showers to soothe tired muscles after workouts; and often choose strong soaps to scrub sweat, grime, and dust off after a game. All these habits strip skin of its natural oils and dehydrate it.

Perhaps the biggest problem with dry skin, besides its mild itchiness and unsightliness, is that it can progress to eczema—a dry, scaly, reddish, and unrelentingly itchy skin condition for which there is no cure (although topical steroids offer eczema sufferers relief and may help to clear up the rash). Some people appear to be more prone to eczema than others, which suggests that there is a family trait or genetic predisposition for the development of the problem.

To avoid aggravating an existing dry-skin problem, avoid long, hot showers and don't soap your whole body—just your groin and underarms. Use a soap substitute, like Cetaphil, Oil of Olay, and Moisturel liquid cleanser or Basis bar, since these remove fewer of your natural oils than do detergent-based soaps. Use a mild shampoo, too, since it will rinse over your body. After your shower, while your skin is somewhat damp, apply a light moisturizer or skin oil.

Finally, if you are eczema-prone and you swim in a chlorinated pool, coat yourself liberally with a hypoallergenic, all-purpose moisturizer before entering the water and once again immediately after rinsing off in the shower after swimming, advises Nelson Lee Novick, M.D., in *You Can Do Something About Your Allergies* (Macmillan, 1994). If additional moisture is needed, says Novick, "You might discuss with your doctor the use of the prescription-strength moisturizing lotion Lac-Hydrin for routine use and before and after swimming."

• *Exercise-induced hives.* If you get hives (a rash of red welts) after beginning strenuous exercise you may be suffering from one of two rare types of allergic reactions to exercise. One condition, cholinergic urticaria (CU) is relatively harmless, while the other, exercise-induced anaphylaxis (EIAna), is potentially life threatening.

With CU, hives crop up in response to a jump in your core body temperature. So you may notice that in addition to getting hives when you exercise vigorously, you are also prone to outbreaks when you take prolonged hot showers, eat spicy foods, and/or run a fever. In CU, your hives are usually small—little pinpoint-size red spots that first appear on the upper body and neck anywhere from two to thirty minutes after beginning exercise. Sometimes, but not always, the hives will spread to other regions of your body. They may be mildly to moderately (not intolerably) itchy, or not itchy at all. As a general rule, a CU reaction disappears as spontaneously as it appeared, usually within twenty to ninety minutes after stopping exercise, according to an article, "Itching in Active Patients: Causes and Cures," in *The Physician and Sportsmedicine* authored by Steven M. Leshaw, M.D., clinical professor of medicine in the division of dermatology, University of California, San Diego.

EIAna, on the other hand, may not be so uneventful. The first symptom is a flush of warmth over your skin, beginning within five minutes of vigorous exercise. From there, large, intensely itchy welts develop—you may experience abdominal cramps, diarrhea, or headache. Sometimes the attack will subside, in anywhere from thirty minutes to four hours. However, if the attack progresses, you may become light-headed and have difficulty breathing. In the worst case scenario, EIAna leads to a loss of consciousness, a dramatic drop in blood pressure, as well as fatal heart and lung failure.

What triggers EIAna? For some, an attack may be triggered by a food eaten in combination with exercise. The foods most associated with EIA are celery, peanuts, and shrimp. These foods are common troublemakers for those prone to food allergies, although little is known about what properties peculiar to them make them more apt to cause allergic symptoms than others. What's more, why these foods would only cause trouble when combined with exercise in some people is poorly understood. One theory is that exercise somehow causes the food allergens to be absorbed more rapidly than normal and thus ignites a quick, dramatic response.

Anyone who has experienced hives during exercise would be well advised to investigate what she has eaten beforehand. Try to identify offending foods and have your suspicion confirmed by an allergist, who will perform a skin-prick test, in which tiny extracts of the suspected allergens are shallowly injected into the skin's top layer. If you're sensitive to a substance, the pricked area turns red and forms a welt within twenty minutes.

Certain medications, when combined with exercise, can also trigger EIAna but sometimes no additional trigger can be found. In other words, exercise, and exercise alone, appears to be what causes the hives and the progressive reaction.

Anyone who experiences hives upon exercising—and has any concurrent symptoms like intense itchiness, faintness, headache, trouble breathing, and so on—should see an allergy specialist immediately. You may be at risk for EIAna, which can escalate into a full-blown attack, without warning, at any time during exercise.

If you are prone to EIAna, you will need to take some precautions. First, when exercising you'll always need to carry with you a dose of self-injectable epinephrine (EpiPen), a medicine that halts the life-threatening anaphylactic reaction. Most experts also recommend that you never exercise alone, since some EIAna reactions can progress at such a breakneck speed that you may need a partner to inject you with the EpiPen.

Luckily, though, most EIAna attacks can be prevented, via a regime of antihistamine use. Antihistamines work by blocking the body's release of histamines, the chemical substances responsible for the allergic symptoms. You'll need to get a prescription for a long-acting, nonsedating antihistamine, then get in the habit of taking it one hour before exercise. If a regime of antihistamines don't prevent EIAna attacks, the corticosteroid medication, prednisone, taken twelve hours before exercise, is usually effective.

• *Hand calluses.* Callused hands are par for the course among certain athletes, such as crew team members, gymnasts, racket sport players, weight lifters. The calluses form as a result of mechanical friction (the pulling of the oars, the gripping of the racket, and so on), and they usually follow on the heels of a lot of blisters and bruises.

"Most calluses are painless and many consider them to be a competitive advantage, since their presence makes the grip 'tougher' and less sensitive," says John E. Wolf, M.D., professor and chairman of the department of dermatology at the Baylor

College of Medicine, Houston. If, for any reason, you want to remove a hand callus, the safest way is to soak your hand in warm water to soften the tissue first, then use an emory board to sand it down.

• *Jogger's nipples.* Another friction-related problem, this condition is caused when your nipples repeatedly rub against something rough, like the seam of a bra or, if you go braless, the stitched logo or coarse fabric of a tee-shirt. Your nipples can become extremely sensitive and painful; in cases where the rubbing has been repetitive for long hours (during the running of a marathon, for example), your nipples may even bleed. Interestingly, this problem is actually more prevalent among men, probably because women often wear soft, protective bras.

You treat jogger's nipples as you would any cut or bruise—apply an antibiotic ointment to help heal and soothe them as well as to prevent an infection from setting in. Obviously, make sure you shield your nipples from any contact with rough or coarse materials and choose sport bras and workout shirts made of soft materials. Some athletes also dab a greasy ointment on their nipples (such as good old Vaseline) or even put Band-Aids over their nipples before competition as an additional safeguard.

• *Poison ivy (or oak or sumac) rash.* As many trail runners and hikers have discovered, you can become allergic to the resins of these plants at any point in your life—just because you were able to traipse around in the woods as a child, seemingly immune, doesn't mean you can't suddenly become sensitive. In fact, it's estimated that 85 percent of all Americans eventually become allergic to these plants.

A poison ivy, oak, or sumac rash may surface anywhere from six hours to three days after you've come into contact with the plant. You may first notice that the affected area is itchy, then becomes red, then forms little fluid-filled blisters (which eventually ooze, then become crusty and scabbed over).

Contrary to what many believe, the blister fluid does not contain resin and scratching the blisters does not spread the rash, notes Dr. Leshaw in *The Physician and Sportsmedicine.* Only contact with resin gives you a poison ivy rash. When a rash appears to be "spreading" what's really happening is that it is just taking time to fully surface. The reason you are advised to not scratch a poison ivy rash is that your fingers can transmit bacteria into the blistered area, leading to infection.

Mild to moderate cases of poison ivy are treated with cool compresses and high-potency corticosteroids applied directly to the affected area. "Occasionally, severe or widespread cases need systemic corticosteroid therapy that requires longer, tapering courses, such as prednisone, 60 mg for five days, decreasing to 40 mg and 20 mg for five days each," writes Dr. Leshaw.

Like so many skin woes, the better course of action is to avoid the problem in the first place. Learn to identify the enemy (most guides to plants have pictures; if possible, ask a knowledgeable friend for an "in-the-field" lesson, too).

If you are not sure you'll be able to avoid the plants completely (if you're doing a trail run in an area unknown to you, for example) several new, over-the-counter lotions, such as Enviroderm's Ivyblock, can be used to create an effective shield against the resins of poison ivy, oak, and sumac.

In addition, if you think you may have come in contact with the resin of poison ivy, oak, or sumac, it's sometimes possible to avoid a rash if you act quickly (within a half hour) to wash off the area. Harsh soaps such as yellow soap, laundry detergent, or dish soap are best at stopping the resin from traveling down under the surface of your skin. You'll also need to thoroughly wash any of your clothing or sporting equipment that may have come in contact with the plants, because the resins do not evaporate and you can get the rash from contact with these things. Beware, too, if your dog went with you on that hike or trail run, since you can get poison ivy from petting an animal who has the plant resin on its fur.

• *Seabather's eruption and swimmer's itch.* Both of these itchy skin irritations are reactions to organisms present in the water.

In the case of seabather's eruption, which may take one to two days to develop, the offending organism may be jellyfish, sea anemone, fire coral, or man-of-war. Sometimes the rash is accompanied by chills, fever, swelling, headache, nausea, and vomiting.

With swimmer's itch, the rash is a reaction to parasites (which may be transferred in the water from waterfowl, such as ducks or geese).

The main difference between the two rashes is that with seabather's eruption, the itchy welts arise in areas underneath your bathing suit after swimming in salt water, while with swimmer's itch, the bumps crop up in areas *not* covered by a bathing suit after swimming in fresh water. You treat the symptoms of both ailments similarly: To help control the itching, you use a combination of topical steroids, antihistamines, and cool compresses. In rare cases of a very severe reaction, you may need an oral corticosteroid to tame your symptoms. Both rashes disappear spontaneously after one to two weeks.

• *Skater's and surfer's nodules.* These are little protruding knots or lumps of thickened tissue in areas where a lot of pressure is placed for a long time. Surfers get them on their knees and on the tops of their feet right below their toes—the two places that tend to be in contact with the surfboard. According to a *Dermatology Nursing* article "They are worn as a badge of distinction by serious surfers, male and female alike, and appear to be seen with equal frequency between the genders."

Dr. Wolf has also seen nodules form on the ankles of professional skaters, probably from the pressure of tightly fitted skates. "Most of the time these things are not a problem. But if they become painful enough to interfere with your activity, they can be treated with injections of cortisone, to reduce the swelling, or they can be removed surgically," says Dr. Wolf. Also, if your activity is seasonal (you only skate during the winter or surf in the summer), the nodules are unlikely to be permanent and will usually disappear slowly once you discontinue the sport.

• *Sun-induced skin injury.* Anyone who has ever suffered a sunburn knows that it's awful. Not only do you look like a lobster, with peeling nose and parched lips, but your skin becomes hot, tender, and exquisitely sensitive to the touch. You may also have flulike symptoms.

First aid for a sunburn involves easing your pain as much as possible by using an over-the-counter cooling, antiseptic spray or cream that is specially formulated for treating sunburns and by taking aspirin, acetaminophen (e.g., Tylenol), or a NSAID (ibuprofen). If you have widespread blistering and/or you have chills, fever, or malaise that lasts more than twenty-four hours, you should see a doctor.

Few athletes need to be persuaded that sunburns are to be avoided—after all, they feel horrible, interrupt your ability to play, and look bad. But when it comes to the advice to avoid tanning, you may need persuading, since a tan doesn't hurt and can even look good.

Still, each time your skin gains some brown pigment it is a sign that the cells and tissues of your skin have been injured. The more frequently your skin becomes tanned, the more broken down its elastic fibers become, leaving your skin more vulnerable to wrinkling, brown spots, roughness, and other attributes that can make your skin look years older than it really is.

But potentially there's an even more serious consequence to sun exposure: Yes, (as you've probably guessed) the danger is skin cancer. It doesn't matter what your sport is, if you play it outside, you're at risk for any of these three different types of skin cancer:

1. *Basal cell carcinoma.* This is the most common form of skin cancer, and is, luckily, also the most highly curable. It tends to develop slowly, often starting as small depressions in your skin with pearly white borders.

2. *Squamous cell carcinoma.* The second most common type of skin cancer, squamous cell carcinomas generally occur on the face, head, shoulders, and arms and may first appear as small sores that do not heal. In general, squamous cell carcinoma is easily cured—although, if left too long, it can metastasize and spread to other parts and organs of your body

3. *Malignant melanoma.* The least common but most deadly type, it usually (but not always) appears as dark blue or black growths and may be flush with the skin or raised. One of the most important signs of a malignant melanoma is a change in the color, size, shape, or texture of a mole. If caught early, malignant melanoma can be removed and cured; however, it can rapidly grow down into the deeper layers of the skin and then spread to your bones, lungs, and brain.

If you use a sunscreen that is oil-based
and greasy or very creamy and thick,
it could inhibit your body's ability to
sweat and cool off.
JOHN E. WOLF, MD, CHAIRMAN OF THE DEPARTMENT OF DERMA-
TOLOGY AT BAYLOR COLLEGE OF MEDICINE, HOUSTON

All these different types of cancer are on the rise—the incidence of melanoma, for example, has been increasing by an average of 4 percent each year since 1973, while basal and squamous cell carcinoma increased 50 percent between 1980 and 1990—and they are also becoming more common in women still in their twenties.

The main reason why skin cancer is becoming more prevalent is increased sun exposure. We all spend more time outside—during recess, after school, and during summers—and from an earlier age than previous generations. We wear less protective clothing, too, when we're outdoors. In addition, the problem is compounded by the depletion of the ozone layer—a layer of protective gas sandwiched between us and the sun that prevents cancer-causing radiation in ultraviolet light from reaching the earth. As the ozone layer thins, so does its ability to shield us from the sun's negative rays.

Clearly, the risk of cancer adds yet another persuasive reason to avoid overexposure to the sun. Yet many athletes with good intentions get thrown when it comes to the usual sun avoidance/sun protection advice.

For example, the advice to avoid being out in the sun when its rays are most intense, between 10 A.M. and 3 P.M., can be pretty restrictive and impractical if you're a tennis or beach volleyball player with a game scheduled at 11 A.M.

Another common complaint is that some sunscreen products cause overheating during exercise.

"That is a real issue," notes Dr. Wolf. "If you use a sunscreen that is oil-based and greasy or very creamy and thick, it could inhibit your body's ability to sweat and cool off. Unfortunately, many of the sunblocks that are marketed specifically for "sport use" do just that—they emphasize sweat resistance, which means they won't run and drip but they may impede your ability to perspire freely."

To this problem, however, there's a solution: Use a gel-based sunscreen (instead of one that is billed as being a lotion, cream, or oil). "The gel evaporates, but the chemical that blocks the sun's rays stays on your skin, so it doesn't have any adverse effect on your ability to sweat," explains Dr. Wolf.

Here, then, are sun protection tips tailored to the special needs and circumstances of active women:

1. Use a sweat-proof sunscreen on your forehead and

around your eyes to prevent it from running into and stinging your eyes.

2. Select a sunscreen with an SPF of at least 15; make sure it blocks both types of harmful ultraviolet wavelength: UVA and UVB.

3. Wear sunscreen even on cloudy days and when in water; when engaging in sports such as skiing, snowboarding, and ice climbing your need for sun protection is especially high, since damaging rays reflect off the snow and can even be stronger than beach sun.

4. Apply 1 ounce of sunscreen for whole-body coverage and remember to apply to the areas many people forget: around the eyes, ears, mouth, and on the head if you have thin hair, recommends a recent article published in the *Physician and Sportsmedicine*.

5. Apply sunscreen at least twenty to thirty minutes before you go outside, then reapply every two to four hours. If you are swimming, reapply every hour. But what if you can't follow this advice—if, like cyclist Brenneman, you are engaged in an event that lasts for more than two to four hours and have no time to stop and reapply sunscreen? Your best strategy is to wear a visor or a helmet equipped with one—a visor will considerably reduce your face's exposure to the sun. If possible, also wear a lightweight, ventilated tee-shirt to protect your shoulders and back.

6. Especially if you have sensitive skin, you may have to experiment with several products to find one that suits you. One ingredient that caused a lot of allergic reactions, PABA, has been removed from the majority of products.

Look for one of the new sunscreens that works by creating a physical barrier to the sun's rays, since these are less likely to be allergenic than a chemical barrier. These sunscreens, which contain titanium dioxide, aren't visible as was the white goo familiar on the noses of lifeguards. Look for words *chemical-free* on the label. In addition, many sunscreens are marketed in a version for sensitive skin and/or for children. If your skin is easily irritated, one of these products often works.

7. Cover up, if possible. A hat with a 4-inch brim will provide additional coverage to your vulnerable facial skin. A lightweight tee-shirt can help shield your shoulders and back. In general, however, clothing is no substitute for sunscreen (a typical cotton tee-shirt offers an SPF protection of about 5 to 9), it just boosts your overall protection. The exception to this rule, however, is clothing made of fabric that provides UVA and UVB protection. L.L. Bean's Tropic Wear line (800-221-4221) uses chemically treated fabric that blocks most of the sun's rays. A company called Sun Precautions (800-882-7860) offers a line of patented clothing and hats called Solumbra that have built-in SPFs of 30 plus. Many of the styles offered are also designed to provide good ventilation during high levels of activity.

◒ Sunglasses for Sport: Three Shopping Tips

  1. Beware of labels that only say "UV protection"—you want glasses that clearly offer 100 percent protection from UV rays.
  2. Check frame fit closely: It can be a major annoyance if your glasses keeping slipping down your nose when you're playing.
  3. Make sure your lenses offer a good field of vision and aren't too dark.

---

8. Don't forget to protect your eyes, since the sun's ultraviolet rays can not only damage the delicate skin around your eyes, but may increase your risk of cataracts (a clouding of the eye's lenses) and macular degeneration (a disease of the retina). Look for models of sunglasses that offer 100 percent protection from UV rays (beware of labels that say only "UV protection"— you want the degree of protection to be clearly specified).

Ideally, your sunglasses should fit close to your face and offer some protection from light entering from the sides. You'll want to pay close attention to how clear your vision is with the glasses on, making sure not to pick lenses that are so dark they obstruct your view (and can thus interfere with your ability to play your best). Fit is very important too, since if your sunglasses are too tight or too loose, they'll be a source of annoyance and distraction during exercise.

If you need to wear sunglasses while playing your sport, you might consider one of the sport-specific sunglasses, made by companies like Nike, Adidas, Reebok, Oakley, and Vuarnet. These tend to be pricey (anywhere from $60 to $200), but they also offer an array of technical design features—like slip-free nose pads, antiscratch lenses, generous lightweight lenses for clearer vision at high velocities—that make them pretty sophisticated, worthwhile pieces of equipment.

COMMON FOOT PROBLEMS

Athlete's Foot

One of the most common infections among active women, athlete's foot or tinea pedis is caused by a fungus. The fungus usually starts growing between your toes or on the bottoms of your feet; the skin of the infected area is often very dry, reddened, and scaly; the area may be itchy, malodorous, and sometimes painful.

Why are the active so prone? The warm, moist environment of your athletic shoes is the perfect breeding ground for fungus. You can also catch the infection by walking barefoot in locker rooms, showers, gyms, and on pool floors, since the microorganisms tend to thrive and multiply in these kind of communal, wet places.

To minimize your chances of acquiring athlete's foot (as well as a similar disease, pitted keratoloysis, in which your feet become very smelly, but not itchy, with a lot of little depressed craters or pits on your heels, balls, or toe pads), wear rubber thongs in the locker room, shower, poolside, or other wet places. Get in the habit, too, of airing your sneakers out after workouts; if possible, rotate between two or three different pairs of athletic shoes.

To treat athlete's foot, there are an array of effective over-the-counter powders and sprays, which usually work after one to two weeks. If your chief complaint is odor, you may also want to try these five measures recommended by Michael L. Ramsey, M.D., an associate in the department of dermatology at Geisinger Medical Center in Danville, Pennsylvania, in a recent *The Physician and Sportsmedicine* article:

1. Scrub your feet thoroughly with an antibacterial soap when showering.

2. Dry your feet thoroughly, making sure to get between your toes. Use a blow dryer if it helps. Spray underarm antiperspirant containing aluminum chlorhydrate or aluminum chloride on your feet to help keep them dry.

3. Change socks frequently. Take an extra pair for changing during the day. (For information on sock materials that wick away moisture, see page 111.)

4. To reduce sweating and odor, soak your feet in black tea, which contains tannic acid, once a day. One method is to brew two tea bags in 1 pint of boiling water for fifteen minutes. Then add the tea to 2 quarts of cool water and soak your feet for twenty to thirty minutes. Some people report great improvement after seven to ten days of daily tea soaks.

5. If your foot odor persists after two or three weeks of trying these tactics, it's time to see a doctor, who can prescribe stronger remedies.

Black Heel

These tiny, little clusters of black dots, like grains of pepper, on your heel are pinpoint hemorrhages. They are caused by friction, according to Dr. Wolf, and frequently occur in women who play sports that require fast stops and starts, like tennis or basketball.

A black heel is rarely painful; it generally disappears by itself after two to three weeks of rest. A felt heel pad placed in your shoe can prevent it from coming back. If you either can't or don't want to rest your heel and the problem persists for weeks on end, it's probably prudent to see a doctor who can rule out the highly unlikely possibility of a cancer. The test isn't complicated or painful—all a doctor has to do to rule out cancer is remove a little surface skin from your heel, mix it with a small amount of water, then perform an occult blood screening test to see if the tissue contains blood (if it does, you've got a simple case of black heel).

Black Toenails

"Black toenails occur when the nail is compressed against the bed that lies underneath it or when the nail becomes separated from its bed," explains Perry H. Julien, D.P.M., assistant medical director for the Peachtree Road Race and Atlanta Marathon and podiatrist in private practice at the Atlanta Foot and Ankle Center, Atlanta. "This results in the formation of a pool of blood in the space between the nail and its bed, which is what causes the black-and-blue appearance."

Any sport in which your toe repetitively jams against the top of your athletic shoe (running, racket sports, skiing, hiking, climbing) can cause black toenails. Anything that intensifies the jamming such as competing at a faster pace, competing for a longer time, or competing in a hot environment (all of which can cause your feet to heat up, swell, and become more tightly packed in your shoes) can cause black toenails.

If your toenail isn't painful, your best bet is simply to leave it alone. The darkened toenail will eventually grow out over the next few months and a new, usually normal-looking toenail will take its place.

If you are experiencing pain in the immediate hours after injuring your toe, it's caused by the pressure of blood building up under the surface of your nail. This pain usually subsides in twenty-four hours on its own, but you can increase your comfort by resting, soaking your toe in cool water, and taking an anti-inflammatory medicine, such as ibuprofen.

A trick used by some doctors: They relieve the pressure by letting some of the blood out. Using a sterile instrument that has been heated, they gently place it on top of your nail so that it melts a hole into your nail, thus allowing the pooled blood to be released. "This procedure doesn't hurt, since your nail is dead tissue. But for it to be of any use, it needs to be done

---

◯ Blister Busters

- Spray an antiperspirant on your feet before exercise to reduce moisture.
- Protect the blister-prone area by taping it with duct tape before workouts.
- Wear shoes that fit properly and socks that are moisture wicking.

within the first hours after being injured. Otherwise, you'll simply be burrowing into dried blood, which isn't going to give you any relief," explains Dr. Wolf.

Finally, anyone who experiences a black toenail should take a good look at their athletic shoes, since shoes that are too short or too narrow in the toebox are often the culprit. (See page 108.)

Blisters

A blister is the result of something rubbing against the skin, causing friction. The friction, in turn, causes the upper layers of skin to separate from the lower layers, creating a space into which seeps either blood or clear fluid.

As with black toenails, the reason many athletes only get blisters when they race is because their feet are subjected to greater friction, heat, and swelling during competition.

The first step to preventing blisters is to wear shoes that fit and socks that offer cushioning and dryness. Keeping feet dry is an important aspect of preventing blisters, too—spraying an antiperspirant on your feet before putting on your socks can help reduce moisture.

However, some women are more prone to blisters than others, no matter how appropriate their shoe gear (it may be that some women have thinner skin than others, although this explanation hasn't ever been proven). Athletes who know they're vulnerable sometimes apply petroleum jelly or Aquafor to problem areas, cover the area with adhesive moleskin or tape the blister-prone zone with duct tape as a preventive tactic.

If you get a blister, home remedies are usually sufficient treatment. If the blister is small and not too bothersome, you can just leave it alone and it should heal by itself within a week to ten days. Larger blisters can be drained: Sterilize a needle, pin, or scalpel by wiping it with alcohol, then puncture the blister near the edge, where it meets the skin. Gently press on the side of the blister to push the fluid out of the opening. Be sure to leave the "roof" of the blister intact, since this provides protection for the sensitive, tender skin underneath. Cover the area with an antibiotic ointment and a clean bandage.

"Generally, blisters are not serious. However, if the area starts to become red and inflamed, swells, develops pus, or remains very tender and painful for more than a day or two, you may have an infection and you should see a doctor," says Dr. Julien. If you have repeated problems with painful blisters, you may want to consult with a podiatrist, who can help you get to the root of the problem. Sometimes padded insoles or orthotics are needed to relieve pressure and get your foot properly positioned in your sneaker. Sometimes, the answer lies with using a prescription-strength drying agent on your foot to reduce friction.

Bunions

A bunion is a condition in which your big toe joint becomes swollen and misaligned: The top of the toe slants inward toward the other toes, while the bone at the base of the toe begins to angle and grow outward. Bunions tends to run in families. Playing your sport doesn't cause them, but wearing shoes that are too narrow in the forefoot and toes can aggravate a preexisting tendency toward bunion formation, according to the American Podiatric Medical Association.

Surgery is frequently recommended to correct bunions. However, if you spot the bunions developing and take steps to intervene, you can often prevent the problem from becoming worse. To minimize the discomfort of a bunion, you might want to try these suggestions, which are adapted from a "Runner's Guide to Home Remedies," an article that appeared in *Runner's World* magazine:

- Apply ice and compression to the bunion, and elevate the foot after exercise. A toe spacer made of sponge rubber will help alleviate discomfort; start with a small spacer between the big toe and second toe, then gradually use wider ones until the toe feels comfortable.
- Wear a doughnut pad over the bony growth to reduce friction, and if your bunion is rubbing hard against the inner surface of your shoe, make a stab incision in the shoe at the point of contact to relieve pressure. For relief from pain and inflammation, try aspirin or ibuprofen.
- Finally, anyone with bunions should avoid any shoes with high heels and pointed toes. You should choose wide shoes for exercising as well as for daily activities.

Calluses and Corns

These growths are protective layers of compacted, dead skin cells. Your body builds them up as a defense against repeated friction and pressure from skin rubbing against bony areas or against an irregularity in the way a shoe fits.

Calluses tend to develop on the weight-bearing portions of your feet, namely the soles and heels. A corn is a concentrated callus—a hard little plug or kernel of dead skin—that occurs at a pressure point, such as under a toe. Either can be painless, in which case there is probably no need to take any action.

But if the pressure of a thicker callus or corn becomes painful, you can usually find relief with some simple self-care tactics. First, soak the affected foot in warm water to soften skin for about five minutes. Then use a callus file, pumice stone, or emery board to file down the dead tissue. Apply petroleum jelly or other high-emollient cream to area, then cover with a bandage or a pair of soft socks. Do this repeatedly to gradually wear the callus or corn away. To prevent them from developing again, wear thicker, padded socks to reduce friction and make sure your shoes fit correctly.

If you've been tempted to cut away your calluses or corns, you've probably been worried by the warning "never cut corns or calluses yourself." But, says Dr. Julien, "I don't think there is anything wrong with trying, as long as you don't have any medical reasons, such as compromised circulation or diabetes, that might put you at special risk. Just be sure to use a clean razor (sterilize it in alcohol first), and if you do cause bleeding, dress the wound with an antiseptic and keep it clean."

Adds Dr. Julien, "The biggest mistake people make when it comes to corns and calluses is to use medicated removers. The acid contained in these products produces unhealthy skin and I have seen at least three significant infections caused by use of these chemical removers. I personally think you are a lot less prone to getting an infection from paring down calluses and corns yourself with a clean razor than you are when you use a chemical agent."

Hammertoes

A hammertoe is a type of toe deformity in which (usually) the second toe becomes permanently bent in a clawlike position. A painful corn may form on the top of the toe, too.

"Poorly fitting athletic shoes may be the cause of irritation to a hammertoe," says Dr. Julien, "but frequently the biggest source of irritation is from a woman's everyday footwear, which often have high heels and a cramped, tight toebox."

Reducing the pain of hammertoes and preventing the problem from worsening usually requires a combination of tactics: switching to shoes that have a toebox wide and deep enough to comfortably accommodate the buckled-under toe(s); wearing roomy, soft socks or panty hose that don't cramp the toes; experimenting with nonmedicated, adhesive pads to find ways to reduce pressure on the affected toe, and sometimes wearing a toe cap—a padded sleeve that wraps around the joint and raises the toe tip. In extreme cases, surgery may be needed to correct a hammertoe.

Ingrown Toenails

Although it is often said that the chief cause of ingrown toenails is improper clipping or trimming of the nails, the truth is that the nail shape you were born with and tight shoes are bigger culprits.

Ingrown nails are caused when a toenail (usually the one on the big toe, although any toe can be affected) becomes embedded in the skin around it. Some people are more susceptible because their nails curve into their skin more naturally. The skin then becomes inflamed, and very often, infected. Minor ingrown toenails don't present much of a problem to people, notes Dr. Wolf. "You can soak your foot in an Epsom salt bath (follow directions on the box), then file away the nail's ragged edge with an emery board."

However, if the problem isn't resolved in a few days and or when an ingrown toenail becomes painful enough to interfere with your activity, it's time to see a doctor. "You probably will need a round of antibiotics to clear the infection up as well as a minor surgical procedure on the nail to remove the portion that is causing irritation," notes Dr. Wolf. To prevent the problem in the future, the offending portion of the nail can be permanently removed. It also helps to keep toenails trimmed and cut straight across. Of course, wearing shoes with a roomy toebox is also essential.

Morton's Neuroma

This is a pinched nerve that usually occurs between the third and fourth toes and is caused by bones and other tissues rubbing against and irritating the nerves. Pressure from ill-fitting shoes can create the condition as can abnormal bone structure.

The symptoms of a neuroma are pain, tingling, and burning or numbness in the ball of the foot or along the third and fourth toes. "You may notice these sensations go away or decrease when you take off your shoes, massage the area, and/or walk barefoot. But the discomfort usually returns when you put your shoes back on and become active," notes Dr. Julien.

A home remedy for Morton's neuroma is to place a cotton ball between the affected toes to spread the metatarsals apart and help relieve the pressure on the underlying nerve. You can also place a metatarsal support pad under the arch of your foot (not on the bones directly below the affected toes—if the pad doesn't feel comfortable, it's a sign you don't have it positioned correctly). "The most effective therapy is an injection of cortisone; it reduces the swelling and takes the pressure off the nerve practically immediately," notes Dr. Julien. However, the problem can recur. In rare cases, the nerve must be removed surgically (this is done on an outpatient basis, although recovery may take six weeks or more).

○ Heel Pain: Practices That Put You at Risk for Plantar Fasciitis

- You increase your running mileage too much, too quickly.
- You increase the frequency and/or intensity of your high-impact workouts dramatically and suddenly.
- You play or run on hard (e.g., concrete), irregular (a banked or crowned road), or very hilly surfaces.
- Your shoes don't provide adequate shock absorption or arch support or don't fit properly.
- Your supporting calf muscles and Achilles' tendons are tight and in poor condition.

Plantar Fasciitis

The word *plantar* means bottom of the foot; *fasciitis* refers to an inflammation of the band of fibrous connective tissue that runs along the bottom of the foot, extends from the heel bone to ball of the foot, and serves to support the arch of the foot.

The initial symptoms of plantar fasciitis may be mild: When you first get out of bed, you may feel acute pain in the forward part of your heel. As you begin to walk and move around, the pain diminishes. The pain may even ease completely during activity, but then get worse afterward. But as the injury becomes more severe, the pain may start to be present anytime you walk or stand, and the bottom of your foot may feel perpetually stiff and achy.

Among the factors that can contribute to the development of plantar fasciitis:

1. a sudden increase in the mileage you run

2. a sudden increase in the frequency and/or intensity of your workouts

3. playing/running on hard (e.g., concrete), irregular (a banked or crowned road), or very hilly surfaces

4. wearing shoes that don't provide adequate shock absorption, arch support, or don't fit properly

5. poor conditioning and stretching of supporting calf muscles and Achilles tendons

The first step in treating plantar fasciitis is to reduce the inflammation in the heel and arch area. You can begin to accomplish this with the usual: taking oral anti-inflammatories, such as ibuprofen, regularly, for at least ten days to two weeks; icing the area for about five minutes (especially after activity), up to five times a day; using an over-the-counter heel cup or heel lift inserts in your shoes; and taping the foot so as to support the arch and take pressure off the fascia.

But perhaps the most crucial element of correcting the problem—and the one that can be hardest for a motivated athlete to adhere to—is rest. If you have caught the problem early, you may be able to stick with your normal workout—just ease up on the distance, intensity, and frequency (and avoid hill running and sprinting completely) for at least four weeks. If you don't start to feel better within two weeks, you may have to reduce your weight-bearing fitness activities or even suspend them completely for a while. "But doing alternate training, such as cycling, swimming, or running in a pool with a flotation device, can allow you to maintain your current fitness level during this time. You need to be patient, which I know is hard, since I'm an athlete myself," says Dr. Julien. "But the reality is that most plantar fasciitis problems require anywhere from two weeks or longer to resolve."

Another component of rehabilitating plantar fasciitis is regular stretching of your calf muscles and Achilles tendon. Tightness in this area prevents the ankle from flexing properly during walking or running and causes the arch of the foot (and the underlying fasciia) to collapse. Stretch gradually and gently after exercise and periodically throughout the day.

Preventing plantar fasciitis is really just a matter of avoiding the factors that cause it. First, don't kick up your training progression too fast—a common guideline is to limit increases in intensity, distance, and frequency to 10 percent a week. So if you are presently running twenty miles a week, you would only increase your distance by two miles the next week—and not increase intensity at the same time. Other aspects of a plantar fasciitis prevention plan include regularly doing exercises to stretch your calves and Achilles tendon, wearing well-cushioned, properly fitted shoes, and avoiding workouts on hard surfaces, especially concrete.

If an athlete is injured anywhere below the waist, I always ask to see their workout shoes, since a poor fit is often part of what incites the problem in the first place.
—JOHN CIANCA, MD, MEDICAL DIRECTOR OF THE HUMAN PERFORMANCE CENTER IN HOUSTON

Plantar Warts

These are warts, all of which are caused by viruses, that grow on the bottom of the foot. They look different from warts that appear on your hands because of the constant pressure that is exerted on them. A telltale sign of a plantar wart is a brownish speck (you may need to place your foot under a bright light to see it) that may be a bit tender.

You can have plantar warts burned off by a doctor (the most expedient option) or you can use over-the-counter wart removers containing salicylic acid (it may take several months for the wart to disappear if you take this route). If the wart doesn't bother you, though, it's safe to just leave it alone.

Sesamoiditis

This refers to an inflammation around the sesamoid bones—two little bones that act as part of the pulley system that moves your big toe. The sesamoids (and the tendons they are embedded in) get injured when too much pressure is placed on the ball of the foot or on the big toe itself—beach volleyball players who play barefoot and crash straight down on their unprotected toes are especially vulnerable. Characteristically, the pain of sesamoiditis is sharp and felt just behind the bottom of the big toe. Your toe may hurt when you flex it upward and when you touch it too.

Icing and the use of oral anti-inflammatories like ibuprofen help reduce the swelling; then you need to take the pressure off the sesamoid bones by padding the area and putting a lot of soft cushioning under the ball of your foot in your shoes. With the area under the sesamoids padded and protected, you can usually resume your activities, if not right away, then within a few days. If the area is too painful to exercise on, even after you have changed to shoes with good cushioning in the forefoot, you should see a doctor, who can rule out the possibility of a sesamoid stress fracture (see page 113).

Toenail Fungus

As many as 10 to 12 million adults in the United States suffer from common toenail fungus, commonly known as *onychomycosis*. And athletes seem to be singled out, according to Dr. Julien "because of the chronic trauma we subject our toes to while exercising, as well as the moist, dark, and warm environment created by athletic shoes and socks, which make for a perfect fungal breeding ground."

As a fungus infects the toenail, it results in a gradual thickening and yellowing of the nail. The nail may eventually become deformed and brittle too. Most of the time, fungus toenails aren't painful, but an athlete may experience irritation because the top of her shoe hits the nail and/or the nail catches on a sock. Usually the biggest problem with fungal toenails, however, is their unsightly appearance.

To treat a fungus problem (although, if you're not in pain, it's perfectly fine to leave the nail alone), there are a variety of over-the-counter as well as prescription topical ointments and liquids. These usually need to be applied twice daily for months and tend to have limited success, according to Dr. Julien.

There are now several oral medications to treat toenail fungus (Sporanex and Lamisil). The success of these medications is much better than that of topical medications, but the risk of side effects, from nausea and rash to serious liver complications, is much higher too. These medications, which you need to take for three months, can't be taken with many allergy or stomach medicines. You may need to have regular blood tests, to check your liver function, too, while taking them.

Another option is to have your affected toenails removed. "This isn't as awful as it sounds—it can be done under local anesthesia in a doctor's office," says Dr. Julien. After the nail is removed, a chemical is applied to destroy the matrix of the nail, so that it won't ever grow back (if the nail grows back, it will just return in the same diseased form). Then a hard, thickened skin surface forms over the nail bed. Especially if you wear nail polish, says Dr. Julien, the skin surface closely resembles a normal nail.

HOW TO CHOOSE THE RIGHT SPORT SHOES AND SOCKS

Even the smallest problem with the fit of your athletic shoes can lead to pain, lowered performance, and problems like blisters, bunions, calluses, corns, hammertoes, plantar fasciitis, and more serious injuries, such as stress fractures.

"If an athlete is injured anywhere below the waist, I always ask to see their workout shoes, since a poor fit is often part of what incites the problem in the first place," says John Cianca, M.D., medical director of the Human Performance Center in Houston and assistant professor of physical medicine and rehabilitation at the Baylor College of Medicine, Houston.

Studies indicate that women, in general, are prone to picking shoes that fit poorly. In a recent study published in *Foot & Ankle International*, of 255 women between the ages of twenty and sixty, 86 percent were wearing shoes that were smaller than their feet in the forefoot area (where your toes are).

There are four steps to matching your foot to the right shoe.

1. *Buy a sports-specific shoe.* You need a shoe that is cushioned and supported with regard to your sport's specific demands.

For example, basketball shoes should have a thick, stiff sole to give you extra stability when running on the court and a high top to provide support (and prevent ankle sprains) when landing from a jump. In contrast, shoes for aerobic conditioning should be lightweight to prevent foot fatigue and have extra shock absorption in the sole beneath the ball of the foot where the most stress occurs, according to the American Orthopaedic Foot and Ankle Society (AOFAS), a Seattle-based association of orthopedic surgeons with special training in the care of the foot and ankle.

Most major athletic footwear companies (Nike, Adidas, Reebok, Saucony, Asics, Fila, Brooks, Wilson Pro) now churn out shoes specifically designed for specific sports and for women. It pays to go to a specialty store that has a large selection of different shoes for your sport. These stores often have very knowledgeable salespeople, too, who can help steer you to the right choices. You'll want to try as many different styles for your sport as are available. (If you are trying a shoe for the first time, buying through mail order or the Internet is probably not the best idea, only because you may find you "settle" for something simply because that's easier to do than make a return. These venues, however, are great if you are already familiar with a shoe that you know works for you).

You don't necessarily need a different pair of athletic shoes for every sport you play, according to the AOFAS. However, you should wear sports-specific shoes for sports you play more than three times a week.

Finally, sports like rock climbing and hiking require very special footwear. The higher your level of expertise, the more vital to your safety buying the proper boot or shoe is (the wrong rock climbing shoe, for example, could lead to a fall or even death). Given that this footwear can also be very pricey, running into the hundreds of dollars, it pays to take a lot of care when shopping for it. Talk to others experienced in the sport and get their recommendations, not only on specific brands and models of boots or shoes that have worked for them, but on stores where there are salespeople knowledgeable about the gear. Also, don't settle for boots or climbing shoes made for men—

there are now good-quality choices designed specifically for women's feet.

2. *Get a good fit.* "Your foot differs from a man's in that it is generally narrower and has a more pronounced difference in width between the heel and the forefoot. And because your hips are wider than those of a man, your heel will tend to move more as your body attempts to maintain its center of gravity. These factors are important to consider when shopping for athletic shoes," according to Carol Frey, M.D., associate clinical professor of orthopedic surgery at the University of Southern California, Los Angeles. Dr. Frey, in an article published in *The Journal of Musculoskeletal Medicine,* offers these tips for choosing a properly fitting athletic shoe:

- Shop for shoes after a workout (since that is when your feet are the most swollen). Wear the socks you wear when working out. If you wear an orthotic insert, bring it along and place it inside any shoes you try on.
- Look for a shoe that has ample midsole and heel-wedge cushioning. If your foot tends to roll inward as you step, look for a harder material built into the inner side of the midsole or heel. A heel counter—a firm cup that is encased in the shoes and surrounds it—also helps by holding your heel firmly.
- Fit the shoe to your largest foot. A recent study of 356 women indicated that 66 percent had one foot larger than the other. Check to see that you can fully extend all toes. Allow a finger's breadth (about ½ inch) from the end of the toebox to the end of the longest toes. The shoe should feel comfortable the first time you put it on.
- Ask for a shoe with a woman's last—a last is the mold on which a shoe is built—that has a narrow heel and a relatively wide forefoot.

In addition, don't rely on the size of your last pair of shoes, since your feet get larger as you age, and be sure to have your feet measured while standing, advises the American Podiatric Medical Association. Adds Dr. Julien: "Take time to put on both shoes and to lace them up fully. Then mimic the activity you plan to do in the shoes. For example, if you play a court sport, move forward, backward and side-to-side in the shoes to see if they give you proper traction, support, and cushioning."

3. *Lace your shoes correctly.* Believe it or not, how you lace your athletic shoes can actually make a difference when it comes to preventing injuries and alleviating pain. Many athletic shoes now come with dual lacing systems (different sets of eyelets, placed at different widths) so as to allow lacing to be adjusted for a custom fit. Especially if you have narrow or wide feet or feet with high arches, this feature can make it easier to find a shoe that fits just right. A description appears on page 112, courtesy of the AOFAS in conjunction with Dr. Frey, of seven different lacing patterns, each of which are designed to meet a specific need.

4. *Wear athletic socks.* "Wearing the right socks can save you from blisters, black toenails, and athlete's foot, among other things. They can also help cushion and support the foot," notes Dr. Julien.

How can a simple sock do so much? A lot has to do with the new materials being used in high-performance socks. For example, Thorlos, a company that makes a whole line of sports specific socks (walking, running, tennis, in-line skating) uses different blends of synthetic fibers that wick sweat away from feet and that increase circulation around them. This means there is less moisture and friction—the two leading culprits in blister formation.

Thorlos (as well as sport-specific socks made by other companies like Wigwam, Nike, Fox River, etc.) are also padded according to where the most impact is placed. For example, the Thorlos tennis sock has dense padding at the ball of the foot and heel to absorb shock on hard court surfaces, with lighter padding over the toes to prevent chafing and blistering. Many of these socks also are ribbed and contoured with Spandex in the arch area to provide support and help prevent problems like plantar fasciitis.

One of the keys to choosing a high-tech sports sock that will help your performance is to pick the right size. Socks that are too big can slip and bunch up, actually causing blisters rather than preventing them. Similarly, socks that are too small can confine your toes and contribute to problems like black

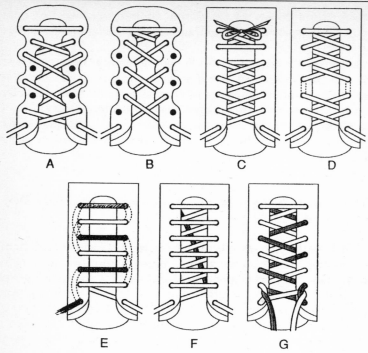

A   B   C   D

E   F   G

A. *Narrow feet.* Consider using the eyelets set wider apart on the shoe. This will bring up the sides of the shoe more tightly across the top of the narrow foot.

B. *Wide feet.* Try using the eyelets closer to the tongue of the shoe. Using the eyelets that are closer together will give more width to the lacing area and have the same effect as letting out a corset.

C. *Narrow heel and wide forefoot.* Use two laces to achieve a combination fit that accommodates the width of the forefoot and tightens around the narrow heel. Use the closer-set eyelets to adjust the width of the shoe at the forefoot and the wide-set eyelets to snug up the heel.

D. *Specific pain.* If you have a bump on the top of your foot, a high arch, a bone that sticks out, or pain from a nerve or tendon injury, consider leaving a space in the lacing to alleviate pressure. Simply skip the eyelets at the point of pain and draw the laces to the next set of eyelets. This lacing pattern will greatly increase the comfort of the shoe.

E. *High arches.* Lace your shoes so that the laces travel in a straight line from eyelet to eyelet. By avoiding the crisscross method, this lacing pattern creates no pressure points at the laces.

F. *Toe problems.* If you have hammertoes, corns, bleeding toes, or toenail problems, consider lacing your shoes so the toebox area is lifted. You can adjust the height of the toebox by pulling on the lace that travels directly from the toe to the top of the shoe.

G. *Heel fit.* To prevent pistoning of the heel in the shoe and heel blisters, the top laces are threaded through each other before tying the shoe, which helps keep the foot snugly in the shoe.

toenail. Use the size of your athletic shoes as a guide to buying and, of course, make sure to wear the sock whenever purchasing shoes.

Regarding what thickness of sock to choose (since many of these high-tech socks come in heavy, medium-weight, or thin versions), if you are prone to blisters, the heavier sock is better. Otherwise, thickness is a matter of personal preference, although many athletes find that medium and lightweight sports socks feel more comfortable in warmer temperatures, while thicker ones feel great in the winter.

OTHER COMMON SPORTS INJURIES AMONG WOMEN (AND HOW TO AVOID THEM)

Unfortunately, your feet aren't the only body part that is damage prone as a result of your sports involvement. To avoid injury to other susceptible areas, it helps to know why problems tend to occur. Also, it's important to recognize early signs of trouble, since there is often a lot you can do to head it off at the pass, before it puts you out of the game.

ACL injury

Sudden cutting (making short stops), planting, and pivoting motions, such as you make when playing basketball, soccer, or volleyball or engaging in gymnastics, martial arts, or skiing are often what lead to injuries to the anterior cruciate ligament (ACL), the ligament that resides within the knee and connects the thigh to the shinbone.

Right now, ACL tears are epidemic among female athletes. Depending on which study you cite (and which sport has been studied), women suffer from ACL tears from two to eight times more frequently than men. The reason women are more susceptible is an issue of intense debate and controversy. Some of the many factors that appear to be involved include physiologic differences, such as wider hips, which place greater pressure on the inside of the knee; looser joints, perhaps because of the presence of the hormone relaxin; and crucial differences between men and women in the "recruitment order" of knee muscles—that is, the order in which muscles around the knee tighten in rapid-fire succession to hold the knee snugly in place and protect it.

Often when the ACL gets damaged, you'll hear or feel a popping sensation, the knee will quickly become swollen and will feel unstable, as if your shin could easily shift away from the knee. Depending on the degree of injury, you may need a brace and a program of physical therapy or, if the ligament is torn, surgery to repair it.

Prevention: In the heat of competition, you can hardly avoid making quick stops or powerful jumps and landings (moves that often lead to ACL tears) if you are going to stay competitive. But you may be able to modify your play technique slightly to reduce your risk. According to one study of two NCAA Division I women's basketball teams, there was a significant decrease in ACL injuries when women were taught to replace the three most common injury-causing maneuvers— plant and cut, straight-leg landing, and one-step stop, with safer ones—rounding off turns, flexing the knee when landing, and the three-step stop.

Another key to reducing your risk of a sudden ACL injury is to develop a balance of muscle power throughout the entire knee and lower thigh region via a strengthening program that emphasizes building the hamstring and quadriceps muscles. Knees are better able to withstand the force of challenging maneuvers if no muscle or ligament has to act alone.

Achilles Tendonitis and Calf Pain

Pain and tightness in the large muscles in the back of the leg below the knee as well as irritation and inflammation of the tendon that attaches to the back of the heel bone can be caused by overuse, inflexibility, and wearing high heels for long hours as well as improper pedaling in cyclists; excessive rolling of the foot in runners; violent stops and starts in basketball, volleyball, tennis, and other court sports. Symptoms usually include pain, tenderness, and/or mild swelling in your calf muscle or Achilles tendon (which is located a few inches above your heel where it meets the bottom and back of your calf muscle).

Prevention: Stretching the calf muscles gently and gradually before and after workouts will ordinarily help alleviate the pain and stiffness, according to the American Podiatric Medical Association. To build calf flexibility (and thus avoid Achilles tendon irritation), stand facing a wall, an arm's-length away, with your hands flat against it for support. Place the leg you are stretching about a foot behind your other leg. Keeping heels to the ground, slowly lean into the wall, bending the knee of your forward leg slightly. You should feel a slight pull in the leg that is straight and furthest from the wall. Hold for the count of ten, then repeat three times on each leg. As your calves become more flexible, you'll need to move the leg you are stretching further back to feel the pull.

Back Pain

Although there are a multitude of causes of sports-related back pain, often weak abdominal muscles are the chief culprit. Athletes in running sports often have strong muscles in their backs, hips, and upper thighs, but undeveloped stomach muscles. Alone, the muscles in your back and hips can't do the job of supporting your spine properly—they need to be bolstered and counterbalanced with a strong abdominal wall. When this strength is lacking, your spine begins to sag and cave in, which puts undue pressure on the tissues, leading to inflammation and pain.

Prevention: There are whole books on how to get your "abs" in shape (keep in mind that your abdominals don't have to be rock-hard to be adequately strong!) and how to beat back pain. But a simple place to start is to add crunches to your workout and to do lower back stretches periodically throughout the day, especially if you sit at a desk for long periods. One safe and easy back stretch: Stand straight, then bend your knees slightly. Lean down and place your hands above your knee caps. Bend at the waist, allowing your head to gradually point toward the floor, pressing your hands into your knees, which should remain slightly bent as you do so. This is similar to the old "touch-your-toes" back stretch, except that it eliminates the risk of you overstretching your back muscles and/or injuring your hamstrings.

Knee Cap Pain

"Pain under or behind the knee cap is often caused by a hodgepodge of problems—hip instability, muscle and strength imbalances, and some basic anatomical vulnerabilities of the knee as it pertains to the demands of the sport," says Dr. Cianca. "It is an extremely common complaint among athletes engaged in sports that involve any sort of running, jumping, or dodging." Skiing, riding a bike with the seat too low, using a stair-climbing machine, and/or taking step aerobics classes are also activities associated with knee cap pain problems.

Prevention: To get good knee stability, the muscles that surround the knee need to be equally strong. When your hamstrings are overdeveloped relative to your quadriceps, for example, the quads can't provide proper counterstrength to keep the knee cap aligned with your leg. As a result, your knee cap slips, slides, and becomes inflamed with use. So if you do leg presses, which is a good all over quad strengthener, it's also important to do hamstring curls.

Shin Splints

Your shin bones are in your lower leg below your knee; shin splints, a catchall term that refers to exercise-related pain caused by injury of the shin's muscles and tendons on the front or inside of the lower leg, are common in high-impact jumping and running sports (basketball, track and field, volleyball) as well as gymnastics and competitive cycling. Be aware that it can be hard to distinguish a shin splint, which is a muscular-tendon problem from a stress fracture, which is a bone injury (and is described next).

Prevention: "The root of the shin splint problem is often your foot—it may be rolling inward too much during movement so that it doesn't support the lower leg and absorb shock properly," says Dr. Cianca. Often all you need to remedy a burgeoning shin splint problem is a stiffer athletic shoe that offers better foot control and stabilization. Arch supports sold in sporting goods stores or custom-made orthotics can also be extremely helpful in correcting this biomechanical problem.

Stress Fractures

A study of stress fractures in 320 athletes, published in the *American Journal of Sports Medicine*, found that, overall, stress fractures represent 10 percent of all sport injuries. This same study found that runners are most likely of all athletes to sustain stress fractures, which account for up to 15 percent of all running injuries.

"Although stress fractures represent true breaks in the bone, they are considered overuse injuries because they are not caused by a single event or trauma, but by a series of repetitive, low grade stresses to a specific area of the bone," explains Dr. Julien.

Stress fractures most commonly occur in the feet and legs of athletes in the running sports, but can also occur in the ribs, arms, and hips. Symptoms tend to come on slowly—gradually you'll begin to feel discomfort or a deep aching in the area but it may wax and wane, depending on what you are doing. For example, the pain may go away entirely at night. Eventually, however, you'll find you can't put in the same performances without experiencing an increase in pain.

Prevention: Avoid doing "too much, too soon" since over-training as well as increasing your training too dramatically are two of the chief causes of stress fractures. Also, women who have eating disorders, are amenorrheic, and/or do not get adequate calcium, protein, and caloric intake are especially at risk for stress fractures since these problems often lead to poor bone health (weak bones with low density are more likely to crumble under repetitive stress). If you find your periods are irregular and/or you feel out of control with your eating habits, get help from a doctor as soon as possible.

Shoulder Soreness

Inflammation of the complex set of ligaments, tendons, and muscles called the rotator cuff that support and cushion your shoulder joint are especially common in players of throwing sports such as softball as well as racket sports, which demand repetitive overhead motions. In swimmers, it is the most common musculoskeletal injury. "At some point in their racing careers, 73 percent of elite swimmers report a history of interfering shoulder complaints," according to a report cited in *Medical and Orthopedic Issues of Active and Athletic Women* (Hanley & Belfus, Philadelphia, 1994). "Symptoms usually include pain or soreness when you try to lift your arm about 90 degrees from the horizontal," says Dr. Cianca, and pain when you roll onto your afflicted shoulder at night.

Prevention: It's important not only to strengthen your rotator cuff, but the entire area that encircles it since strong muscles in your upper back, chest and upper arm all help keep your shoulder stable and secure in its socket. The idea is to have no weak link that might make your shoulder susceptible to stress. Whether you use free weights or a machine, it's important to include exercises for the upper back, chest, and arms as well as shoulders.

Warming up your shoulders with gentle stretches before exercise, then using the same exercises to cool down afterward, may also help prevent problems. Two simple, easy stretches to do five to ten times before and after exercise: Simply stand straight, feet hip-width apart, arms hanging loosely at your sides. Slowly lift your shoulders up (shrug) as high as possible, hold to a count of three, bring them back down and release. In the same position, slowly roll your shoulders up, back, down and forward in a complete rotation. Relax and repeat.

◯ First Aid for Injuries

If the pain is really severe, get to a doctor immediately. If you think the injury may not be so serious, apply the RICE formula for twenty-four to forty-eight hours and see if the injury starts to mend.

- **R**est the injured body area.
- **I**ce it in twenty-minute on, forty-minute off cycles.
- **C**ompress it by lightly wrapping an ace bandage around it.
- **E**levate it, above your heart if possible.

WHAT TO DO WHEN IT HURTS

If the pain is really severe, you can't bear weight on the injured area, you heard or felt something pop, there is a large amount of swelling, or you can't move the injured area, see a doctor right away. However, if the pain and discomfort is less severe, you can often safely treat the pain with an over-the-counter NSAID (nonsteroidal anti-inflammatory) medication, such as ibuprofen (Advil) or naproxen (Aleve) for at least the first twenty-four hours as you apply the well-known RICE formula:

1. Rest the injured body area for 24 to 48 hours.
2. Ice it to limit internal bleeding and keep swelling and in-flammation down. Gently place an ice pack, plastic bag of crushed ice, frozen peas in a plastic bag, or ice wrapped in a towel over the injured area in a twenty-minute on, forty-

minute off cycle for up to two days (taking a break from the routine at night, obviously).

3. Compress the area by lightly wrapping an ace bandage around it, taking care not to pull it too tight.

4. Elevate the affected limb, as often as possible, above your heart to reduce swelling.

If the pain and swelling subside after two days, you can usually begin to resume your activity. If the pain shows clear signs of abating, wait another two days before trying to resume your training and be sure to keep at well below normal levels. If your pain remains strong despite rest and RICE, it's probably time to seek out a physician who is knowledgeable about sports injury and understands your need to get back in the game. If the only advice your doctor gives you is to rest, be wary; most experts feel that some activity versus none at all helps promote healing via increasing blood flow to area.

HOW TO CHOOSE A SPORTS BRA

"When I ran my first marathon in 1977, sports bras didn't exist. So I wore a regular bra and ended the race with bleeding abrasions on my shoulders and rib cage. Right then and there, I vowed I would find a better means of protecting myself," says LaJean Lawson, one of the pioneers in sports bra research and presently an adjunct professor of exercise and sport science at Oregon State University, Corvallis.

In the two decades since that time, sports bras have come a long way. "The sports bra used to be basically one pattern, available in different sizes. One of the really cool things about what's happening now is that companies are coming up with different designs, made specifically to accommodate the different body sizes and shapes of women as well as their different activity levels," says Lawson. As a result, there is not only a greater array of choices, especially for larger-breasted women, but sports bras—as a category—tend to offer better fit and function.

For example, many bras now incorporate breathable synthetic fabrics that wick away moisture from your skin, some encapsulate rather than compress the breasts (so you get support from separating the breasts rather than squashing them into a "mono-boob"), plus there are models that offer wide, adjustable straps as well as front or back closure (so you don't have to pull them over your head).

Of course, there is still room for improvement, according to a study by Julia Alleyne, M.D., medical director of Sport C.A.R.E. at Women's College Hospital in Toronto. In her survey of sports bra use among four hundred active women, Alleyne found that women still have complaints about getting enough support and shoulder strap comfort. In addition, Alleyne feels that sport bras need to be designed for different sports (i.e., a bra for marathoners versus a more protective bra for kick boxing or soccer). "Just as different athletic shoes are made and modified to fit the demands of the particular sport, so should sports bras be."

But do you really need one? "There is a lot of talk about how bouncing can cause the skin and ligaments around the breasts to stretch. But the truth is that this hasn't been well studied or proven," says Alleyne. "In fact, the only two things that have been proven to cause the breasts to droop and sag are malnutrition and multiple pregnancies."

Physiologically, then, the scientific argument for using a sports bra to prevent the stretching of skin and other elastic connective tissue is not tremendously strong. From the standpoint of pure comfort, however, there may be many good reasons to make the investment in one.

"Having your breasts bounce and slap during workouts can be very uncomfortable, plus a lot of women feel very self-conscious about it," notes Dr. Alleyne. "And anything that makes exercise more comfortable for women is positive."

Here, then, is what to look for in a sports bra:

1. *Fit.* "If you don't buy the right size, it doesn't matter how good the bra is, you'll have problems with it," says Dr. Alleyne, who recommends women get themselves sized professionally (i.e., with help of a department store clerk who has been trained in bra fitting). In agreement with this advice is Lawson who says, "As a general rule, women don't buy the right bra size. They don't realize that their body shape may change with age, even if their weight hasn't."

If it is not possible for you to be fitted professionally, be aware that the bra should feel snug but not be so tight that it constricts your breathing. "During vigorous movements, the entire upper body should move as one unit, with limited bouncing of the breasts," writes Bryant Stamford, M.D., professor of exercise physiology at the University of Louisville, Kentucky, in *The Physician and Sportsmedicine.* "Give the bra the jumping-jack test to be sure it meets these criteria."

The wide elastic band around the rib cage should not ride up. Clasp your hands over your head: if the band shifts up, the bra doesn't fit properly.

Check arm mobility too. Mimic whatever arm movements you make in your sport to make sure the armholes are ample enough to allow for unrestricted movement.

2. *Support.* "Minimal movement of the breasts within the bra is important to reduce chafing," notes Dr. Stamford. Larger-breasted women should look for bras that encapsulate the breasts with molded cups, since each breast is then supported separately; a full or Y-back can provide extra support to accommodate the weight of larger breasts. Smaller-breasted women may prefer a compression type sports bra, which works by holding the breasts against the body, with a less constrictive X-back or racer back.

3. *Ventilation.* "Keeping dry is the key to reducing friction," notes Lawson, who recommends avoiding sports bras made of cotton and looking for bras lined with CoolMax or blends of synthetic fabrics made to wick away moisture. If you exercise for more than forty-five minutes at a time, you should also look for ventilation panels in the cleavage area, at the sides, and at the back as well, advises Dr. Alleyne.

4. *Straps.* You don't want them to slip or to dig into your shoulders. Larger-breasted women, especially, should look for wider shoulder straps that provide support. Longer-waisted women should consider adjustable shoulder straps to accommodate their torso length.

For sports requiring a lot of overhead reaching and shoulder rotation, such as aerobic dance, basketball, volleyball, and racket sports, a bra should have adequate stretch in the straps so that shoulders don't become chafed and "cut into," points out Lawson. "But for sports involving mostly leg action or vertical body movement and little overhead arm motion, such as running, walking, horseback riding, or soccer, the bra design should incorporate minimal stretch in the cup and strap areas and should focus on control of vertical motion of the breast rather than strap comfort."

5. *Feel.* The fabric of the bra should be soft next to your skin. "Cups should be seamless (so as not to irritate the nipples) or at least have covered seams," notes Dr. Stamford. Hardware, such as hooks, clasps, or shoulder adjusters should be lined and padded so as to avoid causing cuts or abrasions.

If you are able, it's best to try on a variety of models to see which style feels most comfortable. If, however, you don't have a well-stocked major department or sports store nearby, you can also get guidance from mail-order sources. If you phone the *Title Nine Sports* catalog, which offers a large selection of sports bras, they will give you instructions on how to find the right fit (800-609-0092 or visit its Website. www.title9sports. com). At Enell brand sports bra, a bra designed specifically for larger-breasted women, you'll also get details on how to measure yourself (800-828-7661). You might also want to visit Champion's Jogbra site (www.championjogbra.com) and click on MCR Fit Center, Guide to the Perfect Sports Bra. All of these companies have liberal return policies and allow you to get a full refund if the bra doesn't fit right.

◑ The Four Requirements for Sports Clothing

1. The material used should effectively manage your sweat output. In other words, it should draw the moisture away from your skin so you stay dry.

2. Fabrics should breathe. In the summer, your clothing shouldn't cause you to overheat; in the cold weather, it should keep heat from escaping without causing moisture to collect, making your skin clammy.

3. Styling should emphasize lightness. You don't want to be weighed down by your clothing, either in summer or winter.

4. The fit should be comfortable, allowing absolute mobility and freedom.

WHAT FABRICS TO PUT NEXT TO YOUR SKIN

Old standby natural fibers, such as cotton and wool, may not always make the cut when it comes to being lightweight, breathable, and sweat resistant. A cotton tee-shirt, for example, becomes heavy and sweat soaked with prolonged activity (and what's worse than being wet and clammy when the wind kicks up, chilling you to the bone?).

Newer textile fabrics often function better, since many of the latest high-tech synthetic fibers are designed to conduct moisture and heat away from the surface of the skin. In addition, many of the designs using these fabrics also incorporate an array of features to enhance ventilation, block wind, prevent skin abrasions, and so on.

Of course, manufacturers also design and pattern clothes to match the specific conditions and requirements of different sports. For example, shorts designed for bike racing differ dramatically from those designed for beach volleyball. For details about sports-specific clothes, look up your sport in Part Two, then go to the section on What to Wear.

The list of technical fabrics, below, should give you a sense of how the different fibers being used in today's sports gear perform. Synthetic fabrics used in sportswear are constantly being reengineered, improved, and renamed, according to the Sporting Goods Manufacturer's Association (SGMA), which supplied the information contained in this glossary. But the following mainstays are likely to be around for years.

Aquator. A knit, hybrid fabric that combines cotton and Tactel to create a soft fabric with moisture management. The Tactel on the inside wicks the moisture to the cotton on the outside to be evaporated. *Found in*: shirts, aerobic/running/cycling shorts, tennis skirts.

CoolMax. Designed to keep you cool and dry. It feels soft, is lightweight, and has great moisture management on hot days. It retains fourteen times less moisture than cotton and eight times less moisture than nylon, so it won't cling and feel clammy next to your skin. *Found in*: shirts, jerseys, socks, and as liners and panels in shorts and bras.

Gore-tex. The original waterproof and breathable laminate. Because of its construction, Gore-tex fabric will be totally impervious to rain, but will still be breathable and let water escape as you exercise. It's also windproof and durable. *Found in*: jackets and pants for rainy conditions, some oversocks and footwear.

Microfiber. Called Microfine, Tactel Microfiber, Barrier, Microft, microfiber is extremely lightweight, thin, naturally water resistant (the water beads on the material), windproof, and breathable. Made of nylon, Microfibers will take to colors very well and have a soft feel that will keep the clothing from making noise while you move. *Found in*: Jackets, windbreakers, pants.

Polarsystem fabrics. Fabrics such as Polartek, Polarfleece, Polarplus, Polarlite: plush, fleecy fabrics of polyester that feel very soft and comfortable. They're warm, durable, and often colorful, water-resistant, and breathable. *Found in*: parkas, jackets, vests, long underwear, sweats, hats, gloves, scarves.

Polypropylene. Has very high insulating power. It wicks moisture away from the body very effectively, and is now being seen in warm-weather apparel. *Found in*: lining of shorts, long underwear, cold weather apparel.

Spandex. Also known as Lycra. An elastic fiber that can stretch 500 percent without breaking, it is added to other fabrics to give them optimal flexibility and shape retention. In clothing that contains Spandex, "recovery"—the return of the fabric to its original shape—is maximized. The higher the Spandex content of the fabric, the more the article of clothing will hug the skin. *Found in*: swimming suits, leggings, bike shorts, sports bras (most active wear contains some Spandex).

Supplex. A nylon fiber that is extremely lightweight, strong, durable, but with a cottony look and feel. Quick drying, the fiber distributes moisture throughout the garment for faster evaporation. This means that there's none of the wet "spotting" you normally see with cotton fabrics when you exercise. *Found in*: leotards, bras, shorts, tops, bathing suits.

Tactel. Also Talsan and 24 carat Tactel. A nylon fabric that can feel as soft as cotton or washed silk, depending on how it is constructed, and has the strength, durability, color retention, and wind and weather resistance of nylon. A good moisture manager: wicks sweat away from skin quickly so it can evaporate fast. *Found in*: warm-up suits, cycling and running shorts, tennis skirts, and outerwear, such as rain jackets.

Thermax. Holds in radiated body heat and wicks the moisture away from the body. It's easy to care for and won't shrink as much as polypropylene or natural fibers. *Found in*: socks, long underwear, tops, and leggings.

SPECIAL FOCUS:

⚬ Exercise-Induced Asthma

Eleven percent of the U.S. athletes (67 out of 597) who participated in the 1984 summer Olympic games had asthma; 41 won
medals, including fifteen Gold medals. Clearly asthma is a problem
that can be overcome. But because exercise-induced asthma (EIA)
can strike people who don't have chronic asthma and/or have no
underlying allergies, the real trick for many athletes is to realize
that they are suffering from the problem of EIA in the first place.
For example, Olympic Gold medalist swimmer Nancy Hogshead
had symptoms for nine years before she was properly diagnosed;
she simply didn't realize the coughing she experienced when exercising might be related to EIA.

Some athletes may fail to recognize the symptoms of EIA
because they think that the feeling of being "winded" or "out of
breath" is normal. "Some complain that they are simply 'too out
of shape' to exercise as vigorously as others with whom they
work out," point out Karen K. Maves, M.D., and John M. Weiler,
M.D., in an article on EIA published in *Pharmacy Times.*

Typically, symptoms begin about 5 to 10 minutes after beginning strenuous exercise: you may feel a tightness or pain in your
chest and you may cough, wheeze, and struggle to get enough air
into your lungs. Sometimes, your symptoms may be tolerable—
you may be able "to run through" them. In general, symptoms
usually peak about 15 minutes after exercise; some athletes may
then be symptom-free for a period of two to three hours.

EIA is the result of a tightening of the muscles that surround
the airways in the lungs; things that are known to trigger this
bronchoconstriction or spasm include allergies, air pollutants, viral
respiratory-tract infections and exposure to cold air.

So what can you do to control EIA? Some non-pharmacologic
approaches include warming the air before it hits your lungs by
breathing through your nose rather than your mouth. Wearing a
face mask during exercise in cold, dry weather also serves to
create a warm air environment. Anecdotal evidence suggests that
a long warm-up period, from 15 to 30 minutes, may ward off EIA
attacks, perhaps by preventing dramatic temperature changes in
the lungs. Finally, some athletes actually work to induce symptoms
by engaging in ten to fifteen minutes of vigorous exertion before

a game or event so that they can then enjoy the "refractory period" in which they are symptom free for two to three hours.

As for drug treatment of EIA, a class of medications called "inhaled beta2-adrenegic agonists" are considered first-line therapy for preventing and/or treating EIA, according to an article in *Medicine and Science in Sports and Exercise* authored by Donald A Mahler, M.D., a pulmonary and critical care specialist at Dartmouth-Hitchcock Medical Center in Lebanon, NH. Typically, you would use two puffs of the inhaled medicine at the start of your warm-up exercise or about fifteen minutes to a half hour before the start of vigorous exertion. Your protection should last about two hours. Elite athletes, in particular, find that they need to work closely with their physicians to not only find the right combination of medications they need to control their EIA, but to determine how to best time the use of the medications before and after exercise.

Thermoloft. An all-purpose fiberfill that keeps you insulated and warm even when wet. Also comes in a lighter version called Thermolite and in a version offering extra insulation called Thermoloft XL, which is 40 percent warmer than standard thin insulation. *Found in*: outerwear.

Thinsulate. A lightweight, very thin thermal insulation. It is extremely warm, moisture resistant, and breathable. Because it's so thin, it gives you the warmth of a big jacket in a much less bulky garment. *Found in*: jackets, gloves, hats, hiking footwear.

4

YOUR MIND AND EMOTIONS

The day in 1992 that Donna Weinbrecht, age thirty-two, of West Milford, New Jersey, won the Olympic Gold medal in moguls (an alpine skiing event), she felt joyous, optimistic, and completely focused. "I wasn't thinking at all about proving myself," says Weinbrecht, who clearly savors the memory of how fully "one" she was with her sport that day. "I was totally in the game. Everything was pure harmony. I have never felt more perfect as an athlete."

We have all experienced that wonderful, transcendent feeling that Weinbrecht describes: that moment when your mind and body suddenly come together in sublime unison to make everything go "right." When, without thought or conscious effort, your physical timing and rhythm become perfect, and magic happens—your hands send the ball flying through the hoop, your skates lift from the ice in a perfect jump, you slice through the water in a flawless dive. When you have that totally "in the game" feeling, you know you've got "it."

But what about the days when you don't have "it"? When you slip, fall, miss easy plays, and/or feel gripped by nervousness? Is there some way to get more control over how you perform?

The emerging science of sport psychology is, in its essence, dedicated to answering that question and to helping you find ways to trigger that "in the game" feeling. Specifically, it offers a battery of techniques to help you overcome all the mental and emotional obstacles—such as precompetition jitters, self-defeating trains of thought, lapses in concentration—that might prevent you from spontaneous, free-flowing play.

In fact, for many competitive, high-profile athletes, learning how to play a good "mental" game (i.e., keeping focused, calm, and in control) is as much a priority as training smart and eating right. During the 1997 summer Olympic games in Atlanta, for example, more than twenty American sport psychologists accompanied athletes to the sites to help them cope with issues of "mind over matter."

"Ask any elite athlete and chances are she will insist that the game is 90 percent mental," says Charles A. Maher, professor of psychology at Rutgers University Graduate School of Applied and Professional Psychology, New Brunswick, New Jersey. "In the upper echelons of sports, the players have practically equal talents. There are no big differences in things like strength, speed, ability. That means that who wins is often determined by who has the best mental approach."

Of course, improving your mental game cannot, in and of itself, make you a champion. "You cannot just will yourself to run a sub–four minute mile," says Maher. "Nothing can substitute for proper training, hard work, and natural talent."

But at any skill level, learning and applying psychological principles to your athletic pursuits can help you be your best, given your training and abilities. Perhaps even more important, sport psychology skills can sometimes help you enjoy your sport more; they can also help you weather rough times, like when you're faced with an injury or you feel stale and in a slump.

THE MENTAL SKILLS OF SUCCESSFUL ATHLETES: A CHECKLIST

Mental skills, like training plans, sneakers, and racing strategies, are not one size fits all.

"Whether or not a mental skill serves you is a highly individual matter—so much depends on who you are, how you approach your sport, and how a particular skill fits your personality," says Carole A. Oglesby, Ph.D., health psychology chair for the Association for the Advancement of Applied Sport Psychology and a registered consultant on the U.S. Olympic Committee Sport Psychology Registry. "The bottom line is that what is beneficial for one athlete simply may not be for another."

So consider yourself an experiment of one. Just as you would test out a new racket or pair of goggles prior to a big meet, so should you "try on" different mental skills in training. That way, you'll have a chance to see how they feel and whether they help.

Set Goals

A vital mainstay of sport psychology is goal setting. It is the launching point for all the other skills for several reasons:

1. Goal setting focuses your efforts. When you have a lot of disparate "aspirations" (such as, you'd like to learn to play soccer, become a better runner, try a triathlon, learn how to fly-fish, etc.), you often end up achieving nothing. But when you set specific goals, you are practically forced to establish priorities in order to accomplish them. For example, an athlete who consciously decides her number one goal is to qualify for the Olympics might realize that in order to achieve that goal, she might not be able to pursue graduate school, childbearing, and world travel at the same time. Setting goals, in other words, helps you realize that sometimes choices need to be made in order for you to become more successful.

2. Goals provide you with incentive to sustain your activity. When you have goals, you have a framework into which you can fit things like pain, frustration, boredom, and disappointment—you overcome these negatives because you have a reason to. Goals give you hope; they stimulate you to keep going; they

---

⚙ Goal-Setting Guidelines

1. Make it realistic: Take into account your past athletic achievements as well as how much time you have to devote to achieving your goal.

2. Make it concrete: Be superspecific about what you want to achieve and when you want to achieve it.

3. Make it self-centered: Your goal should be to better or best yourself, not just beat a competitor.

provide you with a healthy perspective so that you can get beyond setbacks.

3. Goal setting can help build self-confidence. If you have a large goal that includes many incremental stepping stones, each achievement can help bolster your sense of mastery, commitment, and confidence.

Steps toward good goal setting. According to an analysis of thirty-six studies of the effects of goal setting on performance in sport and exercise, conducted by researchers from the Department of Exercise Science and Physical Education at Arizona State University, Tempe, the trick to good goal setting is to set moderately difficult (not-too-easy but not impossibly high) long-term and short-term goals that are very specific. Vague generalities, such as "I'll just try to do better," don't really cut it. Instead, goals must be realistic and concrete if they are to create a focus for your efforts and give purpose to your training.

An example of a concrete goal might be, for example, a rower who wants to jump from being at the intermediate skill level to becoming a senior or elite crew member. The questions she must ask herself are: What does being a senior member mean in terms of strength, speed, training, and time commitment? What would I need to do in terms of my athletic development? Do I have at least a 50 percent chance of becoming eligible? How long is it likely to take me? By analyzing these kinds of issues, an athlete can hone in on exactly what her goals are, how achievable they are, and what she'll need to do to attain them. After all, you can't expect to attain your goal if you haven't defined it and defined what you need to do to achieve it.

Beyond being specific, most experts advise you to set goals that target mastery and performance. Your goals, in other words, should be pegged to how well you have done relative to yourself and your past performances. For example, one of your goals might be to better a previous race time, to develop better control over your tennis serve, to improve your soccer kick, and so on.

Research suggests that women don't do as well as men when their goals focus solely on beating the competition—i.e., goals that aim to outperform another athlete. The other problem with win-or-nothing goals is that they are not within your control: for example, you may skate flawlessly, beautifully, the best you ever have, yet a judge could still decide to award first place to another skater.

Having control over your goal outcome doesn't mean you have to set your sights low. It just means you might consider reframing your goals slightly to allow for the unforeseen "uncontrollable." For example, instead of defining your immediate goal as winning the race, you might say, "I want to be in good enough physical form to be in striking distance of the lead and in good enough mental shape to go for the victory if it's at all possible." (For more about how to set your goals, see Special Focus, page 154). Of course, it's important to remember that you may need to be flexible at times. First, you may find your priorities shift—that something you thought wasn't very important suddenly seems so. Also, every plan needs to allow for changes or even crises in your life.

―♒♒―

I don't allow my whole life and
happiness to hinge on every win or
loss. I try to remember that there are
things in life other than racquetball.
—MICHELLE GOULD, 1998 WORLD RACQUETBALL CHAMPION

―♒♒―

"It's important to keep the big picture in mind and realize that there may be days, or even entire seasons in your life when you have to shift, even downsize, your goals," notes Susan Zaro, sport counselor in private practice in Mountain View, California. "Female athletes are often juggling a lot of things in their lives—a job, children, and other family responsibilities. There are bound to be times when the demands of these other activities impinge on her ability to achieve her sport goals."

In other words, be ready to allow for the possibility of setbacks—whether that means you lose a race or miss a scheduled workout. "This is important because it not only frees you from crippling self-recrimination, it frees you to keep trying and striving," notes Zaro.

Michelle Gould, twenty-seven, the 1998 female world racquetball champion, learned this the hard way. "In 1990, I lost the World Championships. I was devastated; I fell into a huge depression. I just couldn't believe I lost—I was the odds on favorite, it was supposed to be my tournament. I felt as if everybody in the whole world knew that I had lost and I believed that everyone thought less of me, looked down upon me, because I lost that match."

After several months of intensive self-exploration, Gould emerged from her depression with an important realization: "I had lost because all I could focus on was how I needed to win—I had become obsessed with other people's expectations. My goals had become superficial and very shortsighted."

Since that time, Gould has reframed her goals: "I now keep playing for myself, to see how far I can go, how far I can push myself. I don't allow my whole life and happiness to hinge on every win or loss. Instead, I remember that there are things in life other than racquetball, and I no longer worry about what other people expect when I play my sport."

The lessons to be learned from Gould's journey are that your goals should be set by you, not superimposed on you by a coach, a parent, an adviser, or the public in general; they should reflect your passions and aims; and they must be expansive so that you aren't crushed by results but can look beyond and learn from each win or loss.

Finally, it's important to remember that every athlete, from the elite to the amateur, needs a break now and then from strenuous training. Sometimes the best thing you can do is set a goal of NOT setting a rigorous goal so as to allow yourself time to properly rejuvenate, mentally and physically (for more about the importance of training breaks, see page 148).

Use Imagery

"The key to being successful in softball is how you perform at the plate—you've got to be a good batter," says thirty-five-year-old Sheila Cornell Douty, first baseman on the 1996 Olympic Gold Medal–winning softball team. "So the night before a game I start to do visuals. I imagine the pitcher of the opposing team on the mound. I'm familiar with most of our opponents, so when I imagine the pitcher, I usually imagine a very specific, real person. Then I feel myself at the plate, locked into the moment, ready for the pitches and ready to aim the ball where I want. I fall asleep picturing all that."

The use of mental pictures or visualization to help enhance performance is a time-honored practice among athletes—a whopping 99 percent of elite athletes reported using imagery techniques, for instance, in a survey published in *Sport Psychology*.

To date, researchers can't really explain why imagery interventions appear to have a positive effect on athletic performance. However, there is some intriguing, preliminary evidence to indicate that the hard-wiring or neuropathways of your central nervous system may actually change in response to your simply thinking about a skill. In other words, when you perceive yourself, in your mind's eye, navigating a steep, technical climb perfectly, your brain may adapt in a way that actually helps your body become a better rock climber.

Douty uses imagery to help get herself focused and primed to play, but imagery is also used in these ways:

• *To help you acquire or refine a skill.* But you don't just think of your racket making contact with the ball, again and again. "When an athlete is trying to work out a specific problem in her technique or learn a specific skill, I tell her to use mental images that are full of detail, drama, and realism," says Zaro.

Let's say you're a swimmer and you've been having trouble executing fast and efficient flip turns during sprint competitions. First, take a few moments to think about what you have been doing wrong. Then, start a visualization exercise by imaging yourself sitting by the side of the pool: conjure up the smell of the chlorine, the sounds of the other swimmers, the blare of the announcers, coaches, and spectators, the filled bleachers, the scores on the board, the sunlight streaming into the gym's windows. Now visualize yourself preparing to enter the pool— don't watch yourself do it, but feel yourself inside your body— feel how the water feels on your skin, how your hand muscles tense and release, how your hips, legs, and feet are positioned. Feel how your whole body readies for the starting gun, then feel your body fly down the lane when it goes off. Imagine the wall approaching, then clock every tiny movement of how you zoom, curl, then torpedo out in a flawless flip turn.

Of course, this visualized performance should be combined with real-life practice. In addition, most sports psychologists recommend you rehearse your skill-enhancing scenario regularly. That shouldn't be hard: all it requires is that you summon as many senses as you can, close your eyes, and let yourself slip into a "succeeding/doing it all right" scenario for a few minutes each day.

- *To help you expect the unexpected.* For example, if your sport and your performance is affected by the weather, you can use visualization to help you prepare for every conceivable weather condition. Sports psychologist John D. Curtis, Ph.D., in *The Mindset for Winning*, (Coulee Pres, 1991) tells this story: "When working with a team of cross-country runners in preparing for major meets, I have the runners visualize the race in all types of weather. They picture themselves running confidently, relaxed, and strong in cold weather, wet weather, sunny weather, snowy weather. They also know that inclement weather often 'psyches out' their opponents while it has no effect on them." Recently, after Curtis worked with these athletes on these images for a week prior to the national meet, the runners finished second in the nation. "They came closer to the national championship than at any time in the history of the school while running the meet in almost a foot of snow on a cold, windy day."

The trick with using mental imagery to help you cope with every conceivable situation is to not let yourself get stuck when imagining a catastrophe—for example, if you're a cyclist, you need to go beyond thinking about the possibility of getting a flat tire to imagine yourself quickly fixing it, jumping back on the bike, and pedaling powerfully to make up for lost time. The idea is that the more you dress rehearse what could go wrong and how you could cope with it, the more capable you will feel of overcoming these situations if they actually occur.

- *To help you see your opponent in new ways so that she doesn't inspire any special fear, awe, or nervousness.* For example, you might imagine that your opponent's positive qualities of self-confidence and strength are capable of flowing to you. You could image yourself absorbing her good qualities, rather than being overwhelmed or cowed by them.

- *To help you cope with precompetition anxiety or other negative feelings.* Some athletes use imagery—or one particular image—as a means to get a grip on their feelings in high-stress situations. A diver who sometimes falls apart or chokes from extreme anxiety during competition, for example, might release some of the tension by flashing an image in her mind of a beautiful gull soaring into the sky, then gracefully swooping toward water. A runner who feels like hanging it up midrace might shake her desire to quit by bringing up a snapshot of her family cheering her on as she crosses the finish line. The idea is to find a picture that combats negative feelings. Then, it's important to get in the habit of evoking that picture so it automatically helps you let go of tension.

Counter Negative Self-Talk

Think about it: If you keep telling yourself you're too slow, too old, too fat, too weak, or too tired, you can't possibly expect to have the mental energy and confidence you need to perform your best. And research backs up the premise that negative self-talk is harmful to performance. In a study of twenty-four competitive junior tennis players, for example, those who muttered things to themselves, while playing, such as "I am really bad," "Wow! My second serve stinks," "I suck," and "You stupid dimwit, you're so dumb!" tended to lose matches.

A running monologue that is negative drains you of confidence, saps you of determination, increases your frustration, and inhibits your concentration. Triathlete Karen Smyers, age thirty-seven, knows this well: "It was in the middle of the bike segment of the 1995 Hawaii Ironman—the year I won—when my chief opponent Paula Newby-Fraser gained a whopping twelve minutes on me. I was so angry that I had let her get away that I sunk into the worst funk and began to berate myself. I just kept saying 'You stink, Karen, what's your problem?' Every once in a while, I would stand up on my pedals and curse. I felt so sorry for myself."

But then a friend and a formidable triathlete himself, Dave Scott, who was volunteering at the race, saw Karen and realized where "her head was at." He yelled to her "Karen, you're doing fine, just concentrate on your own race."

Recalls Smyers: "All of a sudden I realized, that, hey, I might not even make second place if I keep beating up on myself. I snapped out of it. And I began to talk to myself, 'Calm down. Just do the best you can riding, then have a great run. You still have a long way to go, with lots of opportunities to catch up."

Although Scott's words were pivotal in this instance, Smyers has also learned how to "self-diagnose" a negative mindset. "I am often able to catch myself complaining and feeling low during a competition. But the challenge is that I have to realize I'm doing it before I can talk myself out of it."

Exactly. The first trick to countering negative chatter is becoming aware that you do it. Then, when you catch yourself in a negative thought loop, you need to learn how to supplant it with something forceful and commanding. You don' t need to be "falsely positive"—saccharin-coated sentiments like "I'm wonderful" or "You're doing great, don't worry" are unlikely to persuade you from further self-criticism. In fact, aggressively positive affirmations like "I will be a success. I have nothing to worry about, I am optimistic and enthusiastic," may drain your energy and distract you from the real task at hand, which is to marshal your resources so that you can begin to perform well again.

So what should you say to yourself? You might find you just need to chastise yourself a little by saying something like, "Okay, so you've made a mistake, big deal, now just move on" or "Quit it, now get your mind back on the game." Saying a cue word like *stop* or a phrase like "slow down," then taking in a deep breath, followed by a hearty exhalation, can work too.

Nipping negative thoughts in the bud, in other words, doesn't have to be complex: You don't need to probe all the reasons *why* you are so self-critical. Instead, just stop getting down on yourself whenever you feel the urge. It's surprising how effective it can be.

◓ Concentration Is Complex

- Concentrating can mean filtering out all distracting stimuli— such as the cheering of the crowd—so that you can focus on a very narrow task, like sinking a basket.
- Concentrating can also involve the fast, sweeping in of many stimuli: the kind of concentration a soccer player, for instance, must have in order to assess where all the players are on the field so she can quickly know where to best pass the ball.

Concentrate

Concentration is essential to playing sports well—it's something all athletes do, to varying degrees (and with varying success). But if you've ever consciously tried to concentrate, chances are you failed. You were probably so busy thinking about concentrating ("concentrate, just concentrate" yells your inner voice) that you missed the serve, the pitch, the target.

But this doesn't mean concentration is uncontrollable. There are different methods of encouraging concentration, as well as different kinds of concentration. Concentration is not one thing. For instance, sometimes concentrating means filtering out all distracting stimuli—such as the cheering of the crowd, the blaring of the loudspeaker, the internal pressures in your head—so that you can focus on a very narrow task, such as sinking a putt or a basket. In contrast, concentrating can also involve the fast, sweeping in of many stimuli: the kind of concentration a soccer player, for instance, must have in order to assess where all the players are on the field so she can quickly know where best to pass the ball.

Here are two techniques of concentration that are frequently taught to athletes:

The first is a practice derived from Zen Buddhism called mindfulness meditation. Jack D. Curtis refers to it as "the present moment technique."

Unlike the practice of Transcendental Meditation, which requires you to concentrate the mind by fixing your attention on one word or image, with mindfulness meditation you focus your attention on what you are experiencing from moment to moment.

During a gymnastics competition, for example, being "mindful" would simply mean being in the here-and-now so that you become absorbed in your movements on the balance beam. "You don't think about what you are going to do next or what you have done in the past. You just try to observe what is occurring in your mind, your body, and your environment this very moment," explains Robert Stahl, Ph.D., director of awareness and relaxation training at the Stress Reduction Clinic at the El Camino Hospital in Mountainview, California. In other words, what you learn with mindful meditation is not to become distracted by worries about whether you are going to fall or not.

By keeping yourself in the present moment, mindfulness frees you from wandering thoughts about failure, expectations, and pressures; it encourages you to give of your full potential. You learn, to cultivate the ability to have a relaxed awareness, to concentrate on what is happening this very moment, and to seize more opportunities to appreciate and delight in the present.

Donna Weinbrecht—the moguls champion who recalled experiencing that beautiful in-the-flow feeling when she won her gold medal in 1992—has found learning how to be mindful invaluable. In fact, it's one of the keys that has allowed her to stay in her sport.

"My whole world came crashing down after winning the gold. My hometown had a huge party for me, I was on *David Letterman*, and my phone was ringing off the hook with people wanting me to make appearances. I couldn't handle it."

Weinbrecht thinks she experienced a nervous breakdown. "I would twitch and freak out every time the phone rang. My hair began to fall out. I began to put tremendous pressure on myself. I felt I had to be even better than before. I just tore myself apart—I couldn't see the good in anything I did while I was skiing."

Weinbrecht suspects that the devastating knee injury she experienced at the end of the 1992 season was partly precipitated by her forcing herself to try new maneuvers to prove she could be even better. Although her injury put her out of the entire 1993 season, Weinbrecht did eventually make a tremendous comeback, winning six World Cups in a row in 1994. But then, during the 1994 Winter Olympic Games in Lillehammer, Norway, she once again found herself becoming overwhelmed by pressures to succeed. "I couldn't cope with the intensity and expectations that came with the whole Olympic experience. I held back from really getting engaged in my skiing and so I didn't perform well."

By 1995, Weinbrecht contemplated retiring. "I had lost my passion and gotten to the point where I was almost scared to ski, I was so obsessed with making mistakes and disappointing people."

Then she had an epiphany: "I realized I could just let it all go—let go of everybody's expectations, of my harshness toward my performances, of my worries about being on display all the time. I had achieved what I had because I loved my sport and that was what I needed to get back to."

Which she did, partly by relying on mindfulness-oriented practices and thinking. At the 1997 World Championships (where she won the silver) and the 1998 Winter Olympics in Nagano (where she placed fourth in moguls), for example, Weinbrecht says, "I just got so positive. I focused on what a great opportunity it was to be skiing at such an elite level and how beautiful my surroundings were. Instead of thinking about failing—What if I don't hit the jump?—and instead of allowing myself to get unnerved by all the pressure, I just took it step by step, living in each moment."

Here's an example of a mindfulness exercise: The next time you run (or swim, play in a tennis match, bike, spar) notice how your feet hit the ground as you move. Think about what you feel in your legs. Observe the swing and rhythm of your arms. Think about your neck and shoulders and sense whether they are relaxed or tense. Notice whether your breathing is smooth, regular, or forced. Drink in your surroundings, paying attention to how the elements—the sunshine, the air, the breezes—feel on your skin, in your hair. Fill your mind only with your action in the moment, nothing else.

These kinds of mindfulness meditations help you to get grounded in real, here-and-now time, and the payback of it is that your mind and body can communicate and work together at full capacity, free from interference.

Another skill of concentration is self-monitoring, which is sometimes referred to as an "associative" strategy. What is it? It involves a conscious paying attention—concentrating—on how your muscles feel, how your breathing is, whether you need to hydrate, etc.

For example, in a study of elite marathon runners, co-authored by William P. Morgan, professor of kinesiology at the University of Wisconsin-Madison, it was found that most didn't try to distract themselves or attempt to take their minds off their efforts. Instead, these top-level runners tended to pay very close attention to sensations in their feet, calves, and thighs as well as to their respiratory sensations while racing. What's more, they regulated their pace according to these body readings.

What's the point of periodic self-checks? "During training sessions as well as during the heat of a competition they help put you in touch with whether you are overdoing it—or holding back," says Jack J. Lesyk, Ph.D., director of the Ohio Center for Sport Psychology, Beachwood.

Self-monitoring may also help you avoid injuries. "It stands to reason that you are less likely to get hurt if you are paying attention to your body and its responses when you exercise," notes Lesyk.

It may also help you compete smarter: For example, if you know you have a tendency to go too fast in the beginning of a race (then crash by the end), you might be able to avoid this by running through a self-check list in which you inventory how you feel (How is my breathing? How is my stride? Am I pushing too hard?). The answers will help you determine whether you need to put on the brakes.

Similarly, rather than get stuck in a familiar groove in which you finish every meet at a pace that puts you in third, self-monitoring might reveal you have the kick left to make second or even first. (You might ask yourself, "Am I holding back? Could I push and withstand a little more pain for another few minutes?")

Mindfulness meditation and self-monitoring are probably equally useful forms of concentration—your particular situation will determine on which it makes sense for you to rely. Mindfulness, if you're a skater, for example, could help you to focus on the flow of your body over the ice and help filter out self-doubts and fears when performing in front of an audience. Whereas self-monitoring might be just what you need to assess how much further you can push when careening down a steep hill during a bike race.

The only hard part of either practice is remembering to do it. If you listen to a Walkman as you train, stop for a while to help get into the habit of zeroing in on yourself. If you wear a digital watch, program the alarm to go off every ten minutes as a way to remind yourself to "check in." With time and practice, moments of self-monitoring and mindfulness can easily become natural, automatic parts of every training session and competition. And the reward for these brief intervals of concentration is that they snap you away from restless, wandering, even self-defeating thoughts and put you right smack into the heart and soul of your activity.

*I used to jump up and down before races
to rev myself up. But as I've gotten older,
I've found being quiet and relaxed behind
the starting block works better.*
—MELANIE VALERIO, OLYMPIC GOLD MEDAL–WINNING SWIMMER

Dissociate—Sometimes

In direct contradiction to "the power of concentration" is the simple technique that some athletes use to get through the tough parts of workouts or competitions— "dissociating." They use fantasy and thoughts of things unrelated to their body to escape from their unpleasant sensations (of boredom, discomfort, or even pain). "It's a very individual thing—some athletes need to stay locked in to the here-and-now more to compete well, while others need to allow their minds great freedom to wander," says Charles A. Maher.

Some athletes use dissociation in training, but then fiercely "associate" or concentrate during competition. Yet others dabble in both.

"Despite the recognized advantage of employing an associative strategy, there is both research and anecdotal evidence that also supports the judicious use of dissociation during competition," states Professor Morgan in a review of the current research published in *Perspectives in Exercise Science and Sports Medicine* (Cooper Publishing, Carmel, Indiana, 1997).

In other words, it's fine and perhaps even beneficial to let your mind drift into la-la land as long as you don't do it continuously—i.e., you make "judicious use" of fantasy, being sure to intersperse your mental journeys with focused self-checks.

Most of us don't need to practice dissociating during exercise; it usually comes naturally. It can be helpful to build a personal library of positive and rich fantasies, memories, or imaginings that you know work to "transport" you. That way, when you're trying to combat the effects of boredom, disillusionment, or pain during a workout or competition, you can easily enter a script you know will lift your spirits.

Learn Your Zone of Optimal Performance

Everyone has a zone of optimal performance (ZOP), and for each of us, it's different. It's the level of arousal you need to perform at your best. At one end of the spectrum, for example, being too calm before a game can lead to disinterest; you're too blasé to "want it" bad enough to pay full attention to your teammates so that you can respond quickly and imaginatively. The other extreme is that you're so nervous—your heart races, your palms sweat, your muscles tense, and your breathing becomes shallow—that you become too emotionally depleted and overwhelmed to respond and play well during a game.

Finding your ZOP means you learn how to strike the best balance between being psyched up enough so that you are inspired to do your best, but not so overstimulated that you get choked by an anxiety attack.

To determine your best pre-race mindset, think about how you've felt before previous competitions—and how well you've performed. It's important to connect your precompetition feelings to your results. Why? Although feeling anxious may not be an experience you like, the truth may be that it leads you to perform your best. So ask yourself: Have I done better on the days when I'm most collected and "centered"? Does my being revved up seem to result in more kick? Or does nervousness at the start seem to end up in my becoming too wrung-out midcompetition?" If you're new to competition and don't have a track record to analyze, the best thing to remember is that it's normal, even desirable, to feel some nervousness, so long as those feelings don't overwhelm you.

There are all sorts of techniques to help get you into your ZOP. For taming out-of-control anxiety, everything from biofeedback training to hypnosis to Zen meditation is recommended. But here are two easy-to-learn, easy-to-teach yourself techniques from *The Mindset for Winning*. They can be done anywhere: "You don't need to close your eyes, have quiet surroundings, or mentally withdraw from the environment; they can be used any time you feel relaxation or stress control is needed as you prepare for a free throw, line up a putt, or get ready to serve or return the game point in tennis," says Dr. John D. Curtis.

The first is called the "Brief Body Scan Technique." With a total of four normal breaths, you relax your body parts sequentially within twenty to thirty seconds.

Take a deep breath, and, as you exhale from the first breath, allow your jaw to relax, let go, and become heavy. Take a normal breath, and, as you exhale, allow your shoulders to relax. As you exhale from the third breath, allow your arms and hands to relax. And, as you exhale from the fourth breath, allow your legs to relax.

The second, the "Deep Breath Technique," is the fastest and probably the most useful to use during actual competition, according to Curtis.

As soon as you feel yourself losing control, simply take a deep breath, hold it for a count of one to five seconds. As you exhale, feel your body slowing down, letting go of tension, and relaxing.

To get the most out of either of these techniques, practice them whenever you start to feel tension building. That way, your ability to use them and rely on them for stress relief will become automatic during actual competition.

Okay, but what if what you really need is to get yourself psyched up, not calmed down? Although little research has been done in this area, work conducted in part by Daniel Gould at the Department of Exercise and Sport Science, University of North Carolina at Greensboro, seems to indicate that getting yourself mad may be a good way to get your adrenaline pumping. In other words, you think angry thoughts right before you set out, then blow them off by racing hard. You might also try speeding up your breathing a bit, precompetition, and giving yourself an energizing pep talk.

In addition, you should be aware that your ZOP may change over time. "I used to jump up and down before races to rev myself up. I really needed to get my heart rate cranking," recalls twenty-eight-year-old Olympic Gold Medal-winning swimmer, Melanie Valerio. "But as I've gotten older, I've found relaxing behind the starting block works better for me. I get very quiet and focused."

So keep an eye on your ZOP, since you may find time and experience cause it to change.

Put It All Together

"Especially in competition, you need to have a strategy," says Lesyk. "When you have a plan, all the skills you have learned can be directed to helping you implement it."

For example, many first-time marathoners reframe how they think about all the miles ahead as a strategy for avoiding becoming overwhelmed by the total distance. They might divide the first 20 miles into manageable 4-mile segments, only allowing themselves to think "I'm halfway there" at mile 20, then break the last six miles down mile by mile. As a subtext to this sweeping strategy, then, the runner might self-monitor to see whether she should slow the pace, dissociate to help pass time, or use self-talk to snap herself out of feeling discouraged.

Professional runners, on the other hand, often begin a race with a complex strategy in mind, in which they think very carefully about how and when to react to the developments occurring among the front-runners. Not only do they try to become familiar with the race course and the running styles of their competitors, they try to formulate a precise plan for how and when to reel in other runners.

Of course, "strategy" means something different for every sport. In tennis, for example, one strategy might be to wait for the other player to make a mistake. An alternate one might be to play a power game, coming into the net early, fast, and hard.

As you map out your game plan, you should also assess what kinds of risk you are willing to take, says Lesyk, who tells this anecdote: "Race car driver Mario Andretti had a reputation for not finishing a lot of races, even though he is one of the best drivers of all time. His strategy was to push it to the limit. If he spun off course while doing it and didn't finish as a result, it was a risk he could accept. His decision was that he would prefer to win or lose than play it safe and just place."

What if your strategy goes astray—as it is sometimes bound to do? For example, maybe your tennis strategy to play a power game didn't work because your opponent simply wouldn't let you do what you wanted. Let yourself feel disappointed, for a while. Then cull whatever you can from the experience since there surely is some lesson to be learned.

"When things go wrong, you need to pay attention since it's an opportunity in disguise," notes Lesyk. "When you perform below par or lose—and when you honestly examine all the reasons why this happened—you expand your self-knowledge,

---

◐ Twelve Symptoms of Overtraining
- A pervasive feeling of melancholy
- Irritability
- Unusual fatigue
- Sleep disturbances
- Loss of appetite
- Reduced sex drive
- More muscle soreness than usual
- A general feeling of sluggishness and "heaviness" in your body
- Feelings of apathy, a "can't get going" mood
- Anxiousness and inability to concentrate
- Increased incidence of minor infections, like colds
- Menstrual irregularities

which leaves you better equipped to face the next challenge." In other words, don't let yourself wallow too long in feelings of defeat. Instead, think of each loss or misfired strategy as a chance to become more of an expert, on yourself and what you need to be to be successful.

KNOWING HOW MUCH IS TOO MUCH: HOW TO RECOGNIZE AND AVOID OVERTRAINING

It's ironic: The things that make you a good athlete—such as commitment, drive, the ability to tolerate discomfort, and the desire to push limits—are the very same things that put you at high risk for overtraining.

Overtraining, which can affect athletes of all skill, in any sport, is a concern for several reasons. First, it's counterproductive—your performances go flat and you can't improve as a result. You also don't rebound from workouts the way you used to. Plus, it makes you prone to a host of physical and psychological ills (see Twelve Symptoms of Overtraining, page 144).

The Causes

Overtraining, which some experts refer to as "the staleness syndrome," is an imbalance between training and recovery. In a balanced, healthy training situation, you systematically stress your body at increasingly higher levels—you lift heavier weights, run further, take more difficult aerobic classes—and your performance progressively improves.

Overtraining occurs when your body can no longer adapt to the increasing workloads—instead of being built up, it gets broken down. This usually occurs because 1) not enough rest and recovery has been built into the schedule and/or 2) the training volume and/or intensity has been progressively intensified at too fast a rate for the body to be able to adjust.

Unfortunately, overtraining is tricky to predict, since there is no threshold at which all athletes become "overtrained." There is huge variability in how different athletes respond to the stresses of exercise. It seems that while some athletes are more resistant to overtraining, others are quite susceptible. So what might be a healthy, adaptive, performance-enhancing regime for you might lead to breakdown in another athlete.

In addition, one's personal threshold for overtraining may

change. You can perform the same training regime that worked so wonderfully last season to make you faster and stronger, only to find that this season it leads you to become stale. When this happens, the cause is usually an overload of stress in other areas of your life. For instance, if you're not sleeping because you're worried about a chronically ill child, if your emotional equilibrium is being thrown out of whack by a rocky relationship, if the stress on your job is out of control, your vulnerability to becoming overtrained increases.

"You don't have to work out for hours everyday to be at risk for overtraining," explains Susan Zaro, "If you have a lot of stress from other sources in your life, your tolerance for strenuous workouts can get very, very low."

Recognizing the Problem

Clearly, the line between training that leads to peak performance and training that triggers physical breakdown is pretty fine. And once you cross that line, your condition can progressively deepen and worsen if steps to reverse the effects of overtraining aren't quickly taken.

Unfortunately, nipping overtraining in the bud can be a challenge. To date, researchers haven't found any reliable physiologic markers. For example, an elevated morning resting pulse rate is often cited as one of the hallmarks of overtraining. But the measurement isn't accurate if you wake up to an alarm and can easily become skewed by things like heat, caffeine intake, and/or dehydration. Plus, studies simply haven't consistently borne out the contention that an elevated resting heart rate is a foolproof indicator of overtraining.

Similarly, it's not known if some of the other apparent markers of overtraining, such as elevations in the stress hormone cortisol or alterations in certain hormone ratios, actually precede the problem (in which case you could monitor them, via blood tests, to detect the onset of overtraining) or only set in afterward as an result of overtraining.

When it comes to detecting the first signs of overtraining, then, your feelings and moods are probably the best barometer. But self-observation can be trickier and more fraught with pitfalls than it seems for several reasons.

First, athletes who overtrain often have very disciplined, hard-driving natures. They don't give in or give up easily. "One of the insidious aspects of staleness is that when a plateau in performance becomes evident, the response of many athletes is to train harder. This can result in a vicious cycle where the athlete exacerbates the condition by continually increasing training in the attempt to overcome a plateau," notes John Raglin, Ph.D., associate professor of kinesiology at Indiana University in *The Handbook of Research on Sport Psychology* (Macmillan, 1993).

The signs of overtraining are easy to mistake for other syndromes too, such as iron deficiency or hypothyroidism (two things that your doctor can easily rule out by performing a simple blood test). It's also easy to spend a lot of time rationalizing and or denying you have a problem by saying things like "I must just be getting lazy" or "maybe I need to eat better."

Give It a Rest

How is overtraining treated? "It has long been recognized that staleness can be effectively treated with prolonged rest," notes Dr. Raglin. "In many cases, rest periods of one to two weeks are sufficient, but it has been observed that even after six months, some stale athletes still exhibit disturbed neuroendocrine function and have not fully recovered."

The prospect of total rest probably makes you shudder; for anyone who thrives on physical activity, it's a pretty abhorrent prescription. Luckily, except in cases of extreme overtraining, rest rarely needs to be "pure." Instead, a growing number of experts are advocating "active rest." With active rest you usually (1) reduce the overall volume of your training; (2) reduce the intensity of your training; and (3) cross-train (play another sport) to get a break from your primary-sport training.

To what extent you'll need a hiatus of active rest in order to recover from overtraining is a highly individual matter. Complete recovery can take anywhere from two to twelve weeks or more. As a general rule, the more overtrained you are, the longer it will take to recover.

Some experts also recommend medications usually used to treat depression, such as Prozac or Zoloft, for treatment of overtraining, since the symptoms of the two disorders are so similar. The scientific evidence showing that antidepressant therapy, which is usually prescribed for six months or longer, is helpful in treating overtraining is still relatively scant; however, the anecdotal evidence from athletes who have overcome the overtraining syndrome with the aid of antidepressants is often impressive.

One of the most highly publicized examples is that of Alberto Salazar, who won the New York City Marathon in 1982, then experienced twelve years of poor racing in large part caused by overtraining, he feels. Upon taking Prozac, Salazar experienced a tremendous comeback, winning the prestigious 53.8 mile Comrades Marathon in South Africa.

If you are considering taking antidepressants for overtraining, it's important to realize that not everyone responds the same to them. In an article that appeared in *Runner's World* magazine (August 1994) some readers reported the medications renewed their love of their sport while others felt sapped of their joy for running. The side effects of antidepressants tend to be minor, but include nausea, headache, diarrhea, and shakiness.

Be wary of self-diagnosing overtraining, although there is probably nothing harmful about trying a two-week layoff to see if it helps. If it doesn't, consult with your regular doctor to rule out the possibility of other medical conditions. Then consult a sports medicine specialist to get evaluated for overtraining. If you are diagnosed as overtrained, your doctor should help you figure out how long you need to rest and/or whether taking antidepressants might be advisable.

Preventing the Problem

By now, it should be pretty obvious that not becoming overtrained in the first place is clearly preferable to having to recover from it. The key to this, in part, is building more rest into your training schedule. Experts estimate that during a layoff an athlete can maintain her fitness level for at least two to three weeks. So you don't need to worry that taking a few days or even weeks off will lead to an instant slide in your conditioning.

Many coaches insist that their athletes take at least one day off a week. In fact, there's a general trend toward a "less is more" training philosophy, partly because this not only seems to prevent staleness but may help performance.

Many experts also recommend building more active rest—in the form of cross-training—into training schedules as an overtraining preventive measure. The reasoning for this is twofold: First, many trainers and coaches know that their athletes simply won't follow the advice to rest completely; these athletes simply become too depressed when they are forced not to work out when they want to. So the advice to cross-train is a good way to help the athlete feel as if she is doing something.

Second, cross-training can be a way for an athlete to rest one muscle group while getting another, usually neglected, group of muscles in better shape, thus leading to better whole body conditioning. For example, a cyclist, in order to rest her quadricep muscles, might focus on upper body strength training on her cross-training days.

A technique called "periodization training" is sometimes used as a tactic for preventing overtraining. In periodization, you schedule and control the amount, intensity, and frequency of your training (which includes rests) so that you reach your peak condition by the time you are ready for competition. After competition, you take a prolonged break from competing in your sport, although you stay active.

Tapering—the practice of progressively reducing the volume and intensity of your workouts for anywhere from a week to four weeks before a competition—is also believed to be helpful in preventing overtraining. It may boost performance too. According to a French study of eighteen elite swimmers, a three- to four-week taper, consisting of a progressive reduction in the training load, resulted in a 3 percent improvement in the swimmers' competition times.

Finally, keeping a logbook, in which you note your feelings in relation to your day-to-day training, may help you detect overtraining before it really gets brewing, according to research from the Department of Human Movement Studies at the University of Queensland, Australia. A log may help you spot trends, such as a string of training sessions that seem harder than usual or a loss of a sense of fun and well-being when it comes to workouts. You can then respond quickly, before the problem sets in, by resting more and/or cutting back in some aspect of your training so that your body has time to recover properly. As a result of this rest, you're likely to feel more energetic and to be able to perform your best.

EMOTIONAL HEALING: COPING WITH INJURIES

Whitewater kayaker and silver medal winner at the 1997 Slalom National Championships, Rebecca Bennett, age twenty-one, was paddling on a very demanding course when she twisted the wrong way and her shoulder came out of its socket. "At the time, the doctor said I needed surgery, but I remember thinking 'never!' Surgery was just too scary."

So for more than four years Bennett paddled in pain. "I just avoided the whole issue, hoping it would somehow magically get better." Instead her shoulder got worse until finally Bennett was unable to train. "I would go out and try to push myself but it was ridiculous. I finally had to face that fact that if I didn't do something about my shoulder I would never be able to compete again. I was really, really depressed. And nervous. I was very, very anxious about being operated on, about the experience of surgery itself and what might happen as a result of it."

Bennett's surgery revealed a badly torn ligament and worn away cartilage, but it is expected that she will be able to regain full use of her shoulder. But her experience of denying her injury and living in pain for almost four years rather than get sidelined highlights how daunting, confusing, and potentially devastating injuries can be in an athlete's life. There is simply no question that dealing with an injury is one of the biggest psychological challenges an athlete can face.

An injury can leave you feeling desperate because it makes you feel so completely at the mercy of your environment.
—JACK J. LESYK, PH.D., DIRECTOR OF THE OHIO CENTER FOR SPORT PSYCHOLOGY

As an athlete, you thrive on your day-to-day activity. Exercise helps reduce stress, and being unable to participate can make you moody, tense, and unhappy. According to a study of joggers, cyclists, and swimmers from the Sport Psychology Laboratory at the University of Wisconsin-Madison, even brief periods (less than two days) of exercise deprivation can lead to mood disturbances. In another study published in the *Journal of Sport Psychology*, runners who were required to miss workouts experienced a host of negative reactions—irritability, restlessness, guilt, muscle tension, depression, frustration, sleeping problems, and even stomach ills.

Even if your prospects of healing completely are very good, being injured can have a serious impact on how you feel about yourself. As sport psychologists Jean Williams and Nancy Roepke point out in the *Handbook of Research on Sport Psychology* (Macmillan, 1993), being physically fit may give you a sense of personal mastery as well as be crucial to your feelings of being physically attractive. The self-concept that "I am an athlete" may also be very important to your identity—without it, you may suffer a crisis of confidence and be at a loss to define who you are.

Yet another psychological backlash of an injury is that it can leave you feeling helpless and out of control. "If you are like most athletes, you are used to feeling autonomous and in command. An injury can leave you feeling desperate because it makes you feel so completely at the mercy of your environment," says Lesyk.

Finally, for many of us, sports provide an important venue for social interaction. You run with friends, look forward to playing ball with the girls, thrive on the camaraderie of your gym buddies, and so on. When this is taken away from you, you may feel very lonely, not to mention isolated, angry and envious.

Getting Better

It helps to know that your complicated emotional reactions are normal. "You should absolutely allow yourself to feel grieved," notes Zaro. "It's okay to feel mad and angry—in fact, allowing yourself to experience these feelings is an important part of the process of getting better. If you shut yourself off from these emotions or try to intellectualize them away, you're more likely to get 'stuck' and become seriously depressed and self-destructive."

The first step, then, toward healing emotionally after an injury, is often *not* to pretend the injury doesn't bother you. Don't feel pressured to "cheer up" and don't belittle your loss when you hear comments like "Oh, it's just basketball, you can always play some other game" or "You were running too much anyhow, now you'll have time for other things."

Of course, you'll want to come to terms with your initial feelings of shock, grief, and anger so that you can eventually accept your setback—then move on from it. In order to focus your energies on rehabilitation fully, you'll need to rebuild a positive attitude and regain a sense of hopefulness. A good way to do this is to use the same psychological skills, especially goal setting and self-talk, you used for playing your sport well.

Goal setting, for example, not only provides you with a sense of control, but may help you to become more motivated, persistent, and committed, note Williams and Roepke in *The Handbook of Research on Sport Psychology*. Bennett, for example, has her sights set on the 2000 Olympics in Sydney, Australia. "It's why I finally risked having the surgery, so I could get better in time to compete. It's a goal I really want to achieve."

Long-terms goals can lift your spirits and help you have a positive perspective on the future. But having short-term goals that are specific, realistic, and challenging is important, too. For instance, if you have torn the tendon below your knee, one of your short-term goals might be to do static (isometric) quadriceps exercises at least three times daily; a more long-term goal might be to strengthen your quads using a leg press machine, working up so that you can press from a 90-degree bend. The more serious your injury, the more important it is for you to consult with your physical therapist or other health professional when setting these goals.

Since it's so easy to berate yourself when you're feeling down and disillusioned, countering negative self-talk can also be a valuable element in your recovery. The more you can recognize destructive trends in self-talk ("I'll never get better," "This is taking too long" and "I might as well just give up") and alter the running monologue so that it is focused and positive, the more likely it is you will have the energy and drive to stick to your rehabilitation program.

It's also important to keep connected with your sport while you're getting better, says Maher. "Don't cut yourself off from your coaches, teammates, and friends because it will just increase your feelings of isolation and abandonment. Keeping involved not only keeps you active, it will help you to feel supported and valued." So attend practices, team meetings, and competitions and help out any way you can. Even if your sport is very individual—if you're a runner, for example, volunteering at meets and races can be a good way to contribute as you maintain your ties with the sport.

Getting Back in the Game

The biggest risk is that you'll try to get back too soon and as a result get reinjured. "I tell athletes to try to take it a step at a time and to use their mental skills of 'staying in the moment' to quell their anxiousness about the speed of their progress," says Maher.

Sometimes, though, you've been given a clean bill of health, yet you're still not confident about returning to your sport. You may be worried that you're not fully healed, worried about getting injured again, worried that you won't be able to perform well, and so on.

"If you're hesitant because your accident was terrifying, it helps to carefully take the traumatic event apart, piece by piece, and really figure out what happened and what can be learned from it," says Dr. Lesyk. "Sometimes you can discover that the accident can be attributed to a changeable circumstance—if you were injured on a day the slopes were particularly icy, for example, you can decide not to ski on days like that anymore."

However, many times you can't attribute your injury to any outside force. "In that case, you need to accept that this was always a risk inherent in your sport and always will be a risk," continues Dr. Lesyk. "What you need to do is to build up your confidence so that you can embrace the risk again. What I usually suggest is that the athlete go several steps backward in her sport, relearning her skills, so that she works her way up to a greater self-confidence." For example, a skier might begin on gentle slopes and then gradually work her way up.

"I have seen other athletes who have been injured come back to paddling changed—their style is less aggressive, more cautious," says Bennett. "But I know that if I expect to compete on the Olympic level I can't become timid. I'll need to work past my fears and learn to overcome them somehow."

Finding Meaning in a Career-Ending Injury

Although most athletes can overcome their injuries to play again, the reality is that not everyone is able to. For some, being barred from their sport is like suffering a divorce or death in the family. What's more, many injured athletes who can no longer participate suffer serious clinical problems such as depression, alcoholism, drug abuse, and suicidal tendencies.

"The first thing I do when working with an athlete who is suffering from a career-ending injury is to encourage her to look back at what she accomplished and to drink in how far she came. I want her to celebrate where she started, what she became, to look at what she gained, what she will always have

SPECIAL FOCUS:

◯ Make Your Goals Real by Writing Them Down

Here's a goal setting exercise adapted from one described by John Syer and Christopher Connolly in their book *Sporting Body Sporting Mind* (Cambridge University Press, 1984). You'll need four sheets of paper. On the top of one write "Life Goals;" take five minutes to write down as many of these as you can think of— from which races you want to enter, what sports you may want to learn, which competitions you want to win to whether you want to get married, have children, achieve a certain level in your profession. Write down anything that comes into your head, aiming to find a dozen or more.

Take a second sheet and write "Three Year goals" at its head. Take five minutes to write down anything that comes to mind without worrying what you wrote on the previous sheet.

On the third sheet of paper, write "This Season's Goals." Enumerate as many things as you can think of, no matter how trivial they may seem. On your fourth sheet of paper, write "One Month Goals" and repeat the procedure.

Return to your first sheet of "Lifetime Goals" and reflect on which ones are really important. Choose the three that are the most significant and put a check beside each. Go through this process of choosing the three priorities that are most important on each sheet of paper you filled out.

As you survey your check marks, think about it—do your goals clash or intersect? Ideally, your one-month goals should mesh with your season's goals which should mesh with your three-year goals and so on: Each goal should intertwine with the others so that the smaller achievements combine, in a step-by-step way, to produce a cumulative effect.

Also, reflect on how well you are working toward achieving your one-month goals. Your season's goals? Your lifetime goals? What steps do you need to take to get closer to achieving them?

Consider keeping a logbook. The good part about putting your intentions and plan of action down in writing is that it helps further clarify and reinforce your goals, plus gives you a concrete blueprint to follow to implement them. List everything you need to do to move closer to your goals. Set dates, times, and deadlines. Then use the logbook to chart your progress and take notes on what's going right, what's not working.

as a result of her sport experiences and what she can take from it," says Zaro.

Many sport psychologists encourage athletes to use a "grief response model" to understand their loss and the process of coming to terms with it. These models—the most famous of which is the five-stage model outlined by Elisabeth Kübler-Ross in her book *On Death and Dying*—identify typical responses in the normal process of grief and typical stages you go through in order to reach acceptance. For example, Kübler-Ross says the first stage in the grief process is denial: when you first hear the bad news, your response is "No, not me, it can't be true." From there you move to the second stage of grief, which is anger: "Why me?" And so on until you reach the fifth stage, which is acceptance. Perhaps one of the most valuable aspects of applying a grief model to the experience of coming to terms with a sports injury is that it helps you feel that what you are experiencing is not only normal, but necessary.

Of course, to accept a career-ending injury completely, you need to find a new and satisfying career. One of the things athletes often have, without realizing it, is a well-honed set of decision-making skills and, if they have played team sports, collaborative skills. These skills can often be transferred and put to good use in other occupations, from coaching and sports administration to any number of businesses.

Finally, most experts feel that it's important to keep active. You may not be able to play soccer competitively, for example, but you may still be able to swim, racewalk, or strength train. The idea is to redefine yourself as an athlete, taking as much good as you can from your past and using it to enrich your future.

5

YOUR PREGNANCY

Member of the U.S. women's bobsled team Alexandra Powe-Allred, age thirty-three, of Westerville, Ohio, was four months pregnant with her second child when she muscled a 325-pound bobsled to a gold medal victory in the first-ever-for-women U.S. National Push Championships. Powe-Allred trained for months to prepare for the 1995 event, regularly power lifting, sprinting, and performing plyometrics (powerfully explosive jumps and movements designed to increase muscle power and speed) at high intensities.

"I worked like a dog—really, really hard. I would be drenched with sweat after workouts," says Powe-Allred, who was monitored throughout her pregnancy by one of the top experts in the United States on exercise and pregnancy, James F. Clapp, III, M.D., a professor of reproductive biology at Case Western Reserve University in Cleveland.

While she was training, Dr. Clapp literally studied Powe-Allred. "There was nothing dignified about what I did," recalls Powe-Allred. "I was hooked up in all kinds of ways while I was exercising—I had to wear a rectal thermometer, a monitor over my stomach for the baby, and a monitor over my heart too. But I felt great. Instead of the workouts getting harder and more difficult as the pregnancy progressed, I was getting stronger. I was training with two other women who weren't pregnant, and I was beating them in everything we were doing. So I felt, this must be okay, my body must be telling me it is okay," recalls Powe-Allred, who gave birth to a healthy girl.

Other athletes have quite a different pregnancy experience. Angel Martino, age thirty, who won two Gold and two Bronze medals in swimming at the 1996 Olympic Games in Atlanta, recalls "My doctor never said 'Don't exercise.' But he did advise me to listen to my body. And in the first weeks my body was saying 'I'm tired!' Whenever I was a passenger in a car, I'd fall asleep; at home, I slept for the longest stretches. I could hardly keep awake!"

Martino also didn't have the desire to push things to the max. "I needed a break from intense training after the Olympics," says Martino, who also admits she worried about miscarrying. "I had several friends who had miscarried early on in their pregnancies and so I tried to be really careful. I quit swimming. Eventually, though, I realized it didn't make sense to get scared off from exercising completely."

Martino ended up doing a combination of different exercises—a little running, weight lifting, swimming, Stairmaster, and Nordic track—throughout her pregnancy. "It was actually very enjoyable. I would switch from one form of exercise to another whenever what I was doing started to feel uncomfortable. I quit running completely in my sixth month, because I would get too hot. And I always did things at a pretty moderate intensity," recalls Martino, who gave birth to a robust baby boy in May 1997.

Luckily for Powe-Allred, Martino and every other athlete who becomes pregnant in this day and age, doctors and other experts no longer consider pregnancy, training, and even competition to be mutually exclusive. Over the past several years, exercise prescriptions during pregnancy have become increasingly more liberal. This is largely owing to the mounting body of evidence that indicates exercise is safe—and may even be beneficial—during pregnancy.

Still, every woman's pregnancy is as individual as her baby-to-be. And there are some risks you should be aware of, as well as safety rules, training realities, and of course, rewards. This roundup of all the latest scientific evidence on exercise during pregnancy, postpartum, and breast-feeding should give you the information you'll need to tailor your training during and after pregnancy wisely.

IS IT RISKY TO EXERCISE WHEN YOU ARE EXPECTING? (THE GOOD NEWS: MOST WORRIES ARE UNFOUNDED!)

For years, experts thought exercise during pregnancy must be risky because studies on pregnant women who worked in jobs that required long hours of standing and other strenuous work often found that these women had babies who were small for gestational age, premature, or low in birthweight. In addition, pregnant research animals forced to undergo chronic exertion often gave birth to unhealthy offspring.

With the fitness boom of the 1970s, researchers finally began to study pregnant women who were actually engaged in sports—not expectant mothers stressed out working on assembly lines or lab rats. What many of these researchers expected to find was trouble—i.e., that women who worked out would have a higher rate of miscarriage, preterm birth, or many other problems.

Instead, they often found the opposite—that exercise did *not* increase the risks and in many cases even reduced them. "It has become increasingly clear that the fit pregnant body has an amazing ability to adapt so as to protect itself as well as the fetus. There are all kinds of compensatory mechanisms that get triggered during pregnancy that help make exercise safe," notes Barbara Sternfeld, Ph.D., research scientist at Kaiser Permanente Medical Care Program of Northern California, Oakland.

For example:

• Exercise does not seem to increase the risk of spontaneous abortion. In a study headed by Dr. Clapp of more than two

---

◇ Warning!

Exercising during your pregnancy may not be safe if you have any of these conditions:
  • a history of two or more miscarriages
  • vaginal bleeding
  • premature rupture of membranes
  • symptoms or history of premature labor
  • intrauterine growth retardation
  • heart disease
  • diabetes
  • anemia
  • multiple pregnancy

hundred recreational athletes who continued a regular (three or more times a week) program of endurance exercise (thirty minutes or more of running, biking, aerobics, swimming, cross-country skiing, or stair-stepping per session) at or above a conditioning intensity (greater than 50 percent VO2max), the women who continued vigorous exercise miscarried at a rate of 15 percent in the first trimester compared to 17 percent in the women who were sedentary.

• There's no evidence that exercise increases the risk of birth defects. Studies performed on pregnant animals have suggested that sharp elevations in body core temperature can increase the risk of birth defects in the offspring. Partly as a result of this animal research, there has long been a concern that women who exercise vigorously may overheat and that this rise in body temperature might lead to congenital malformations or birth defects in the fetus.

Yet no link between overheating during exercise and birth defects has ever been demonstrated. And experts think this is because athletes who enter pregnancy in a trained state have an increased efficiency when it comes to dissipating body heat. In other words, the body of a fit mother-to-be becomes better at thermoregulation, thus providing protection for the fetus.

Backing up this theory is an influential study published in *Obstetrics and Gynecology* that found heat storage in fit women did not increase as a result of exercise. In another study of pregnant recreational runners, the capacity to dissipate heat during exercise actually seemed to become more efficient as pregnancy progressed.

• Exercise during pregnancy doesn't lead to fetal hypoxia (oxygen deprivation). For a long time, the worry was that by diverting blood flow to the muscles, exercise might reduce the flow of oxygenated blood to the uterus, placenta, and baby.

But the fit pregnant body and fetus appear to have several mechanisms by which they compensate for this potential effect. First, the pregnant uterus becomes more efficient at extracting oxygen from the blood during exercise, thereby canceling out the problem of a reduced delivery of it. During exercise, blood flow to the uterus is also diverted to favor the placenta, ensuring the fetus gets a constant supply of oxygen and nutrients. Finally, according to Dr. Clapp in *The Journal of Sports Medicine,* "by late pregnancy the recreational athlete's measured blood volume is about 20 percent greater than that seen in nonexercising women. This increase in blood volume should decrease the need for flow redistribution away from the fetal supply lines during exercise, thereby maintaining the availability of oxygen to the fetus and placenta."

• Exercise does not seem to starve the fetus of a continuous supply of glucose (blood sugar), which the fetus depends on to synthesize fat and protein.

Since glucose is also one of the chief fuel sources for exercising muscles, it has long been feared that exercise would compromise glucose delivery to the fetus. But according to one study, when pregnant women exercise they draw more on their fat stores for energy and less on glucose, thus sparing the glucose for the fetus. In other words, it appears that a mother-to-be's body changes its process of fuel metabolism during exercise in order to protect the fetus.

• Pregnant women who exercise do not experience a higher rate of preterm labor. For example, in a University of Northern Colorado study analysis that included 2,314 pregnant women, women who exercised were at no greater risk for preterm labor than sedentary women. In another study conducted by Dr. Clapp, the incidence of preterm labor—9 percent—was similar in the exercising and nonexercising group. Finally, a small study published in the *American Journal of Obstetrics and Gynecology* found that running and stationary biking didn't stimulate or increase uterine activity—an important precursor to preterm labor—in the last eight weeks of pregnancy.

• Babies born to exercisers aren't underweight. One study of eight hundred prenatal patients found that the pregnant women who exercised heavily had heavier babies. Yet other research has found no difference in birth weights at all in the babies born to those women who exercise compared to those who don't. To further confound things, there have been a few studies that have shown that the babies of moms who exercise weigh on average 300 to 500 g less than the babies born to sedentary moms.

"I think when you really look at the literature, it mostly comes down on the side of there being no relationship at all," says Dr. Sternfeld. "In other words, when it comes to birth weight, exercise doesn't appear to have a negative or beneficial effect."

Especially important to note is that even the studies that found a link between exercise and lower birth weights did not find that the babies of exercisers suffered from actual Low Birth Weight (LBW), an outcome associated with a long list of short- and long-term health complications (LBW babies weigh less than 5.5 pounds). Instead, the babies of the exercisers were just on average a little lighter than the babies of the nonexercisers— they weren't underweight, LBW, or unhealthy in any other way.

- There have been no reports of increased injury rates in pregnant women. The concern: As pregnancy progresses, there is an increase in the hormone relaxin, which serves to relax the ligaments and joints of the pelvis in preparation for giving birth. If relaxin also loosens the knees, ankles, shoulders, and other joints, the speculation has long been that a pregnant woman's risk for sprains and other joint injury might increase. However, this has never been substantiated. What's more, there is some data to suggest that fit pregnant women get injured less and have fewer muscle and joint complaints during pregnancy.

THE RULES

Even the formerly conservative American College of Obstetricians and Gynecologists (ACOG)—which in 1985 warned pregnant women to limit exercise to a maximum of fifteen minutes per session, no more than three times a week and never to exceed a heart rate of more than 140 beats per minute—states in its most recent (1994) technical bulletin on exercise during pregnancy that "there are no data in humans to indicate that pregnant women should limit exercise intensity and lower target heart rates because of potential adverse effects."

In essence, female athletes have been given the green light by ACOG when it comes to continuing their aerobic activity during pregnancy, as long as they keep in close contact with their doctors. This is an especially important guideline for elite athletes since less is known about the safety of high-intensity exercise (most of the research has been conducted on recreational athletes). Although there is nothing yet in the data to suggest that elite athletes must necessarily reduce their training, the higher your level of training the more important it is you discuss your athletic life frankly with your obstetrician.

"You need to have a relationship with your doctor that allows you to tell the truth. This may sound very basic, but a lot of athletic women hide the fact that they exercise intensely from their obstetricians because they are afraid they will be criticized," says Julia Alleyne, M.D., medical director of Sport C.A.R.E. at Women's College Hospital in Toronto.

Finding a doctor who can provide guidance around exercise issues can be a real challenge, especially for the more high-level athlete. Many physicians simply tell all women to ease up and back off, partly because they want to err on the side of safety (and probably out of fear of malpractice lawsuits).

"Many physicians simply don't know that much about exercise, during pregnancy or otherwise," says James M. Pivarnik, Ph.D., a professor in the department of kinesiology and osteopathic surgical specialties at Michigan State University, East Lansing. "My universal recommendation to pregnant women whose doctors won't give them personalized guidance is to find another physician, although I know this isn't always easy."

Be forewarned, though, that even experts who are very knowledgeable about exercise during pregnancy may not support you if you desire to compete. "I don't feel we really know yet what the effects of severe intensity exercise are on the baby-to-be," says Michelle Mottola, Ph.D., associate professor of anatomy and kinesiology at the University of Western Ontario. "I feel women should err on the side of safety. Elite athletes in particular are accustomed to pain and they can easily ignore what their bodies are telling them, which can lead them into trouble. My advice to women is to leave the competition until after the baby is born and drop back to a moderate level of intensity while you're pregnant."

When Dr. Alleyne has a patient who wishes to continue to train at a high level during pregnancy, she first informs her, "I can't give you 100 percent reassurance that exercise does no harm since we have so little data on elite athletes and exercise. Still, I'd like to help you." She then works with the athlete and performs these additional health checks throughout the pregnancy:

• Glucose tolerance test for gestational diabetes. (Some doctors only perform this test in women over thirty.)

- Fetal kick counting, starting at twenty weeks.
- Frequent urine dips (to check for the presence of protein, which can signal a problem with the kidneys), blood tests (to check for anemia), and weigh-ins.
- More frequent prenatal appointments may be—but aren't always—required. It depends on how your pregnancy progresses.

In addition, the following safety guidelines apply to all active pregnant women (for sport-specific safety guidelines, see pages 171 to 175):

- After the fourth month, don't exercise lying flat on your back, since your expanding uterus may compress the vena cava, the vein that carries blood back to your heart. This could interfere with normal blood flow to the uterus.
- Do not use a steam room, sauna, or Jacuzzi bath while pregnant. There is some evidence to suggest that when you are passive (i.e., lounging in a hot tub) and your body temperature becomes raised you don't dissipate heat effectively (as you do when you are active during exercise), thus the risk of fetal injury from overheating is increased.
- Be especially vigilant to keep properly hydrated when exercising in hot, humid weather. Wear cool, breathable clothing and protect yourself properly from the sun's rays. If you feel overheated or dizzy, stop.
- According to many obstetricians, the key to exercising safely during pregnancy is to be flexible. If you don't feel better after a workout, it's probably a sign you are overexerting yourself. Learn to quit if you're feeling worn out or an exercise feels uncomfortable. Remember, every pregnancy is different—just because Powe-Allred, for example, was able to work out "like a dog" throughout her pregnancy doesn't mean you can or should be able to.

Keep in mind, too, that the standard benchmark for determining exercise intensity, your target heart rate (which involves either wearing a monitor or measuring your pulse, then factoring in your age) isn't very reliable during pregnancy. Why? Increases in blood volume and oxygen consumption kick up your resting heart rate and just generally invalidate most standard exercise prescriptions and formulas.

A growing number of sports-knowledgeable obstetricians feel that the best way to keep exercise intensity levels safe is by using a rate of perceived exertion (RPE) scale.

It's the ultimate "listen to your body" test: Using a scale of 0 to 10, you simply assess what you are experiencing during workouts—how physically pushed, fatigued, winded, or stressed you feel—to determine if you are in a comfortable range. In the Borg Scale of RPE, 10 is very, very heavy (you're taxing yourself to your absolute maximum), 4 is somewhat heavy and 1 is very light exertion.

Some experts feel a level of exertion in the 3 to 4 zone— moderate to somewhat heavy—is safest. "I advise women to stay in this zone and also to monitor their exertion by using the 'talk test'—if you can easily carry on a conversation while you're exercising, then you're working out at a safe level. If you are breathless and can't speak full sentences, then you are pushing too hard," says Dr. Mottola.

Although other doctors feel you can safely work out at higher levels of perceived exertion (since no adverse effects have been found to date), if your workouts regularly go into the heavy to very heavy range you should make sure your obstetrician is monitoring your pregnancy for any potential detrimental exercise effects.

- Keep an eye on how your athletic shoes (and street shoes too for that matter) fit, since feet often expand, in width and length, during pregnancy, and you may need to buy larger sneakers.
- Keep properly hydrated to encourage your body to dissipate heat. One rule of thumb is 8 ounces of liquid before exercise, then another 8 ounces for every fifteen minutes of working out. Sports drinks are fine and may even be preferable during pregnancy, since they may help supply your baby with glucose. Adequate fluid intake is especially important in the last trimester, since dehydration can trigger premature labor.
- Pregnancy requires an additional 300 calories a day; women who are active need to pay particular attention to eating enough calories to ensure adequate weight gain (as much as 20 to 30 pounds is usually recommended).
- Stop exercising until you see your doctor if any of the following symptoms crop up: pain, fever, bleeding, dizziness,

shortness of breath, faintness, back pain, pubic pain, persistent headaches, failure to gain weight, absence of usual fetal movement, sudden swelling, difficulty in walking, or tachycardia (abnormally rapid heartbeat after exercising).

THE REALITIES

The good news is that the complex set of physiological changes you experience during the course of nine months won't necessarily effect your exercise performance in a negative manner. For example, in a Finnish study of thirty endurance athletes who had been at national top level in cross-country skiing, running, or speed skating, sixteen (53 percent) did not notice any change in their exercise performance during their pregnancies, three (10 percent subjectively felt themselves to be in a better physical condition, and seven (23 percent) felt they were in worse condition during pregnancy.

In terms of specific changes in your heart function, lung power, metabolism, etc. none seem to have any great impact on your ability to exercise strenuously. For example, according to the results of a study of twenty well-conditioned recreational athletes, your VO2 max—your maximal aerobic capacity—is maintained and may even be improved if you continue to exercise.

There has even been speculation that certain changes that occur early in pregnancy may improve your performance. During the first twelve to fifteen weeks of pregnancy—before you begin to be hampered by too much extra weight and/or your enlarging uterus—your blood volume increases by as much as 35 to 45 percent and you have a greater red blood cell mass, too. This means your blood has an increased oxygen-carrying capacity, which could, theoretically at least, lead your performance to improve.

Of course, the catch is that this is just a theory. Also, if you experience any of the nausea or fatigue characteristic of the first trimester, any advantage you might gain would easily be canceled out.

Which brings us to the bad news: Even though physiological changes in your cardiovascular and respiratory system may not, per se, prevent you from performing well during pregnancy, there are other pregnancy-related changes that might, such as morning sickness—a queasy feeling often accompanied by vomiting that can strike at any time of the day and that affects up to 50 percent of all pregnant women, usually during the first trimester—or later in your pregnancy dyspnea—short-windedness caused by the crowding of the diaphragm by the growing fetus and your expanding uterus.

In addition, Ralph W. Hale, M.D., and Leslie Milne, M.D., in a *Seminars in Perinatology* article, "The Elite Athlete and Exercise in Pregnancy," note that many women find their performance is impeded by one or both of these pregnancy side effects:

1. *Weight gain.* As pregnancy progresses, your increasing weight will gradually decrease your ability to attain the same exercise level of speed, endurance, and intensity. "Although the amount of weight gain in the elite athlete may be less than the nonathlete, it still creates an added burden," note Dr. Hale and Dr. Milne.

Of course, what's crucial here is that you don't try to limit your pregnancy gain by severely restricting your diet. Instead, keep in mind that the weight you gain is serving to build a healthy baby. In addition, your extra weight may ultimately produce a training effect of which you'll reap the benefits postpartum. Here's how and why: Being heavier makes your body work harder; when your body works harder, it increases your physical capacity. According to studies conducted by Dr. Clapp, this increased physical capacity doesn't vanish when you lose the pounds postpartum, which provides, according to Clapp, "objective support for the anecdotal reports that have suggested that physical capacity and competitive endurance may be improved by pregnancy."

2. *Alterations in your posture.* Another change that might impede your athletic pursuits, according to Hale and Milne, is the shift in your center of gravity: "As the pregnancy reaches the fifth to sixth month, there is a progressive lordosis of the vertebral column associated with a forward tilt of the pelvis. This results in a change in the center of gravity and a tendency for the athlete to pitch forward. In stop-and-go training regimens, this tendency can be a source of injury. I have personally witnessed an elite tennis player charge the net, be unable to stop,

and fall over the net. Fortunately, no harm came to her or the fetus, but the potential is present."

In addition, runners—or women who engage in sports that demand a lot of running—often report that they feel more at risk for injury by the last trimester because their balance, and thus their foot strike, gets out of whack. This may largely explain why a study headed by Dr. Sternfeld found that of the fifty-seven women who entered pregnancy as recreational runners, only one woman continued running or jogging into the third trimester. However, most of these women didn't give up exercising completely—they just switched to an activity that felt better. For example, the percentages of women participating in swimming in the Sternfeld study increased from 9.8 precent prepregnancy to 16 percent, 19.6 percent and 25 percent in the first, second, and third trimesters respectively. Obviously, many women found that as their pregnancies progressed, working out in the water—which helps support your added weight and takes the stress off your swollen legs and stressed back—was more comfortable than exercising on land.

◐ Five benefits of exercising during pregnancy

If you stay active, you may be
- less prone to common pregnancy discomforts like swelling and shortness of breath,
- better able to tolerate labor pain,
- more energetic over your nine months,
- less likely to have a Cesarean or forceps delivery,
- happier with your body image.

THE REWARDS OF KEEPING ACTIVE DURING YOUR PREGNANCY

You're probably athletic because you like the way exercise makes you feel. Well, during pregnancy you stand a chance of reaping these additional benefits if you stay active:

- *Fewer pregnancy discomforts, such as nausea, fatigue, leg cramps, swelling, shortness of breath, and backache.* In a study from East Carolina University's School of Nursing of one hundred pregnant women, for example, the group that continued a regimen of brisk walking throughout their pregnancies had 50 percent fewer complaints of common discomforts compared with the women in the sedentary group.

Similarly, in a study headed by Dr. Sternfeld of 388 women, the more active women reported experiencing fewer symptoms of pregnancy overall than less active women. An additional finding of this study was that the more a woman sustained her activity, both prior to and during pregnancy, the better she was likely to feel as her pregnancy progressed: "The data clearly showed that women who exercised more in the three months before pregnancy felt better in the first trimester, and those who exercised more in the first and second trimesters felt better in the third trimester," notes Dr. Sternfeld.

- *Lower risk for multiple types of medical intervention during delivery.* In a study conducted by Dr. Clapp of 131 well-conditioned athletes (runners and aerobic dancers), those who continued to exercise regularly at or above 50 percent of their preconceptional level throughout pregnancy had only a 6 percent risk of cesarean or forceps delivery (compared to a 30 percent risk of cesarean or a 20 percent risk of forceps delivery in the group who discontinued exercise). The women who continued exercising also had half as many episiotomies (46 percent vs. 81 percent) as compared to the women who discontinued their regimes during pregnancy.

- *Shorter labor!* In Clapp's study, active labor was 30 percent shorter on average in the exercise group. Dr. Clapp speculates that exercise at moderately intense levels lasting thirty minutes each session, three or more times a week in late pregnancy may have a positive effect on how well and fast the cervix ripens and the uterus contracts, thus leading to a shorter, more "efficient" labor (yet not leading to premature labor). "In fact, three subjects initially qualifying for the exercise group were excluded from analysis because labor was so short that they entered the labor suite at or near full dilatation and were delivered before adequate assessment could be accomplished," wrote Dr. Clapp in the *American Journal of Obstetrics and Gynecology*, which published the study results.

Specifically, the active labors (defined as 4 cm dilated to delivery) of the exercising women included in Clapp's study lasted anywhere from four hours, forty minutes to two hours, forty-eight minutes compared to the labors of the discontinued exercise control group, which lasted from six hours, thirty-six minutes to four hours, fifty-eight minutes.

In addition, labor began on average five days earlier (but not prematurely) in the exercising group.

• *Better stamina and pain endurance during labor.* In Clapp's study, only 29 percent of the women who continued to exercise used epidural anesthetic versus 41 percent of the discontinued exercise group. This finding seems to provide some support for the commonly held (but far from proven) belief that women who stay active tolerate labor pain better than sedentary women. Some speculations about why this may be? Active women may develop higher pain thresholds via their hard workouts and/or they may go into labor with greater confidence and a more positive attitude about their own strength and stamina.

• *More energy.* According to studies conducted by Dr. Pivarnik, a fit pregnant woman has more economical ventilation than an unfit one. Essentially, that means that fit pregnant women breathe better and more efficiently, so "the energy cost of breathing is probably much less in fit women," according to Dr. Pivarnik.

This may account for the anecdotal reports of how women who exercise seem to be less exhausted by the end of their pregnancies. They don't have to huff and puff their way up stairs and they generally seem to have more energy as well as endurance.

• *Better emotional state.* Studies have shown that women who continue to keep active throughout their pregnancies feel better about their bodies, have greater self-esteem, and sleep better. In a University of Miami study, for example, pregnant women who exercised rated their attitudes toward their body build, facial complexion, physical stamina, muscular strength, and overall energy level higher than the nonexercising group. The active women also felt little change in regard to their sex lives, whereas the sedentary women had an increase in negative feelings about sex.

In addition, exercise is one of the few things that can help you feel in control of your life and body—at a time when things can seem pretty out of control.

- *Better baby?* The babies born to the women in Clapp's study who continued exercising experienced 50 percent fewer instances of abnormal heart rate, meconium-stained fluid, and entanglement in umbilical cords—all signs of stress—at birth.

What about beyond birth? The babies of exercisers may actually turn out to be slimmer and smarter.

For five years after birth, Dr. Clapp (in another study published in *The Journal of Pediatrics*) followed the offspring of two groups of twenty women. The two groups were individually matched in a huge number of variables—marital stability, number of months of breast-feeding, body size, type of child care, diet, birth order, education, and more. The only difference was that one group of women exercised vigorously (three or more times a week, for more than 30 minutes a session, at an intensity greater than 55 percent of their maximal capacity in activities like running, aerobics, cross-country skiing) throughout their pregnancies. The other group was physically fit but stopped all sustained exercise other than walking while pregnant.

The findings: At five years of age, the children born to the vigorous exercisers have less body fat than the children of the walkers. But, noted Dr. Clapp, "it is not that the offspring of the exercising women are unduly lean at age five years, rather that the offspring of the control subjects are a bit on the fat side."

In addition, the exercise offspring performed significantly better on the Wechsler scale of general intelligence and tests of oral language skills. Motor, integrative, and academic readiness skills were similar in the two groups.

Although Dr. Clapp is ready to admit that there might be some unknown variable, such as time spent with grandparents, that might factor into why the exercisers' offspring performed better in language skills and intelligence, he also speculates, "it is just possible that some stimulus associated with exercise (e.g. intermittent stress, vibration, sound, motion, fast heartbeat) may alter neurodevelopment in utero in a beneficial way."

Although still considered preliminary, these findings certainly are reassuring for active women who wish to continue vigorous exercise during their pregnancies.

SPORTS FIT—AND NOT FIT—FOR TWO

Here's a rundown of how to keep your participation in your chosen sport safe—plus a look at the activities experts think are too risky to engage in.

Aerobics

Most experts frown on high-impact workouts, but approve of low-impact. Still, as your pregnancy progresses, keep tabs on how your knees and back feel; avoid leaps, sudden twisting, quick turns, or other jerky power moves.

If you do step aerobics, you may find you feel more coordinated and less strained if you lower the step to 4 to 6 inches.

Box aerobics (and boxing) is fine too, as long as you limit yourself to shadow boxing—fighting or contact with other participants should be avoided.

Basketball

There are several potential problems with continuing to play into and beyond your second trimester. First, as your center of balance shifts, it can become very hard to make short stops and quick turns safely and effectively. Second, forceful vertical leaps and jumps as well as a direct hit in the abdomen by a basketball could cause your uterine wall to bleed and could potentially increase your baby's risk of brain damage. ("The worry is that the baby's brain may strike, then reverberate against the uterus, leading to a hemorrhage," explains Dr. Alleyne.) Finally, as with any aggressively played team sport, you simply can't predict the actions and movements of other players—so no matter how careful you are, there is always the risk that a player will crash into you or knock you over. Of course, this doesn't mean you can't shoot baskets or play a modified version of the game that is less intense and less likely to involve collisions.

Biking

Because it is non–weight bearing (thus there's no risk of impact-related joint injury) stationary biking is considered an ideal activity to engage in for all nine months.

Road and mountain biking, however, are considered risky beyond the first trimester (when the uterus becomes more vulnerable to direct traumas) because the risk of falling may increase owing to the changes in your weight distribution and body balance. If you are an experienced cyclist who is determined to keep riding outdoors, increase your safety margin by lowering your speed and choosing low-traffic routes that are smooth surfaced.

Karate and Other Martial Arts

No sparring, no fighting, no body contact. Aggressive kicks and leaps should be avoided during your last months. Otherwise martial arts appear to be safe during pregnancy.

Racket Sports

Tennis, badminton, racquetball, handball, and squash, especially if you play in a closed court, all pose a risk of getting hit in the abdomen with a fast-moving, hard ball.

In your third trimester, making fast lateral moves as well as short stops may become difficult, and you may be more prone to falls. To reduce this risk, start by playing less aggressively (i.e., don't rush the net, don't choose partners who bring out your most competitive side); consider playing doubles and/ or half court, if possible.

Running

It's safe, as long as you feel well while doing it.

Swimming

Many women find this the most comfortable activity to engage in during late pregnancy because it doesn't place stress on joints and muscles and helps relieve some of the swelling that often strikes women in their last months.

A few rules: make sure the body of water you swim in is clean and safe; avoid crowded pools or swim areas, since you could be inadvertently kicked or hit; ideally, water temperature should be around 82 to 84 degrees. If you have been doing the butterfly stroke, aquatics expert Jane Katz in *Water Fitness During Your Pregnancy* (Human Kinetics, 1995) advises you eliminate it from your workout: "Since the butterfly is very strenuous and requires an arched back, it is a poor choice for pregnant women. Some advanced swimmers may use the butterfly stroke into their pregnancies, but they will have to stop during their third trimesters."

Finally, Katz advises women to avoid jumping or diving

into bodies of water since the impact could potentially cause uterine trauma. When entering a pool, carefully climb down the ladder or stairs or enter by sliding gently into the pool from a sitting position.

Hiking or Mountain Climbing

Besides watching that you don't lose your balance as you go downhill and choosing terrain that isn't unpredictable (i.e., choose the beaten not unbeaten path!), the other safety rule is not to hike above a 8,250 foot elevation if you are not acclimated, since it could result in your fetus being deprived of oxygen. To get acclimated to higher altitudes, Dr. Renate Hutch, a professor in the department of obstetrics and gynecology at University Hospital, Zurich, Switzerland, offers this advice in a *Seminars in Perinatology* article:

1. Do not exceed altitudes of 8,250 feet in the first four to five days.
2. If exercising directly after altitude exposure, do so at a lower altitude in the first few days. Preferably, however, pregnant women should err on the side of caution by spending a few days at rest after exposure, to allow for effective adaptive mechanisms to come rapidly into play.
3. The more intensive the exercise, the lower the altitude at which it should be performed.

Team Sports: Hockey, Soccer, Rugby, Volleyball, Softball

How potentially risky any of these sports are depends, to a large extent, on how competitively and aggressively you play them. If the whole team plays at a relatively low-key recreational level and you avoid wildly diving for balls, you might be relatively safe. However, whenever a ball or puck is involved, there is always the risk of direct uterine trauma. Obviously, you should, at the very least, avoid playing certain positions—such as goalie in soccer or catcher in softball—in which there is a higher risk of someone else's body crashing into yours.

Weight Training

Lower weight, higher reps may be preferable as your pregnancy progresses. Don't lift weights lying on your back; avoid the Valsava maneuver in which you hold your breath while lifting since that can impede blood flow to the fetus.

Waterskiing

Skip it until after you deliver: High-speed falls can not only cause blunt abdominal trauma, but also forceful entry of water into the vagina (possibly precipitating miscarriage or preterm labor).

Rock Climbing

Since the risk of a fall is great, especially given your changing body shape, most experts advise you avoid rock climbing after the first trimester.

Rowing

Whether you use a machine or are on a crew team, it's probably safe as long as your abdomen doesn't get in the way, your back doesn't feel strained, and/or you're able to get in and out of your shell comfortably.

Scuba Diving

Not recommended since the fetus is not protected from decompression problems and is at risk for malformation and gas embolism after decompression disease, according to Enrico M. Camporesi, M.D., a professor in the department of anesthesiology, SUNY Health Science Center, Syracuse, New York, and the author of a paper on diving and pregnancy published in *Seminars in Perinatology*. If you made a dive before you realized you were pregnant, there is a good chance that your fetus wasn't harmed since several normal pregnancies have been documented, according to Dr. Camporesi.

Snorkeling can be practiced safely.

I started paddling again about nine days after birth.
—DEANNE HEMMENS, FIVE-TIME NATIONAL CHAMPION AND OLYMPIC COMPETITOR IN FLATWATER SPRINT KAYAKING.

Skating (In-Line and Ice Skating)

There is always the risk of a fall and subsequent abdominal

trauma. You need to judge these risks against your skill level; also, you can increase your safety by avoiding tricky maneuvers, keeping to lower speeds, and not skating in crowds. In-line skaters should also avoid hills and rough surfaces.

Skiing

You'll be hard-pressed to find a doctor who supports downhill skiing past the first trimester since no matter how skilled you are, you can't control all the variables, such as hitting an ice patch, having another skier slam into you, and so on. Cross-country is considered safer. Don't ski above 8,250 feet unless you're acclimatized.

Other Sports Considered Too Risky

Stock car racing, sky diving, hang-gliding, surfing, horseback riding, and snow-mobiling (although it's okay to leisurely tour) are not considered safe.

YOUR POSTPARTUM WORKOUTS

"I started paddling again about nine days after birth," says DeAnne Hemmens, age thirty-four, a mother of a toddler and a five-time National Champion and Olympic competitor in the sport of flatwater sprint kayaking. "My doctor said I should probably avoid the water because my cervix wasn't fully closed and there was a risk of a bacterial infection, but I knew I wouldn't fall in and I felt great."

◓ Rules for Resuming Exercise Postpartum

- If you had a normal, uncomplicated vaginal delivery, you can begin working out after two weeks.
- If you had a C-section, ask your doctor when you can begin exercising.
- Pick up at about 50 percent of where you left off at delivery (i.e., if you were running 20 miles a week during your last month of pregnancy, you can start doing 10 miles a week postpartum, then gradually increase your mileage if you desire).
- If exercise triggers excessive vaginal bleeding, cut back on your routine's intensity.

Hemmens needed to be in shape within eight weeks of her son's birth in order to compete at the U.S. Canoe and Kayak Team national trials. "I came in fifth at those trials, which I was happy about. I had definitely lost some speed, but my endurance was fine."

Jackie Paraiso, age thirty-two, a mother of a four-year-old and the number two ranked racquetball player in the United States in 1998, needed to get back in shape for an important tournament by six weeks postpartum. "I had gotten back to my prepregnancy weight with almost no trouble and had managed to train almost every day within a week after my daughter's birth. So I thought I was ready when I entered the tournament."

But when Paraiso began to play hard and competitively, she began having a lot of pain in the area where an episiotomy had been performed (she had a forceps delivery, which requires a larger-than-usual incision). "I knew I would have to forfeit. It just hurt like mad. It was just too soon after delivery. I never knew you used those muscles as much as you do until I began to play that day," says Paraiso. Still, after another few weeks of recuperating, Paraiso was back playing, less than two and a half months postpartum.

Even if you don't have an important competition you need to get ready for, you may be anxious to get back in shape as soon as possible. Yet many doctors will advise you to wait anywhere from three to six weeks before resuming a vigorous regime, even if you had a normal vaginal delivery. However, this recommendation isn't based on much solid research or evidence that says starting back to exercise earlier is dangerous.

"Most elite athletes will want to resume high-intensity training as soon as possible after delivery," note Dr. Hale and Dr. Milne. "In the uncomplicated pregnancy this may be as early as two weeks postpartum. Currently there are no known maternal complications to resumption of exercise in the immediate postpartum period for the athlete who has been exercising throughout her pregnancy."

In other words, there's no reason to avoid vigorous exercise soon after birth if:

1. You had a vaginal delivery. If you had a C-section, you need to give your incision time to heal, and so you'll need more time to recuperate. Talk to your doctor.
2. You start back at about 50 percent of where you left off

and increase your workouts gradually. In other words, if you ran 20 miles per week until delivery, you can probably start running 10 miles per week after the second week postpartum. However, if you stopped running during your last trimester and began brisk walking instead, don't try to go back to running right away in the immediate postpartum period. Instead, progress gradually into a more strenuous routine.

3. You listen to your body and realize that it may take time for your body to recuperate. Although some women recapture their prepregnancy stamina and energy right after birth, in a study conducted by the Melopomene Institute for Women's Health Research, only 53 percent of the runners and 60 percent of the swimmers felt fully recovered or back to "being themselves" after two months.

If exercise triggers excessive vaginal bleeding, you should cut back on the amount and intensity of your routine and give yourself more time to recover. Another warning sign of overdoing it is plugged ducts or mastitis—conditions in which your breasts become hot, heavy, hard, and painful. You may experience fever and chills too.

As a general rule, if your episiotomy site is really sore or you're exhausted from having paced the floor with baby all night, a hard workout may not be the best prescription. Sometimes just taking a walk, or even a nap, with your baby is a better restorative. In fact, if you push yourself too hard to work out when your body is resisting, you may find you become more prone to illness and more likely to be forced to take to your bed. The trick is to find the right balance between rest and activity.

When not done to excess, studies have shown that exercise can play a positive role in reducing postpartum depression. For example, a University of Wisconsin, Madison study of twenty women who had given birth within the previous four to twelve weeks found that the women who exercised for an hour at an intensity of 60 to 70 percent maximal heart rate compared to those who sat quietly in a room free from distractions for an hour experienced a significant decrease in anxiety and depression as well as a significant increase in vigor.

But if you let yourself get buried in self-induced pressures to get back into shape too soon after birth, you may find that trying to schedule workouts and/or perform at a certain level becomes a source of frustration, additional pressure, and anxiety. You may even begin to experience burnout and become so worn out by all the pressure that you veer toward just giving up entirely. A better alternative is to learn how to be more flexible, to shift away from aggressive short-term goals if the new circumstances of motherhood are making them too hard to achieve.

BREAST-FEEDING AND EXERCISE DO MIX

Cory Sertl, age thirty-nine, a sailor on two Olympic campaign trials and Yachtswoman of the Year in 1995, breast-fed her second child for six months. During that time, if she was involved in a race, she would sometimes run off the boat during breaks to nurse her son. If she needed to be in her boat all day, she brought a cooler and her breast pump along and pumped her milk and stored it. "It was pretty funny, since there wasn't much privacy on the small boats I was sailing and my teammates weren't moms—I'm sure they were looking at me pumping and thinking 'oh my god, that's gross!' But I was very motivated to feed my baby breast milk. And I pretty much have the attitude that if it is something I want to do, I can find a way to do it."

As Sertl's experience illustrates, most of the problems athletes face with breast-feeding are logistical. Once breast-feeding is successfully established, which takes about six to eight weeks, the problems are rarely physiological.

"Many of the worries about how exercise might negatively affect a mother's milk volume have turned out to be unfounded. Today, most of the evidence indicates that athletic women, even those who are competitive soon after delivery, can produce enough milk to successfully nurse their babies," says Dr. Alleyne.

Recently in *The Journal of Nutrition* a review article of different studies found that even when exercise was combined with moderate caloric restriction (dieting) during lactation, there was no significant change of milk volume, nursing frequency, or infant weight gain among the group of women who exercised and dieted and the group who just dieted. Even short periods of more rapid weight loss (such as you might experience with an increase in your training) is not harmful to lactation according to other data (although longer periods of fast weight loss might be harmful).

Another recent study published in the *New England Journal of Medicine (NEJM)* found no difference in breast milk volume in nonexercising nursing mothers versus those who exercised forty-five minutes per day, five days per week for twelve weeks beginning six to eight weeks postpartum. This study found no differences in the composition of the milk of exercising versus nonexercising women either.

Still, some research has found that maximal (versus more moderate) exercise has an impact on the content of breast milk. For example, a study from the University of New Hampshire found that the milk of women who exercised on a treadmill up to maximal oxygen uptake (100 percent VO2max) increased in lactic acid content—a by-product excreted by muscles after hard workouts. Higher concentrations of lactic acid may make milk sour tasting, which in turn may affect how willing a baby is to nurse.

Other research on the effect of exercise on the immune properties of human milk, published in *Medicine & Science in Sports & Exercise*, found a reduced concentration of substances known as immunoglobins, which help fight infections in babies, especially newborns, during exercise and for about an hour after maximal treadmill exercise. Within sixty minutes postexercise, however, the concentrations of immunglobins had returned to normal levels. In addition, researchers suspect that more moderate levels of exercise may have little to no effect on immunoglobin levels.

"I think the lesson here is that the timing of exercise appears to be important," says Dr. Alleyne. In other words, breast-feed first, then exercise. Not only are your workouts bound to be more enjoyable if your breasts are not uncomfortably heavy with milk, by the time of your next feeding your milk should regain its normally sweet flavor as well as regain its normal levels of immunoglobins.

If you think your baby will need to feed before an hour's lapse after exercise, you can also collect your milk via expression to give at this feeding. Whether this is really necessary or not, however, isn't clear since not all babies will refuse postexercise milk, and there is nothing in the research that suggests occasional feedings of milk with reduced concentrations of immunoglobins compromises a baby's overall immune status.

―――

The basic rule for fluid intake is that every time you breast-feed you should drink eight ounces of fluid and that for every fifteen to twenty minutes of vigorous exercise you should do the same.
—JULIA ALLEYNE, M.D., MEDICAL DIRECTOR OF SPORT C.A.R.E. AT WOMEN'S COLLEGE HOSPITAL, TORONTO

―――

A few other practical pointers for mixing breast-feeding with exercise:

- In the first weeks postpartum, wear your nursing bra for exercise (instead of your sports bra) and place protective nursing pads inside it. Why? "Especially during high impact exercise, it's common for new mothers to experience an involuntary letdown response, which means you could end up leaking milk rather profusely in the middle of a workout," explains Dr. Alleyne. After a regular nursing pattern has been established, usually after eight to twelve weeks, you'll find this is less likely to happen.

- When you combine nursing with exercise you need to make a concerted effort to stay properly hydrated. "The basic rule for fluid intake is that every time you breast-feed you should drink eight ounces of fluid and that for every fifteen to twenty minutes of vigorous exercise you should do the same," notes Dr. Alleyne.

- If, because of an upcoming competition, you anticipate having to be separated from your baby, you don't necessarily need to wean or have your baby fed formula during your absence. Instead, consider expressing your milk for a week or two before leaving to build a supply in your freezer; that way your baby can get your milk while you're away. For comfort and to keep up your supply, pump your milk during your travels. You'll probably just want to discard this milk, rather than trying to deal with storing it properly.

Finally, the American Academy of Pediatrics recommends that all mothers nurse their babies for a full year, if possible.

This can be a very hard prescription for competitive athletes, in particular, to fill. Single mom Charlene Johnson, age twenty-four, a player on the 1998 National U.S.A. volleyball team who is currently living and training at the Olympic Training Center in Colorado Springs, Colorado, for example, simply found that her breasts remained so big and she experienced so much leaking that it interfered with her ability to play volleyball well. As a result she weaned her son at three months. "It was an emotional bond that was hard for me to give up. I knew it wasn't the best for him nutritionally, but it was best for the situation."

Jackie Paraiso weaned her daughter at four months for similar reasons: "My breasts would become so large and uncomfortably filled with milk that I would often have to run to a bathroom between matches to pump." Then the pumping began to cause nipple soreness and abrasion. She finally decided to wean when she knew she would be away from her baby for a ten-day stretch. "I was pretty bummed that I wasn't able to nurse her longer. When I was with her, nursing was wonderful, it went so easily. But the constant pumping finally became too much of a problem. It hurt and I just couldn't juggle it."

If you are forced to give up breast-feeding for your sport before you are really ready, it helps to know that many athletes are forced to make similar compromises. But any time you invest in breast-feeding serves to benefit your baby, so rather than view yourself as a failure because you were unable to nurse for a full year, you should garner a sense of accomplishment from succeeding as long as you did.

LIFE AS AN ATHLETIC MOM

Keep in mind that your body is only one part of the equation—your emotions and lifestyle need time to recover, too. Adapting to having a baby in your life is no minor life change, after all. Pre-baby you could probably take an extra half hour to work out without a lot of forethought, but post-baby, there may be myriad considerations, from whether the babysitter can stay longer to whether your baby will need to breast-feed. There will be days when you can't work out because your baby is sick, your husband or other support caregiver is away, or you simply feel too guilty to leave your baby again for several hours.

"It can be a real challenge to juggle everything," admits Charlene Johnson. "In the first few months after my son's birth, I would be up several times a night breast-feeding, then I would get up early to attend classes, then I would do some strength work in the gym and then I would go to volleyball practice. There have definitely been times when it is hard to maintain my focus on volleyball." Johnson feels that once she finishes the field work necessary to complete her bachelor of science degree in therapeutic recreation, things will ease up for her. "I can do two things, be a good mother and play volleyball, but going to school too has been a real strain."

In addition, Johnson realizes that there may always be some tension when it comes to her responsibility and emotions toward her son and her participation in her sport. "When my son was about two years old, I went to Japan for a month to play with the U.S.A. team. When I came back he didn't recognize me at first and it broke my heart. It just devastated me. I want to be with him and yet I want to play volleyball. It helps that my parents are the ones who care for him when I am away, but still it is so, so tough at times."

Powe-Allred agrees that athletes who are moms have to cope with much more stress than other athletes. "When you don't have children, you only have to think of yourself. If you hurt yourself, you only worry about how it might put you out of the action for a while. A teammate of mine, for example, had a really bad crash while bobsledding and broke her arm and the first thing she said was, 'Oh my god, how am I going to pick up my baby?' "

Still, Powe-Allred has a lot of positive thoughts on how motherhood can actually help you become a better athlete. She feels that the experience of labor helped her discover depths and inner resources she didn't know she possessed. "It showed me how much strength I really have and how capable I am of enduring discomfort."

In addition, Powe-Allred says having children has forced her to get more out of her workouts. "Before I had children, there were days when I would give my workouts half an effort because I wasn't in the mood. But now that I'm a mom I have to fight to make time to work out, so that when I get to the gym, I really cherish the opportunity and knock myself out to make the most of it. I think that when you have to struggle for something, you appreciate it more. I care more deeply about

SPECIAL FOCUS:

◖ A Crucial Caveat

Any discussion of the fine points of exercise during pregnancy makes one very big assumption: That you are healthy, are experiencing an uncomplicated pregnancy, and have no special risk factors. The following medical and obstetric conditions are absolute contraindications to exercise:

- A history of two or more miscarriages.
- Vaginal bleeding. Early in a pregnancy, vaginal spotting and/or bleeding may be a symptom of an impending miscarriage (although it may also simply stop on its own in a day or two, after which your pregnancy progresses as normal). Later in a pregnancy, vaginal bleeding can be a sign of premature labor or other problem. In any case, bleeding is a signal to discontinue exercise and to contact your doctor. Of course, if the bleeding stops and your doctor feels any danger has passed, you may be able to resume your workouts.
- Premature rupture of membranes (PROM). The spontaneous breaking of the amniotic membranes—i.e. when your water breaks—before you have gone into labor is not only time to stop exercising, but to call your doctor.
- Symptoms or history of premature labor. The symptoms of premature labor include achiness in the lower back region; mild pelvic soreness or cramps akin to what you might feel before a period; painless tightening and/or pressure in your lower abdomen; noticeably more frequent bowel movements or diarrhea; markedly increased vaginal discharge and/or discharge that is mucusy, watery, or blood-tinged; contractions, especially ones that occur with any kind of regularity (every twenty minutes for instance) and/or last for more than thirty seconds.
- Intrauterine growth retardation (IUGR). This means your baby is lagging in growth. There's no evidence that exercise causes IUGR, but your doctor will want you to stop to be on the safe side.
- Other problems, such as a history of heart disease, pulmonary disease, diabetes, anemia, being pregnant with triplets or being very underweight or overweight may not prevent you from playing altogether, but you'll need to work closely with your physician to modify your exercise regime. Then, you'll need to be closely supervised to avoid any problems.

what I am doing because I realize what a gift it is to be able to do it."

I often look at younger competitors who don't have kids and say to myself, 'Boy, you have no idea what it took to get here!'
—CORY SERTL, 1995 YACHTSWOMAN OF THE YEAR

Cory Sertl says, "Once you're a mom, you have to do so much organizing in order to compete. You need to plan who is going to drive the kids to the baby-sitter, who is going to pick them up, what everyone is going to have for dinner when you're away . . . all that stuff. I often look at younger competitors who don't have kids and say to myself, 'Boy, you have no idea what it took to get here!' "

But, adds Sertl, "Once you're out there you enjoy and appreciate your time so much more. I sail with some other women who are moms and we say,'Wow, this is amazing, we have this whole day to just sail.' And we really work hard, hang out with each other, and savor everything about the experience."

Becoming a mom also helps many athletes gain a healthier, more balanced perspective on their involvement in their sport. "I still strive to be my best, and racquetball is still a priority in my life. But it's not my everything anymore. Losing doesn't mean life falls apart, because I always have my daughter. This realization has been very positive for me. It really takes the pressure off and gives me peace," says Jackie Paraiso.

There's no doubt that it takes a lot more effort to get to the starting line once you're a mother. But most athletic women, even if it takes longer than they planned, manage to find a way to get there. As a reward, many (just like Powe-Allred, Sertl, and Paraiso) discover that motherhood makes playing their sport a far more special and rewarding experience.

WHAT TO EXPECT AS YOU AGE

"Turning forty was a wake-up call for me, it really shook me up. I didn't want to believe that my age might slow me down. So I went all out, really gave it my best and had a great year. I was faster at age forty-one than I was at thirty-five," says Missy Le Strange, now forty-six, a Visalia, California, resident who was the top-ranking female triathlete in the United States in her age group (forty-five to forty-nine) in 1997.

Still, as she has entered her mid-forties, Le Strange has had to face certain realities of aging. "I am not getting my period regularly anymore. More than anything else, losing my period is a definite statement that I'm starting menopause and getting older. And I've started to get hot flashes. The hot flashes are as if my blood suddenly starts to boil; they come in rapid-fire succession, sometimes every six minutes. I don't drip with sweat, but I find them uncomfortable."

Some of the other changes Le Strange has noticed is a loss of clear vision (she now needs glasses), increased stiffness, and a need for more recovery time between workouts.

"I realize I am running out of time to achieve a goal I have—to break ten hours in the Hawaii Ironman," says Le Strange, whose fastest time is ten hours, five minutes. "I refuse to give up. I don't like to use the word *old*." Yet I realize there are some issues I really need to explore. I'm not sure if I should take hormones and I have a lot of thinking to do about what I want to achieve in my sport as I get older."

Le Strange is clearly at a crossroads. She is at the age when the question, "What will happen to my body and to my athletic performances as I move into midlife?," starts to seem more pressing with each passing birthday.

To help you answer that question, this chapter will provide you with a preview of the biological changes you can expect to experience as you enter midlife. As an athlete, you'll be happy to hear you are probably already doing a lot to optimize the way you age. You'll also find "the active woman's guide to menopause," which details steps you can take to get through this transition in a positive, problem-free way.

ATHLETES AGE BETTER

Your physical performance eventually will decline with increasing age. That's the bottom line. If this weren't true, you would see sixty- and seventy-year-old women regularly winning Olympic Gold medals, big-money marathons, and the like.

"The body is made to wear out. There is no way around this fact," points out Joseph Bernstein, M.D., director of sports medicine service and Women's Sports Medicine at the University of Pennsylvania Orthopedic Institute in Philadelphia.

◗ Active Women Live Longer

And they have a lower risk for the following diseases:

- breast cancer
- osteoporosis
- heart disease
- stroke
- high blood pressure
- diabetes
- colon cancer

Still, as understanding increases of what constitutes "normal aging" in athletes (as opposed to "abnormal aging," which would include chronic, degenerative diseases), it has become clear that women who stay active can significantly forestall many of the negative aspects of aging that sedentary women often experience. Women who are inactive, for example, are at high risk for an entire array of age-related changes, such as muscle weakening, weight gain, and loss of energy and endurance that more active women can often avoid for decades.

"Athletes start to age from a higher, more advantageous point: their heart, lungs, legs—their entire bodies—are in better shape. So they not only do better healthwise as the years pass—staying vital for more years—they enjoy themselves more," notes Dr. Bernstein.

Specifically, when you enter your middle years as an active athlete you reduce your risk for a panorama of problems and diseases. Among the benefits you reap:

• *You'll live longer.* In a study that included over seven thousand women ranging in age from twenty to eighty-eight years, published in the *Journal of the American Medical Association* (*JAMA*), the women with the highest fitness levels had a 48 percent to 67 percent lower risk of premature death than less fit women. Even when fit women had two or three other risk factors, such as high cholesterol or high blood pressure, they still had an almost 50 percent lower death rate than less fit women with no additional risk factors.

• *Your risk of breast cancer is lower.* In the largest study to date of over 25,000 Norwegian women ages twenty to fifty-four, who were followed for about fourteen years, women who exercised regularly for at least four hours a week were found to have a 37 percent reduction in the risk of breast cancer. The study, which was published in the *New England Journal of Medicine*, found that the protective effect of exercise was greatest among lean women and women who exercised continuously for at least three to five years. One leading hypothesis about why exercisers may be less likely to get breast cancer is that they experience less exposure to estrogens, which are believed to promote the growth of breast cancers, in their lifetimes. Exercise may reduce the amount of estrogen the ovaries produce each month and/or decrease the number of estrogen-producing menstrual cycles you have in your life. Exercise may also reduce your fat stores, which contain a form of estrogen.

• *You have better bone health.* As your estrogen levels decline during and after menopause, so does your bone density. But being an athlete may give you a natural edge when it comes to this decline of bone. Exercise puts stress on bones, which stimulates them to build and become stronger. In a small Australian study, for example, female athletes with twenty years of consistent training in a weight-bearing exercise had significantly greater whole body and leg bone density than sedentary women and athletes (namely swimmers), who engaged in non weight-bearing activities. A review of a wide array of studies on whether a lifetime of exercise can lead to a lowered osteoporosis risk, conducted by researchers from the Medical College of Georgia at Augusta, concluded that "Older people who have been active for years seem to exhibit generally enhanced bone density."

•   *Your risk of heart disease, stroke, and high blood pressure are lower.* Several studies have documented the relationship between exercise and better cardiovascular health in women. As a rule, the women who exercise the most have the least risk.

Some of the reasons for this: Exercise helps elevate your levels of HDL (high-density lipoprotein) cholesterol. This "good" kind of cholesterol helps dissolve fatty deposits that clog your arteries and increase your risk of coronary heart disease. Exercise may also have a directly beneficial effect on your artery walls and the size of your arteries. For example, researchers at the University of Washington in Seattle who examined over one thousand women age sixty-five or over found an inverse relationship between exercise intensity and signs of thickening of the inner and middle layers of the carotid arteries in the neck, a vascular situation that is associated with stroke.

•   *You may avoid getting diabetes later in life.* In a study of over five thousand women ranging in age from twenty-one to eighty years old, the nonathletes had three times the risk of developing noninsulin-dependent diabetes as the women who were formerly college athletes. Noninsulin-dependent diabetes is the kind that develops during adulthood; exercise may reduce your risk by improving your body's ability to metabolize glucose or blood sugar.

•   *Your chances of colon cancer are less.* Women who are active—at least walk at a normal or brisk pace for an hour a day—have a 46 percent reduction in their risk of colon cancer, according to data from the Nurse's Health Study, which has over 67,000 participants, published in the *Journal of the National Cancer Institute.*

- *You're at lower risk for uterine prolapse.* Exercise can fight the atrophy of the muscles and ligaments of the pelvis that sometimes occurs with the decline in estrogen during menopause, according to a *Physician and Sportsmedicine* article by Kathleen M. Hargarten of the Medical College of Wisconsin in Milwaukee. Atrophy can increase the risk that your uterus will prolapse (sag and stretch), an uncomfortable condition that can lead to urinary incontinence.

---

*I am without doubt, faster, better,
stronger, and more limber than I
was ten years ago. I have improved
tremendously in my game.*
—JOANNA G. KENYON, AGE SIXTY-FOUR, U.S. WOMEN'S
RACQUETBALL CHAMPION IN HER AGE GROUP

IT'S NOT ALL DOWNHILL

What's more, the rate at which an athletic woman's performance declines over the years appears to be relatively modest. A study based on data from masters swimmers, from the University of Colorado at Boulder, found that peak performance was maintained until age forty to forty-five. Then there were small increases in swimming times (an indicator that performance declined) until age seventy-five to eighty. The rate and magnitude of the decline, on average, was only about 5 percent in total during these years. After age seventy-five to eighty, there was a larger drop-off in performance that increased with each passing year.

In a study of rowing performance of 1,615 women ages twenty-four to eighty-four, conducted at the University of Texas at Austin, average performance time declined about 1.2 percent per year in elite women. This decline was steady and gradual until about age seventy-five when it became steeper. Studies of runners and cyclists have produced similar findings, although one study found that there was a relatively larger decline in running performance somewhat earlier, in the sixties.

As a rule, then, athletes who remain active don't experience dramatic drop-offs in performance until quite late in life.

What's more, many of the factors that affect your performance as you age are highly individual. For example, some aspects of how you perform may be preprogrammed into your genes. Just as your genetic gifts partly determined how talented an athlete you were when young, experts suspect there is a genetic component in how you respond to training later in life. In other words, some of us will be able to train hard, remain uninjured, and maintain high-quality performances better than others in our later years simply because of good genetic luck.

But heredity isn't fate. Even those who find they have "low" trainability thresholds—i.e., they have a greater requirement for recovery, a higher risk of injury, and less natural endurance as they age—can usually get around these problems with a well-designed training program.

In fact, your training habits, your competitive desire, and your commitment to being an athlete have as much to do with how you perform as age alone.

A perfect example of this is sixty-four-year-old Joanna G. Kenyon, a Tallahasseee, Florida, resident who is the U.S. Women's racquetball champion in her age group. She feels that her performances today are better than her performances ten years ago, when she was fifty-four. "I am, without doubt, faster, better, stronger, and more limber. I have improved tremendously in my game," she says.

Why has Kenyon improved? "I began to learn what kind of discipline and dedication it would take to become a national champion. I realized I needed to do more than just get out and hit the ball around. I needed to pay attention to getting my whole body fit and conditioned. So I became more aware of the nutritional content of all sorts of foods and changed my diet. And I began going to the gym three times a week for two hours each time—I do the rowing machine, stationary bike, treadmill, and I do strength-training too. I made a conscious effort to get the whole machine in good form."

Kenyon is proof positive that there is nothing etched in stone that says *your* performance, in particular, will decline from one year to the next. Your aging timetable is not only partly personal, it's partly in your power. As you'll see in the following rundown of the body changes most likely to effect your athletic performance as you get older, there are a lot of steps you can take (or may already be taking) to minimize the impact of aging.

THE SPECIFIC IMPACT OF AGE ON FITNESS AND PERFORMANCE MARKERS

Your Aerobic Capacity

According to a study of sixty-seven female athletes between the ages of eighteen and sixty-nine, published in the *American Journal of Physiology*, even highly trained athletes experienced a 4.2 percent decline in aerobic capacity per decade after age fifty. That means that if a sixty-year-old were matched to a twenty-year-old in things like height, weight, training regime, and racing times, the sixty-year-old would still have a reduced aerobic capacity.

Your aerobic capacity is usually measured as VO2max, the maximal amount of oxygen that can be removed from circulating blood and used by working tissues during a specified period. In essence, your aerobic capacity is a marker of how fit and efficient your entire cardiovascular system—your lungs, heart, and circulatory function—is.

There are several plausible explanations for why your heart's ability to pump oxygenated blood to your muscles is inevitably reduced with age:

1. Especially after age sixty, your lungs start to lose elasticity, which means you can't move air in and out of them with the same efficiency.
2. Your chest cavity decreases in size, thus your chest wall isn't able to expand as much, which in turn impedes your lung capacity.
3. Your arteries become less elastic and so can't supply your muscles with oxygenated blood at the same speed as during your younger years.

What you can do. All the evidence indicates that if you train at relatively high intensity levels now and continue to do so, you'll only start losing your present level of aerobic capacity after age forty-nine. Even at that point, the losses may be so minimal as to have little or no effect on your performance for quite some time. That's because there's evidence suggesting that even though you may have lower VO2max values as you age, your body may compensate for this deficit in a number of ways. One study, for example, found that the hearts of aging athletes actually change in structure and function, becoming more efficient in response to physical conditioning. Yet other research has found that aging athletes may be able to work closer to their VO2max for longer periods than younger athletes, thus explaining why master athletes can often perform as well as younger athletes despite their lower aerobic capacities.

What if your sport doesn't include a lot of regular continuous aerobic exercise? It is possible to build aerobic fitness, no matter what your age. You can improve your VO2max as you age by doing more "cardio" workouts (brisk walking, running, biking—exercises that keep you breathing hard, huffing and puffing, for extended periods). A study of fifty-seven women aged sixty to seventy-one, from the Washington University School of Medicine in St. Louis, Missouri, for example, found that after six months of endurance exercise training, the women were able to increase their aerobic capacity by 20 percent and bring their level of cardiovascular function to a level typical of women twenty years or more younger.

The American College of Sports Medicine recommends a minimum of thirty minutes of moderately hard to hard aerobic exercise three times a week to offset a dramatic cardiovascular decline. Other experts feel slightly harder, longer (forty to forty-five minutes) and more frequent (four times a week) workouts are necessary to protect your aerobic capacity from the deleterious effects of aging.

Your Muscle Strength and Endurance

Here's what happens to the muscles of the average sedentary woman: Between the ages of thirty and eighty muscle strength drops by as much as 60 percent; muscle endurance—the ability of muscles to sustain power without becoming fatigued—diminishes by about 50 percent. These losses are partly attributable to a decline in muscle cells as well as a decrease in the muscles' ability to process oxygen. But it is also clear that disuse is a big culprit in muscle degeneration: Not using your muscles speeds up the progressive loss of muscle power and encourages muscle enzymes, cells, and capillaries to atrophy. When you don't use your muscles, your body assumes you don't need them and so responds by allowing them to shrink.

What you can do. Keep playing—when you play a sport you use your muscles, which is the single best way to keep them from weakening. Also, consider adding strength training to your regime to balance out your program. There is an over-whelming body of evidence that shows that strength training can forestall declines in strength and muscle mass for decades.

In fact, the American College of Sports Medicine advises every woman to include strength training in her fitness regime. The benefits of keeping your muscles strong as you age via strength training are multiple: It bolsters bone density, promotes healthier connective tissues, and lowers your risk of injury and fractures; it gives you more energy, since the effort required to perform tasks like putting your skis on the roof rack or carrying your kayak around a dam is less tiring when you are strong; and it helps control your weight. Lean muscle tissue burns more calories than fat tissue, so the more lean muscle tissue you have, the larger the number of calories your body burns, both while exercising and while at rest.

No matter what your age, research indicates you can easily get stronger and reap the benefits of strength training. In a study from Tufts University in Boston, of thirty-nine healthy postmenopausal women ranging in age from fifty-one to sixty-eight, significant strength changes were seen after training only twice a week for three months.

Athletes should focus on strengthening the parts of their body they tend to use least: runners, for example, need to focus on upper body strength, while swimmers might need to do more leg work. Strength training can be as simple as doing push-ups or investing in a pair of 5- or 10-pound weights, then following a weight-training program illustrated in a fitness magazine or book. Or, it can be as involved and structured as meeting a personal trainer at a health club and learning to run through the circuit of exercise machines that control resistance. Whatever route you decide to take, most experts recommend you strength-train twice a week and that you gradually increase the load you lift as your muscles develop. Lifting the same 5-pound dumbbell year after year will maintain your muscle mass but will not result in any improvements.

Your Body Composition

In a University of Maryland at Baltimore study of highly trained competitive women athletes ranging between eighteen and seventy, the older athletes did not lose fat-free mass (muscle) or gain body fat across the age span. In other words, the athletes were able to maintain a good lean tissue to body fat ratio as they aged via high levels of exercise training.

However, the study also found that as women aged, their resting metabolic rate—the rate at which your body needs calories to maintain your present weight—inevitably declined despite the continued vigorous exercise. That means that keeping fat tissue in check can definitely become an uphill battle the older you get.

Besides staying lean leading to a better body shape, you'll want to keep your lean tissue to body fat ratio healthy since it influences your aerobic power. According to a study of 409 women ranging in age from twenty to sixty-four, all of whom were employed at NASA/Johnson Space Center in Houston, almost 50 percent of the decline in aerobic power that many of the women experienced with age was strongly linked to an increase in the ratio of body fat to muscle tissue. The link appears to be both direct (i.e., the fewer muscles you have consuming oxygen, the lower your aerobic capacity) and indirect (the more fat tissue you have, the higher the probability that you are exercising less).

What you can do. The key to maintaining your lean-to-fat ratio is simply to continue to exercise and strength-train as you age. That ensures you maintain muscle mass (which burns calories and counters fat-tissue gains) and your metabolic rate stays boosted (which counters calorie-need declines). Even though you maintain a steady exercise level, there is still the chance that over the years you may put on a few pounds, owing to the inevitable decline in resting metabolic rate. The way around this: either escalate your activity to compensate for the metabolic decline and/or eat somewhat less, so you have fewer overall calories to burn. Yet another option is to shift your focus away from the number on the bathroom scale and not become overly concerned about slight increases in body weight. As long as you are starting out lean, your activity level is high, you regularly strength-train, and you eat a fat-reduced diet, there is no evidence to suggest that putting on 10 pounds or less over the decades is health risky. Also, remember that muscle weighs more than fat, so it's possible you may gain a few pounds simply because you are getting stronger.

Your Flexibility

As you age, cellular changes in your joints and connective tissue lead them to become stiffer and less elastic. As a result, you can slowly lose the ability to move your limbs through their full range of possible motions. Exactly how much flexibility you lose over time and when you start to lose it appears to be highly individual. It's partly dependent on how good your range of motion was when you started out: If you tend to be naturally flexible, the odds are good that over the years you will remain more flexible than a woman who was always tight and stiff. Yet retaining your flexibility is also linked to how well you maintain it: If you don't routinely put your limbs through their possible motions, their capacity to do so will eventually be diminished.

As an athlete, the main reason to stay flexible with age is to avoid injury. If you can't bend down to pick something up without pulling a muscle, you are far more likely to spend a lot of time sitting on the sidelines. But whether stretching, per se, can help you avoid specific athletic injuries and/or if it will improve things like speed, agility, and overall performance is a matter that is hotly disputed.

What you can do. Although experts continue to debate the benefits of stretching for athletes and argue about how much to do and what type, there is a consensus that if you don't practice range of motion, you will lose it. Which means you should stretch regularly. This doesn't mean you need to practice yoga, master the splits, or be limber enough to touch your nose with your toes (an endpoint some stretching methods advocate). Everyone should be flexible enough to perform their daily tasks without risk of straining a muscle. From there, how much stretching you need depends a lot on your sport and the range of motion required for it: a gymnast, for example, needs to be a lot more flexible than a cyclist.

Whether you stick with a simple, quick, sports-specific stretching regime or decide to enroll in a full-body stretching program, it's important to distinguish between stretching and warming up, two things people often confuse. Warming up refers to getting your blood flowing to your muscles; most experts recommend you warm up by easing into your activity (by running slowly for a while before picking up your speed, for example). Stretching refers to elongating the muscle, something you should only try to do after you're warmed up. If you try to stretch cold muscles, the risk of tearing or pulling the muscle is quite high. In fact, many experts feel you should only stretch after workouts, when your muscles are clearly warmed up enough to be stretched safely. An easy-to-use guide to stretching is *Stretching* by Bob Anderson (Shelter Publications). This book has been in print for over twenty years and includes short stretch routines for different sports.

Your Vision

When you're around forty-two, the lens of your eye loses its flexibility and some of its focusing ability.

What you can do. In any sport requiring visual acuity, from the racket sports to cycling, it is important to recognize this change as soon as possible. Glasses or contact lenses can easily correct the problem.

At age fifty-five you can't train in the same way you did at age twenty-five.
—HELEN M. SCHILLING, M.D., MEDICAL DIRECTOR OF HEALTHSOUTH REHABILITATION INSTITUTE, HOUSTON

Your Reflexes

"The older you get, the slower your reflexes are," explains Dr. Bernstein. "Let's say you are running and you step on something funny, a rock or a small hole. When you're young, you react quickly and automatically to throw your weight off that foot, thus avoiding an ankle sprain. As you get older, your reaction time slows and in that same situation you may very well end up with the sprain."

What you can do. You can pay more attention to the surface of the road you are running on, for instance, or avoid risky ski maneuvers that require split-second timing. Becoming aware that your reflexes aren't as acute is half the battle because you can then take steps to avoid ordinary injuries.

WHY YOU NEED MORE RECOVERY TIME AS YOU GET OLDER

Exercise is essentially a continual process of tearing down and building up muscle tissue. This process occurs on a microscopic, cellular level. When you are young, the rebuilding process tends to be swift and efficient. What happens as you age is that your cells' ability to repair muscle tissue as well as cartilage, ligaments, and soft connective tissue slows and requires more time to build up than before. The result is that it takes longer for tissues to repair and recover, especially from hard workouts. Sometimes it takes twice as long as it used to.

The real challenge for an aging athlete is to recognize that she needs more recuperation time. Many athletes try to hammer away at their same old routine and become frustrated, injured, and/or burned out when they find that their training doesn't result in them performing the way they used to.

"At age fifty-five you can't train in the same way you did at age twenty-five," notes Helen M. Schilling, M.D., medical director of HealthSouth-Houston Rehabilitation Institute in Houston. "You need to build in more rest time because you are at a much higher risk for overuse injuries as you age."

You don't necessarily have to lower the intensity of your playing or workouts. Getting older doesn't mean you suddenly have to compromise the way you engage in your sport. You simply need to allow for more recuperation time in order to bounce back in good form.

Most athletes find that more rest results in better performances.

"I'm sure that another one of the reasons my game has excelled over the years is that I've learned to let up a bit," explains racquetball champion Joanna Kenyon. "I used to overtrain, get injured, then lose a lot of playing time recovering. But as I've learned to respect my body and faced the fact that I need more rest time built into my training program, my playing has improved tremendously and I don't get injured as much."

There's no surefire formula for how much rest you need—it's highly individual. But if you find your motivation is flagging and your performances are stale it's a clear signal that your training regime is in need of an overhaul. Start by playing your sport fewer days each week—instead of playing five days a week, cut back to four or even three. Make sure at least one day of the week is pure idleness—you may need to walk the dog and haul the groceries, but don't engage in any athletic activities. On your other rest days, you can substitute activities that work muscle groups different from the ones you normally use. For example, find an activity that works your upper body if your primary sport requires a lot of leg muscle. But don't go all out in your secondary sport; take it easy, keeping in mind that one of your goals is to get rest.

You might also consider working with a coach or masters group, if you aren't already. Training with others your age and older can often help you gauge how to strike the right training balance of hard work and rest.

THE ACTIVE MENOPAUSE

Ardeth R. Mueller, a fifty-six-year-old masters swimmer who has set forty-six world records, won seven world championships, as well as sixty-four national championships had very few complaints when she experienced menopause. She had a few hot flashes between the ages of forty-nine and fifty. "I didn't even really know I was going through menopause until my doctor did a blood test and told me I was going through it."

According to Mueller, going through the "change" didn't change her performances. "I can pretty much handle the same workout load I have always handled. I can work out at the same intensity as I did ten or fifteen years ago. I need more recovery time and my times have gradually gotten a little slower, but I partly attribute that to age. Menopause just wasn't a big deal. In comparison, I recently went through a divorce—the stress and personal turmoil of that had a much bigger impact on my training and times than any symptom I experienced during menopause," she says.

Mueller's experience highlights an important point: Meno-

◗ Athletes Have Fewer Hot Flashes

During menopause, active women may also reap these benefits:

- less spontaneous night sweating
- fewer mood swings
- sleeplessness may be less of a problem

pause isn't something that should fill you with dread and trepidation. Irrespective of age, menopause in and of itself has never been linked to an inevitable decline in your performance. (Medically, "menopause" refers to your last menstrual period, but it is more commonly used to refer to the years that comprise this whole era of a woman's life).

Although every woman experiences it differently, fewer than 10 percent of all menopausal women find it to be a major disruption to their lives, according to Anne W. Moulton, M.D., co-founder of Women's Health Associates in Providence, Rhode Island, and co-author of *The Complete Book of Menopause* (Perigee Books, 1994). "The reality is that most women thrive during their menopausal years. Sure, they have some symptoms which may bother them, but these either pass or can be treated."

For example, contrary to what is often reported, not all women find hot flashes horribly distressing. "When they get hot flashes, some women's reaction is " 'Oh, this is kind of cool. Isn't this interesting!' " says Dr. Moulton. "Of course, others think 'God, this is uncomfortable. I don't like this.' But what's important to remember is that women's reactions are very varied and you shouldn't assume you will experience major discomforts."

Athletes, in fact, appear to have several advantages compared to sedentary women when it comes to how they experience the symptoms of menopause. Among them are the following:

- *Active women may have fewer hot flashes.* In a Swedish study of over 1,300 women between the ages of fifty-two and fifty-four, menopausal symptoms of moderate to severe hot flashes and spontaneous sweating were only half as common among the physically active women as compared to those who didn't exercise.

It may be that physical activity itself somehow alters the chemical mechanisms that induce menopausal symptoms. It may also be that women who are physically active are better able to deal with symptoms associated with menopause. In general, your participation in sports may give you a higher tolerance for bodily discomforts like hot flashes than someone who has not regularly challenged their body to perform.

- *Menopause-related mood swings may be less frequent.* Estrogen has a mood-elevating effect; the ebbing of estrogen during menopause may explain why some women experience sudden bouts of irritability or nervousness during the menopausal years. But exercise may help counteract these mood swings because it activates another set of mood-altering chemicals in the brain called endorphins, which affect one's sense of general well-being, reducing muscle tension and anxiety.

• *Sleeplessness may be less of a problem.* "Menopause's effect on sleep can be exactly like that of having a newborn baby—in other words, it can be awfully disruptive in some women," notes Dr. Moulton. Regular exercise is a well-known insomnia reliever; many researchers think it is also helpful specifically for menopausal sleep problems.

Athletes as a group are more likely to have an easier, healthier menopause than women who are sedentary. Still, that doesn't deal with the specifics—namely, about how you as an individual feel and about whether you should opt to take hormones during and after menopause.

SHOULD I TAKE HORMONES?

There are two reasons why any woman, athletic or otherwise, would consider taking hormone therapy at menopause. The first is for treatment of short-term symptoms—as a way to garner relief from hot flashes, night sweats, vaginal dryness, or other menopausal discomforts. The other reason women consider taking hormones is for long-term health protection against things like osteoporosis, heart disease, Alzheimer's, and a variety of other illnesses.

There are two types of hormone therapy: estrogen replacement therapy (ERT) is simply estrogen, given alone. It is prescribed for women who have had a hysterectomy (surgical removal of the uterus and sometimes the ovaries). The more commonly prescribed therapy is hormone replacement therapy (HRT), which consists of a combination of estrogen and progestin. When estrogen is given alone, it may cause an overgrowth of the lining of the uterus, which can lead to cancer. Progestin helps protect against this and so is prescribed for women who still have their uteruses.

Short-term HRT or ERT—the Pros and Cons

Let's say you're having a hard time putting up with certain menopause symptoms and you want some relief right now.

One option is to take HRT, since it provides almost immediate respite (within two weeks) from unpleasant menopausal symptoms in most women. "I think it's important for women who choose estrogen therapy for relief of hot flashes or night sweats not to feel that this is a bad choice," writes one of the most outspoken critics of routine estrogen therapy, Susan Love, M.D., in *Dr. Susan Love's Hormone Book* (Random House, 1997). "No studies have found that short-term use of estrogen is dangerous, and it certainly can improve the quality of your life." The one caveat: any woman who has had breast cancer or is at especially high risk for it because of a family history of the disease should approach any hormone therapy with caution.

Short-term hormone use is usually defined as anything under three years. As mentioned, the pros of short-term HRT therapy are that it is effective at relieving symptoms and doesn't appear to pose any increased disease risks.

The cons? HRT can bring back your period. The usual HRT regime consists of twenty-eight days of estrogen with an overlap of ten to fourteen days of progestin, which almost always triggers some bleeding for a few days a month in the first year you are on the regime. The alternative, taking both hormones every day, may cause unpredictable light bleeding or spotting during the first year. "What determines whether you continue to have periods on HRT is your estrogen levels. As you get older, your levels increasingly decline," explains Dr. Moulton. "If you are athletic and thin, you may not have high estrogen levels and so you may be able to take both hormones every day and not experience any bleeding."

In addition, some women find that HRT causes a variety of side effects, such as nausea, headache, depression, weight gain, and bloating. Mueller, for example, tried hormones on and off for two years but found they caused more side effects than they cured. "It relieved the hot flashes, but it caused lots of heavy bleeding and bloating. I didn't want to have periods." Another problem is that short-term HRT does not always provide a permanent cure for your symptoms; they can come back when you stop HRT. Sometimes you can wean yourself off HRT slowly to prevent this from happening.

"Any woman who opts for HRT should know that there is no such thing as 'one size fits all,'" says Dr. Moulton. "There are lots of different formulations of hormones today, in all sorts of doses and combinations. A woman should insist on working closely with her doctor so they can tinker with the dose of HRT and tailor it to find the dose that delivers the least side effects for the most benefits.''

There is no evidence to suggest that HRT *directly* aids or hurts your athletic performance. In other words, it has never been shown that athletes who take estrogen postmenopausally are stronger or faster (or weaker or slower, for that matter) than those who don't opt for HRT.

It's important to note that HRT is not the only option when it comes to treating menopausal symptoms. There are other nonhormonal prescription drugs for treating symptoms as well as an array of nontraditional, alternative therapies. Remifemin, a capsule containing extracts of the herb black cohosh, is a hugely popular remedy for hot flashes in Germany, for example. The herb vitex is often used to treat irregular or heavy bleeding, a common but usually transient effect of menopause. Of course, there is very little research to prove these alternatives and herbs are truly effective. Probably the most comprehensive, detailed source of information about alternative treatments is Dr. Love's book, mentioned previously.

◑ How Hormone Replacement May Benefit You

- relieves unpleasant menopausal symptoms almost immediately
- protects against heart disease
- guards against osteoporosis
- may help prevent colon cancer
- may fight Alzheimer's disease
- may prevent wrinkles

Long-Term HRT Use

Long-term HRT is advocated as a way to prevent diseases that result from the loss of estrogen. It is a complicated subject steeped in controversy. Very broadly, the pros of estrogen use are said to include the following:

- *May prolong life.* Various studies show that estrogen users live longer
- *May protect against heart disease.* Estrogen users have been shown to have as much as a 60 percent lower risk of coronary heart disease.

- *May guard against osteoporosis, which makes you more susceptible to fractures, especially of the hip, as you age.* Estrogen is instrumental in building and maintaining bone mass; when your estrogen levels decline postmenopausally, your bone mineral density also declines. But hormone therapy slows bone thinning and may even promote rebuilding. Estrogen users appear to have 50 percent lower fracture rates than nonusers.
- *May help prevent colon cancer.* A woman's risk may be reduced by over 20 percent.
- *May fight Alzheimer's disease.* In one study of over one thousand women, only 2.7 percent of the women who had used estrogen developed Alzheimer's versus 8.4 percent who had not used it.
- *May prevent wrinkles.* One study from the University of California at Los Angeles found that HRT users developed fewer wrinkles, but these results haven't been widely duplicated.

The cons of ERT and HRT include:

- *May increase your risk of breast cancer.* Numerous studies indicate that older women who take hormones for over ten years after menopause may increase their risk of breast cancer from anywhere from 10 to 40 percent. A decade or more of taking HRT or ERT extends and lengthens your lifetime exposure to estrogen, a hormone believed to stimulate cancer cell growth. This may explain why, unlike the birth control pill, it seems to increase your risk of developing breast cancer. (When you take the pill, you slightly increase the dose of estrogen you are exposed to when young—you don't increase the number of years your breast tissue is exposed to estrogens.)
- *Women who take estrogen have twice as much risk of developing gallbadder disease as nonusers.* Liver problems may also increase with estrogen use.
- *May slightly increase your risk of uterine cancer.* Although progestin is largely effective in protecting the uterus against the effects of estrogen alone, there is some data that suggests HRT users do have a very slight increase in risk for cancers of the uterus.

- *May increase your risk of ovarian cancer and asthma.* Evidence of these links is considered very preliminary.

Increasingly, experts are acknowledging that every woman's situation needs to be evaluated individually. There is no blanket recommendation that is right for everyone—your particular family history, lifestyle, athletic history, medication use, and psychological comfort level with taking HRT all must be considered when making a decision.

◯ The risks of long-term hormone replacement

- increases your risk of breast cancer
- doubles your chances of developing gallbladder disease
- may increase the risk of uterine and ovarian cancer
- may also increase the risk of liver problems and adult-onset asthma

---

LOOK FORWARD, NOT BACK

There is no doubt that making decisions about whether to opt for HRT or not and coming to terms with getting older in general can be difficult. But staying active can help you weather the rough times, bolstering your body confidence and self-confidence too.

Still, how do you face the reality that at some point you will reach a plateau in your primary sport—you'll achieve the best you ever can? Ardeth Mueller simply accepts that her times may fall off, then continues in her sport because she loves it. "If I worried about my times and allowed myself to become really upset when they fall off, I wouldn't still be in this sport," says Mueller. "Of course I try to do my best and I am momentarily disappointed if I haven't reached my goal. But my disappointment truly doesn't last more than ten minutes. That's the beauty of getting older. You have less to prove, you can take setbacks in stride, and you just enjoy the *doing* of the sport without getting overly concerned about the *winning* of it."

Other athletes deal with the issue of declining performances by switching allegiances from one sport to another and finding new challenges in new activities.

"I don't compare my performances from decade to decade because I keep learning new things and changing my focus," says Becky Sisley, age fifty-nine, who is the world record holder for indoor and outdoor pole vault in her age group (fifty-five to fifty-nine) as well as professor of physical activity and recreation services at University of Oregon in Eugene.

At age forty-two, Sisley ran her first marathon. At age forty-three, she set the goal of running a 10k race (6.2 miles) in forty-three minutes (her age). At age forty-nine, she started competing in the track events of high jump, triple jump, and javelin. She holds the American records for those events (in the age group fifty to fifty-four). At age fifty-five, she took up pole vaulting.

"Each time I learn a new event, I enter a new learning curve," says Sisley. "I don't start out so well because I don't know much and I haven't mastered the technique. But then I start to see progressive improvements. That's a real psychological boost—it keeps me involved, challenged, and motivated. Right now, my high jump is declining and I suspect my javelin is as good as it is ever going to get. But in my newest event,

SPECIAL FOCUS:

◯ Bone Check

To find out how high your risk of developing osteoporosis is, you need to have a test called dual-energy X-ray absorptiometry (DEXA). "This is quite an accurate test and can help you weigh your needs and alternatives," advises Helen M. Schilling, M.D.

If your bone mineral density is very low, hormone replacement therapy for at least five years is the treatment of first choice, according to a recent article published in *The New England Journal of Medicine (NEJM)*. But if your bone loss is only moderately low, there are options other than HRT you can explore. For example, there are nonhormonal drug treatments for protection against bone thinning, such as the drug Fosamax. Or, if your problem is very mild, you might opt for other remedies that have proven effective, such as taking a daily dose of 1,500 mg dietary calcium, 400 to 800 IU of vitamin D, and simultaneously adding more high-intensity strength training to your regimen.

pole vaulting, I am still getting better and better and that is very exciting."

Other athletes find that the key to staying in the game with age is to "get social"—to train with a group, volunteer at events, and/or mentor a younger athlete. Reaching out in this way can keep you from becoming isolated and depressed, especially if you're having a hard time grappling with the change in your performances.

Clearly, one of the keys to weathering the changes and transitions that come with age is to abandon comparisons with the past and to reach out to the future for new goals. Only then can you discover how being an older athlete has its own rewards.

PART TWO

Your Sports Resource: An Alphabetized Directory of Forty Activities

INTRODUCTION

Sports aren't just about staying in shape or getting faster or winning; they're also about playfulness and joy and simply having a good time. And a great way to recapture those feelings about playing a sport is to try a new one.

That's one of the points of the alphabetized sports directory that follows. Its purpose is to make it easier for you to explore a new activity by giving you all the details you need on how to get involved, from clear descriptions of how a sport is performed to lists of organizations you can consult for information on local lessons, clubs, tournaments, etc.

Of course, fun isn't the only reason to take on a new activity. Other benefits:

• *Your self-esteem and sense of mastery get a nice little boost.* Whether you're trying to learn how to dribble a basketball or stand on a surfboard, it's a challenge to try something new. And the reward for meeting that challenge—when you find out you can do it—is personal growth.

• *It wreaks havoc on ruts.* Although there is often a well-deserved place for monotony in a workout (after all, it can be quite soothing and meditative to do a familiar workout), being too single-track in one sport can backfire, leaving you stale, disenchanted, and without much zest or motivation to do your workouts. When you get involved in another sport, you always have another ace in your pocket—another option on days when you don't feel like doing your primary sport. This can help prevent you from becoming burned out.

• *It can, oddly enough, reinvigorate your involvement in your favorite activity, too.* Trying a new sport not only breaks up the mental tedium you may be experiencing, it can also serve as a foil or contrast that helps to remind you of why you fell in love with your primary sport in the first place.

• *It can help you become more flexible and less "season-dependent."* If the only thing you do is play squash, you're out of the action if you can't find a court to play in. If you're only a mountain biker, certain weather conditions, such as a heavy snowfall, will throw a major monkey wrench in your workout plans. Obviously, having exercise alternatives so that you're not too dependent on club operating hours or weather whims makes a lot of sense, especially if you have a busy schedule. Being flexible— being able to take a run instead of playing squash or being able to snowboard instead of cycle—helps ensure that you'll overcome obstacles to get in your workout and thus stay fit.

• *It can help your whole body be in better shape.* Most sports whip certain areas of your body into good shape, while failing to get other areas into condition. Running, for example, does wonders for your heart, lungs, and legs, but it does almost nothing for your upper body and your overall flexibility. Playing more than one sport can be a great way to counter this imbalance (see What's Your Workout Missing? page 213).

• *It can offer a welcome change of scenery.* You might be surprised at how exhilarating it feels to move freely in the fresh air on a bicycle or on in-line skates if you're always working out in the confines of a gym (in an indoor aerobics, swimming, or general gymnastics class, for example). Or if your tennis game or running routine always keeps you land bound, you might find the liquid landscape you are exposed to when rowing or windsurfing opens up your mind to all sorts of new meditations and pleasures.

• *It gives you alternatives for the days when your body needs a break from your primary sport and/or if you get injured.* Especially as you get older, you may find your body needs a longer rest between hard workouts. But you may not want to be completely sedentary on those days. Having other activities can help you stay in shape at the same time you are resting the overtired parts of your body. Similarly, if you get injured, you may be able to perform in your secondary sport while you recuperate.

THE CROSS-TRAINING DEBATE

By now, you're probably wondering why the words *cross-training* haven't been mentioned. Today, the term tends to refer to a specific concept of training—it's a tool used by many coaches and athletes that involves training in a secondary sport or sports as a means to *improve* performance in the primary pursuit. In other words, cross-training does not simply refer to "taking a break from your favorite sport to sample something different."

Despite its widespread popularity and despite what many books and articles might lead you to believe, cross-training has not actually been proven to be effective as a training technique. A few studies, most of which looked at male runners who also engaged in high-intensity cycling, did find that extensive training in two sports (running and cycling) boosted performance to the same extent as extensive training in just one (running). It is not known whether these findings will apply to women, to athletes other than runners, and to other forms of secondary exercise.

In addition, it has never been established that training in two or more sports improves your performance to a *greater degree* than training in just your primary sport. Most experts suspect this will never be proven: They believe that specificity is extremely important and that the best way to train for a sport is to do that sport.

In fact, there is some evidence to suggest that certain kinds of cross-training may have some drawbacks. In a study of female collegiate swimmers who were followed for more than seven years, published in the *Clinical Journal of Sports Medicine,* cross-training caused as many injuries as swimming did. The cross-training injuries were sustained under the supervision of a coach, who had designed a cross-training program that included intensive running, sprinting, and stadium step climbing. Not surprisingly, most of the injuries involved bones, tendons, and muscles of the leg and foot (parts of the body that may be weak in a swimmer). Part of the problem is that no one really knows what the exact content of an appropriate cross-training program should be for a given athlete. The concept of cross-training is still quite new and there isn't an abundance of evidence from large studies to back up recommendations.

For example, many coaches and experts feel strongly that strength training should be included in the regime of every athlete. Yet many studies have found no significant association between strength training and improvements in things like VO2max (the maximal amount of oxygen your heart can pump) or lactate threshold (the point at which lactic acid builds up in your muscles and causes fatigue).

Even so, many experts have a strong hunch or intuitive belief that the stronger you are, the more likely it is you'll be able to reach a high-level performance. And there is certainly no doubt that strength training is an essential component of total fitness—it helps make you fit all over. It helps replace fat with muscle, halts bone loss, speeds up your metabolism, and sculpts your body shape. It's also a great way to ensure you have good strength to perform everyday carrying and hauling tasks. But given the state of current research, it's premature to assert that clocking time in the weight room will actually improve your speed and/or endurance performance.

◓ Stretching the Truth About Stretching?

As you get older, gentle stretching can help you maintain your range of motion and your ability to bend and reach. But contrary to common lore, it is far from proven whether stretching can do more—i.e., actually prevent injuries and improve performance. For example, a study of nineteen competitive male distance runners, conducted at the University of North Carolina at Greensboro, found that the runners who were *less* flexible, especially in their hips and calves, were 47 percent more economical in their running. The researchers speculated that inflexibility might be desirable when it comes to running performance because it minimizes the need for "muscle stabilizing activity and increased storage and return of elastic energy."

Of course, it may be that future research will find that a program of regular stretching boosts the performance of athletes in one sport (such as gymnastics) but not another (like running). But more studies on the benefits of stretching are needed before these kinds of conclusions can be drawn.

SPECIAL FOCUS

◒ What's Your Workout Missing?

If you need help finding activities that offer conditioning components missing in your primary pursuit, the table, below, offers a variety of suggestions.

If your sport . . .	Consider . . .
works your legs, but neglects your arms (cycling, running, ice skating, snowboarding, snowshoeing)	*getting your upper body involved* (rowing, swimming, basketball, volleyball or a racket sport)
doesn't have a strong aerobic/cardiovascular conditioning component (general gymnastics, diving, softball, or downhill skiing)	*something that gets your heart rate up and keeps it up* (badminton, skating, in-line skating, cycling, running, cross-country skiing, snowshoeing, or soccer)
doesn't work out your bones (cycling, swimming, canoeing, or kayaking)	*a bone-bolstering weight-bearing activity* (aerobics, basketball, cross-country skiing, running, downhill skiing, skating, snowshoeing, volleyball, or a court sport)
works your upper but not lower body (swimming, canoeing, or kayaking)	*a sport that targets your leg muscles* (cycling, running, in-line skating, skating, cross-country skiing, snowshoeing, or soccer)
tends to increase muscle tightness (running, triathlon, rowing)	*a practice that promotes range of motion* (aerobics, general gymnastics, or yoga)
involves joint-jarring impact (aerobics, basketball, volleyball, any racket sport, downhill skiing, or running)	*giving your joints a break* (cycling, in-line skating, swimming)

COMMONSENSE RULES

So, as researchers sort out what's effective and what's not when it comes to cross-training regimes, you'll just need to rely on common sense. If you are a competitive athlete, your coach may have a cross-training regime she has used with good results in the past. It's probably a good idea, however, to make sure this regime hasn't resulted in a lot of injuries. For example, the common cross-training routine of running stadium steps has never been shown to improve the performance of any athlete, but it does damage the knees, according to a report in *The Physician and Sportsmedicine*. Ask questions and, most important, self-monitor to make sure your cross-training activities are helping, not hindering, your progress and performance.

If you are a recreational athlete training on your own, a good rule of thumb is to start by *substituting* workouts in your primary sport with ones in your new one. If you start adding (instead of substituting) really strenuous cross-training sessions you may increase your risk of injury. Instead, allow yourself sufficient time to adapt before piling on extra playing time. Ease into the new activity gradually: start with very short sessions, at an easy to very moderate exertion level. Pay attention to any signs of overtraining: If you start to feel more tired than usual, you may be doing too much.

As for how hard or intensely you should play your new sport, it all depends on what you are trying to achieve. If you are training for an important event in your primary sport and/or are supposed to be having a rest day in your training schedule, it makes sense to go easy in your secondary activity. But if everything is equal, you can be flexible—as long as you have become adequately adapted to your new sport, there's no reason not to play as vigorously as you want.

AEROBICS

In its essence, aerobics is calisthenics set to music. Usually performed indoors in groups, with music playing in the background, you follow the directions of an instructor who guides you through movements designed to get your heart rate cranking as well as your muscles strengthened, lengthened, and toned.

There are several broad subcategories of aerobics:

Floor aerobics: This is the most traditional type of aerobics, done with no equipment. You just stand on the floor and follow your instructor. High-impact routines include jumps, hops, skips, and kicks. Low-impact aerobics, in which you keep one foot on the floor at all times, is designed to minimize the stress to your back, knee, and other joints.

Step aerobics: This aerobics movement is similar to low-impact floor aerobics, except that you also use a small bench, usually 2 to 3 feet long and adjustable to different heights off the floor.

Sport aerobics: Also called "competitive aerobics," in this sport athletes compete in mixed pairs, men's, women's, and team categories, performing two-minute choreographed routines set to music. Using the 10-point system prevalent in a number of Olympic events, judges score each athlete on technical merit, artistic merit, and degree of difficulty. There are national and international World Aerobic Championship competitions.

Boxerobics, aerobox, cardio kickboxing, taeborobics, **etc.:** All of these movements are a marriage of fast-paced aerobics and basic boxing or martial arts moves such as punches, boxing jabs, and karate kicks. These classes are often taught by former boxers or martial arts black belts.

Within these broad categories, aerobics presents a world of variety. Aerobics' choreography, for example, ranges from simple and easy-to-follow to intricate, balletic, and quite complex; the pace can be fast and furious or slow and steady; the maneuvers can be limited to basic athletic moves like knee lifts and arm raises or include wild mambo-like gyrations, stylized arm waving, or intense power hops and lunges. The musical approach might include anything from a medley of fifties oldies to live African percussive music. Every gym has its own roster of often idiosyncratic offerings, but you should expect classes to be carefully geared for different levels of fitness and expertise.

How It's Done: Most classes, no matter what variation of aerobics you are doing, have roughly the following format:

Warm-up (five to ten minutes): Full body movements and stretches designed to increase blood flow to the muscles are performed first. You might march in place some of the time or do step repeats.

Aerobic segment (twenty to fifty minutes): The intensity of the aerobic segment will vary, depending upon the fitness level of the class. The types of movements you do will depend on the style of the class. Some aerobics classes employ complex dance patterns to get your heart rate up, while others depend on simpler things like light jogging and jumping jacks.

Cool-down (five to ten minutes): Involving slower, less intense movements of the large muscles as well as stretching exercises, cool-down brings your heart rate back to normal.

Muscle toning/strength training (ten to fifteen minutes): This segment is often included at the end of an aerobics class. May include work with weights and/or exercises like abdominal crunches, leg lifts, squats, bicep curls, and so on.

Key Physical Requirements: A beginner needs to realize that everyone feels uncoordinated at first; it will take a few sessions for you to become familiar with the basic movement patterns used in most aerobic classes.

Most classes will improve your cardiovascular endurance, flexibility, muscular endurance, muscular strength, coordination, and balance. Obviously, the more advanced the class, the more challenging the physical effort will be.

Equipment need: Good, rubber-sole aerobic shoes are recommended. You'll need a towel or exercise mat for the floor work. Bring a water bottle too. When choosing a class, find out what kind of floor the gym has. A suspended or cushioned hardwood floor (such as you find in most school gymnasiums) is fine. What you want to avoid is a concrete slab, because even if it is carpeted, it will still be murder on your joints.

What to Wear: A leotard and tights, or shorts and a tee-shirt.

To Find Out More:

You can get a referral to a certified aerobics instructor from the following organization:

Aerobics and Fitness Association of America
15250 Ventura Boulevard, #200
Sherman Oaks, CA 91403
PHONE: 800-446-2322
FAX: 818-990-5468
WEBSITE: www.afaa.com

www.turnstep.com is a well-designed website that includes a dictionary describing the array of aerobic moves available; it also has links to most other major aerobics-related sites.

To find out more about competitive aerobics, contact:

Association of National Aerobic Championships Worldwide
8033 Sunset Boulevard, #1420
Los Angeles, CA 90046
PHONE: 800-NOW-JUMP or 213-850-3777
FAX: 213-850-7795
E-MAIL: NACUSA@aol.com

Books to Check Out

Lynne G. Brick, *Fitness Aerobics* (Champaign, Ill.: Human Kinetics, 1996).
The first part of this book gives advice on how to select the right clothing, equipment, and music, how to assess your current fitness level and how to warm up and cool down properly. The second part contains descriptions of 42 progressive aerobic workouts that vary in intensity and training focus.

Tamilee Webb, *Tamilee Webb's Step Up Fitness Workout* (New York: Workman Publishing, 1995).
Authored by the instructor-star of the popular *Buns of Steel* exercise videos, Webb maps out low-impact workouts for all fitness levels. Each workout is composed of seventeen key step patterns that demonstrate weight use, warm-up, muscle sculpting, stretch, and cool-down.

◒ Aerobics Lingo

Around the World: A pattern of sixteen movements that circles over and around a step bench and may include lunges, jumps, and stretches

Rocking Horse: An eight-part move used in step aerobics that includes knee lifts and hamstring curls

---

BADMINTON

Competitive badminton is as different from the game you play in your backyard with toy store equipment than a jog around the block is from running an ultramarathon. "Real" badminton is a serious sport that is physically demanding, requiring stamina and speed. It also requires considerable skill and subtlety to play well.

Still, the basics of badminton are easy to learn. Most first-timers on the court find hitting the shuttlecock isn't difficult—and is a lot of fun.

How It's Played: The game can be played by two people (singles) or four (doubles). Although it's possible to play outdoors, tournaments officially sanctioned by the United States Badminton Association (USBA) are played indoors, on regulation-size rectangular courts.

The object of the game is to serve and return the shuttlecock (sometimes called a bird or shuttle) strategically across a net so that your opponent is unable to return it. Unlike a tennis ball, a shuttlecock will not bounce, so it needs to be kept airborne in order to remain in play.

The flight of a shuttlecock is quite unlike that of a ball, notes authors Herbert S. FitzGibbon II and Jeffrey N. Bairstow in *The Complete Racquet Sports Player* (Simon & Schuster, 1979): "The bird can move very rapidly through the air and then drop agonizingly slowly, giving a receiver time to set up for the return. Or the bird can be flicked gently over the net to die before the opponent can race up to retrieve the point. So badminton calls for considerable skill in shot-making."

Only the server can score points; the serve shifts to the

opponent when the server misses a shot or commits an error. Games are played to 11 in women's singles. After each game, you change court sides with your opponent. The winner is the first to win two games.

Key Physical Requirements: Stamina agility, and power are the main qualities of a badminton player.

Fast feet: The court is small, so you don't have a large area to cover. But you do need to be quick in your stops, turns, jumps, twists, and stretches. You may only move four or five steps each time you return the shuttlecock to your opponent, but you need to move with agility, lightness, and power.

Endurance: One of the main distinctions between badminton and all other racket games is the length of the rallies (the exchange of shots). The bird can cross the net a dozen or more times before a point is finally won. That means, during the approximately fifty minutes that it takes to play an average set of games, you'll be running, jumping, and turning constantly. As FitzGibbon and Bairstow note, "Badminton is so demanding that it is almost a game of attrition, where the objective is to tire the opponent and so win the match."

Flexible wrist: Unlike tennis, a stiff wrist is not used in badminton. In fact, just the opposite is required. "A well-timed whip of the wrist supplies explosive power to a badminton stroke. Proper wrist action is vital to success in badminton, as it is in baseball. In fact, if you grew up batting and throwing, you are already tuned in to the wrist snap that badminton demands," notes Steven Boga, author of *Badminton* (Stackpole Books, 1996). "Some coaches tell their players to imagine they are throwing the head of the racket at the shuttle. Others have them imagine their wrist bending like that of a house painter wielding a brush."

Equipment: Besides a playing court 17 feet wide by 44 feet long (or 20 feet wide by 44 feet long for doubles) divided by a net that is 5 feet, 1 inch in height, you need a racket and shuttlecocks. Rackets are about 26 inches long, lightweight (weighing under 6 ounces), and start at about $25. The most important consideration when selecting a racket is the size of the handle, it should feel comfortable—not too small or too large—when you grip it.

Competition-grade shuttlecocks must weigh less than ⅙ of an ounce and can be made from natural or synthetic materials. Especially if you're a beginner or just practicing, it pays to keep in mind that the plastic and nylon shuttlecocks tend to be less expensive and more durable than the feathered versions.

What to Wear: Tennis whites are traditional for tournament play, although any loose, comfortable clothing is fine for recreational play. Athletic shoes designed for tennis are ideal; because badminton requires so many quick stops and changes of directions, the game puts you at high risk for blisters. The best way to avoid this is to wear thick, shock-absorbing socks (see page 113). Bring an extra pair to change into between sets to ensure your feet stay dry.

To Find Out More

The USBA can help you locate a place to play badminton in your area as well as direct you to instruction and training camps:

United States Badminton Association
One Olympic Plaza
Colorado Springs, CO 80909
PHONE: 719-578-4808
WEBSITE: www.usabadminton.org

Books to Check Out

Steven Boga, *Badminton* (Mechanicsburg, PA.: Stackpole Books, 1996).
Written in a very conversational, highly readable style, this is

---

◓ Badminton Talk

Flick: A very quick snap of the wrist—and almost no arm movement—that causes the shuttle to fly high and far into the rear of the opponent's court.

Kill: A hard, tight, down-driving shot that can't be returned.

Smash: A fast, powerful overhead shot that is badminton's key attacking and point-making stroke.

a great beginner's guide. It will also be a useful resource as you improve your game, since it contains many hints and advice from top players on how to get better.

BASKETBALL

There's a lot more to basketball than getting it through the hoop, something virtually all of us have at least tried to do at some point in our lives. "Basketball is a complex game filled with graceful and sneaky moves that rely on psychological cunning as well as physical bearing" was how journalist Rebecca Johnson, writing in a 1996 *Women's Sports & Fitness* article, perfectly described this artful game.

Playing a good strategic game of basketball means being willing to inflict and tolerate a certain amount of pushing, shoving, and physical contact with other players. It's not a hands-off game, although it's not boxing or wrestling either. But you do need to be comfortable with, in basketball lingo, "laying a body" on an opponent.

Playing a good game also requires mastering an array of surprisingly subtle and varied skills. There are dozens of ways to make a good shot, there is an arsenal of tactics you can use to defend your court, and there are dozens of ways to dribble the ball. For example, the crossover dribble, in which you switch the ball from hand to hand, is low and is used when you are directly facing an opponent. A speed dribble is usually one-handed, fast and high, and is used to get you across the court as quickly as possible.

Virtually every basketball skill serves a tactical purpose in a specific situation. So although you might perform a lot of drills on your own in an empty court to master the moves, the real test is playing in a game——that's when you learn to combine your technical expertise with thinking on your feet.

How It's Played: In official play, basketball is played by two teams of five players on a rectangular court approximately 94 by 50 feet. The court is divided into two equal areas so that each team has a front court, where its own basket is located, and a back court, which has the basket it defends (the opponent's basket). The purpose of each team is to score into the opponents' basket and to prevent the other team from securing the ball or scoring.

Play times vary but usually consist of two twenty-minute halves with a fifteen-minute intermission. Whoever has the highest score at the end of regulation playing time wins.

Key Physical Requirements: Here are the qualities you need in order to become a good player:

Flexibility: So that you can easily stop, start, change directions, bend, crouch, and contort while doing maneuvers with names like the crab dribble, you need to be loose and flexible.

Upper body strength: You use your back, shoulder, and arm muscles whenever you hurl the basketball effectively toward the hoop. Being strong also gives you a psychological edge on the court: "Strength gives you confidence to go out and match up with any player—big or small," note Nancy Lieberman-Cline and Robin Roberts, authors of *Basketball for Women* (Human Kinetics, 1996).

Endurance: You need to be able to easily sustain a lot of nonstop running for approximately forty minutes. If you don't have this kind of energy, your performance will flag toward the last crucial minutes of the game.

Jumping power: Being able to jump high and quickly are essentials of basketball. Professional players do specific work and exercise training to hone their jumping abilities.

Equipment: You need a standard basketball, a hoop, and a court. What's great about basketball is that you don't necessarily need a gym with a standard-size wooden court and two hoops. You can play outdoors and you can play with one hoop. Most local parks, schools, and recreation areas have at least some sort of a setup for playing basketball, which makes it easy to find "pickup games"—impromptu gatherings of people looking to play.

What to Wear: Most women wear loose-fitting shorts and sleeveless shirts, so as to allow for good freedom of movement and sweat ventilation. Pay particular attention to your shoes— you want ankle support to brace your jumps, cushioning to soften your landings, and traction to allow for quick changes in direction. Most of the major athletic shoe companies now manufacture basketball shoes designed specifically for women.

To Find Out More

Your local YMCA, YWCA, or similar recreation center is the best place to look for a local adult league. If you are interested in learning how to play the game or in honing your skills, there are many camps and instructional programs although the majority of them are directed at women of high school and college age. The following group offers ten-week clinics or evening courses and weekend camps for players of all ability levels and all ages throughout the country:

Never Too Late Basketball Camps, Inc.
P.O. Box 235
West Medford, MA 02156
PHONE: 781-488-3333 or 888-NTL-HOOPS
WEBSITE: www.nevertoolate.com

Books to Check Out

Nancy Lieberman-Cline and Robin Roberts, *Basketball for Women: Becoming a Complete Player* (Champaign, Ill.: Human Kinetics, 1996).
This is a great book, with many specific drills, practices, and strategies; however, it does assume you have a basic knowledge of the rules of the game and how it is played.

◐ Basketball Talk

Block: Personal contact that impedes the progress of an opponent with or without the ball.

Lay-up shot: Made while the player is running, the shot is tricky since it is made practically from under the basket or at least at a position very close to it, from the front or either side.

Screen: Also "set the screen," an offensive technique used to prevent an opponent from going where she wants to go on the court.

Mark Vancil, *NBA Basketball Basics* (New York: Sterling Publishing, 1995).
Besides explaining the fundamentals of dribbling, ball handling, shooting, and so on, this book outlines some fun shooting games that can be played with as few as two players.

CANOEING AND KAYAKING

Paddlers tend to be attracted to their sport because they share a deep appreciation, affection, and fascination for waterways; not surprisingly, many paddlers and paddler organizations are deeply involved in river, lake, and ocean conservation and ecology issues.

When you participate in canoeing or kayaking as a "sport" and/or for fitness on a recreational or competitive level, there are an array of basic moves, paddling strokes, boat control maneuvers, and self-rescue techniques you need to learn. In addition, you need to learn the fundamentals of how a river flows (or the ocean if you plan to sea kayak), river safety, as well as river-running strategies. In other words, renting a canoe then leisurely tooting around on a placid lake for an afternoon is really not what paddle sports are about.

What's Involved: What distinguishes paddling from rowing is that the paddler faces forward without the paddle being supported by a fulcrum on either side of the vessel. The main difference between canoeists and kayakers, according to the United States Canoe and Kayak Team, is this:

- Kayakers sit down with their legs extended in front of them, and the vessel is covered or decked. A kayaker uses a double-bladed paddle.
- Canoeists paddle from a kneeling position with a single-bladed paddle in a relatively open vessel.

Canoes or kayaks can be single (manned by one woman) or double. There are also four-women kayaks and competitions.

Canoe and kayak racing has a long tradition; distances can be as short as 5 miles or as long as an ultramarathon of 250 miles. In addition, there are two Olympic disciplines for canoe and kayak:

- Whitewater slalom, in which paddlers negotiate a twenty-five-gate course suspended over stretches of whitewater rapids 300 to 600 meters long. The athletes attempt to negotiate the series of upstream and downstream gates as quickly as possible without accruing time penalties for touching poles (two seconds) or missing gates (fifty seconds).
- Flatwater sprint, which is a contest of speed, strength, and endurance in which athletes compete head to head on calm bodies of water.

Key Physical Requirements: A prerequisite for becoming involved in any paddle sport is an ability to swim at a moderate level.

All the paddle sports require a good deal of upper-body strength—good muscle power—combined with endurance and aerobic strength.

Boaters must do a lot of lifting, so strength in the lower-back muscles and the antagonistic abdominal muscles is important, according to Jackie Johnson Maughan, author of *The Outdoor Woman's Guide to Sports, Fitness and Nutrition* (Stackpole Books, 1983).

If you canoe, the arms are worked the most, says Maughan. Next comes the back, abdomen, chest, and shoulders, in that order. When kneeling in an open canoe, your thighs and hamstrings will get a workout too.

In kayaking the demands are greatest on the arms and shoulders. To prepare for paddling distances, Maughan recommends a training regime that combines swimming, working out on a rowing machine, and weight training.

Equipment: Most paddling outfitters and schools will provide the "big stuff" basic equipment, including a boat, a paddle, a life jacket, and a spray deck (which is worn around the waist of a kayaker and serves to close around the cockpit of the kayak to keep waves and spray from filling the boat). A helmet is also necessary for most types of kayaking.

What to Wear: You need to plan on getting wet and probably being completely submerged. So it ultimately depends on what season and in what temperature waters you plan to travel. In cold weather and/or waters, you would be well-advised to wear a wet or dry suit, for example. Before setting out, ask your outfitter what kind of clothing is best. Specifically, find out if you should have a waterproof hooded jacket, rain gear, gloves, hat, visor, and/or sunglasses. Find out what kind of foot gear is usually worn. And see if you need to come equipped with a first aid kit and a dry bag (a waterproof sack for things like your identification, money, and camera).

To Find Out More:

The American Canoe Association (ACA) promotes and sponsors events in virtually all paddle sport disciplines. The association supports hundreds of local competitive and recreational events; it certifies instructors in the paddle sports and can help you find a qualified teacher or school; it also offers a wide selection of instruction manuals and videos in canoeing, river or whitewater kayaking as well as coastal and sea kayaking and river rescue. *Paddler* magazine is provided as a benefit to ACA members (it costs $25 a year to join ACA).

American Canoe Association
7432 Alban Station Boulevard, Suite B-226
Springfield, VA 22150
PHONE: 703-451-0141
FAX: 703-451-2245
E-MAIL: acadirect@aol.com
WEBSITE: www.aca-paddler.org

If you think you might want to compete in a paddling sport, you should consider joining USA Canoe/Kayak, the membership division of the United States Canoe and Kayak Team (USCKT), since that will give you access to USCKT's Resource Center for information about training, competing, coaching, and officiating as well as a USCKT membership card, which you'll need to be eligible to compete in USCKT sanctioned events.

United States Canoe and Kayak
P.O. Box 789, 421 Old Military Road
Lake Placid, NY 12946
PHONE: 518-523-1855
E-MAIL: USCKT@aol.com

Books to Check Out

The Beginner's Guide to Canoeing and Kayaking is an excellent compilation of articles from *Canoe & Kayak* magazine on how to select the best gear, find a club, a good instructor, and so forth. The guide is updated annually and can be ordered via the publishers of the magazine (which is also a very good resource):

Canoe & Kayak Magazine
P.O. Box 3146
Kirkland, WA 90883
PHONE: 800-692-2663
FAX: 425-827-1893
WEBSITE: www.canoekayak.com

◔ Paddler's Lingo

Blade: The wide part of the paddle that is placed in the water.

Chute: An area where a river's flow is suddenly constricted, which causes the current to become quite strong and concentrated in a narrow channel of water.

Eskimo roll: A form of capsize recovery in which you use your body weight to completely roll your inverted kayak over, so that it turns upright again.

CROSS-COUNTRY SKIING

Also known as Nordic skiing and XC skiing, cross-country skiing attracts about 4 million participants each year, 52 percent of whom are women, according to the Cross Country Ski Area Association (CCSAA).

The distinctions between downhill (or alpine) and cross-country skiing are often quite pumped up, but the truth is that the two sports can be quite similar in terms of speed, tricky turns, and thrilling descents. In one variation of XC skiing, known as Nordic downhill or telemark skiing, skiers snowplow, kick turn, and do virtually every other maneuver downhill skiers do.

Still, there are some important distinctions between the two sports:

- on cross-country skis, your heel is free (only the front of your foot is clamped into the ski), which allows you to stride on level land as well as go uphill and downhill. In alpine skiing, your whole foot is secured to the ski.
- XC is more of an "all-terrain" sport. Unlike downhill, which is done on groomed slopes, XC can be done on unbroken snow, on trails, or in the wild. "Backcountry" cross-country skiers, for example, learn how to cross fences without removing their skis.
- Cross-country skiing makes a strong claim to being an endurance sport. Whereas a downhill skier can often spend the better part of the day waiting in line to ride the lifts, once a cross-country skier has on her skis, she can tour nonstop if she wishes. Also, where a ski lift pulls a downhill skier up, a XC skier must do it herself and push herself up the slopes.
- Cross-country skiing equipment is less elaborate than downhill and is easier to use. Innovative micro skis (ski length is only chest high) in particular have reduced the learning curve for XC skiing.
- By all accounts, the sport is less expensive, too—you don't need the complex boots and bindings required for downhill, and you don't necessarily have to XC ski at a resort (you can ski out your back door if there's snow).

How It's Done: The many variations of cross-country skiing include:

- *Classical or traditional XC:* This is the type about which people say, "If you can walk, you can cross-country ski." Its movements are similar to an aggressive power walk, and it involves sturdy, diagonal, forward-gliding motions and use of two poles.
- *Freestyle:* This style is more similar to skating or roller blading than to walking, since skiers use the inside edge of their

ski to get traction and work up speed. It's a faster form of XC skiing than classical and often involves no poles.

- *Nordic downhill or telemark:* Telemarkers tend to live for steep descents, since that's where they can practice their trademark maneuver, telemark turns, which are described as ''a curtsy-like move'' that involves a ''distinctive raising and lowering of the body'' by Laurie Gullion in *Nordic Skiing: Steps to Success* (Human Kinetics, 1993).

- *Ski racing:* Cross-country ski competitions (which are similar in character to road races and are of varying distances) are held in most cold weather regions in the United States, and most are open to competitors of all ages and abilities. The premier ski race in North America is the 55k American Birkebeiner held in Wisconsin. It attracts over eight thousand skiers from around the world. (Contact: American Birkebeiner Ski Foundation, P.O. Box 911, Hayward, WI; phone: 715-634-5025; www.winaona.com/birkie.)

Key Physical Requirements: It's a fact that most of the best XC skiers are also very good runners or bikers. That's because they have already built up the strong leg muscles and endurance needed for XC skiing. But unlike running, XC skiing can result in better conditioning of your arms and whole upper torso if you ski using poles. Poling requires you swing and pump your arms vigorously, forward and backward, simultaneously but in an opposite direction with your feet.

Equipment: Basically, you need skis, bindings, poles, and boots. But you'll want to match your equipment with the type of skiing you want to do. For example, telemark skis tend to be fat and heavy to facilitate turning in deep snow and navigating over steep terrain. Classical XC skis are lighter and skinnier. Then there are decisions on whether to buy skis with waxable or waxless bases. As general rule, waxable skis glide and grip better; however, waxless skis are easier for beginners to just strap on and use, and you don't have to learn the rather considerable nuances in theory concerning the proper waxing of skis.

If you've never XC skied, consider renting skis the first few times you go out. That will give you a feel for what level and what kind of involvement you are likely to want to have in the sport and will thus help steer you to the right choice of ski.

What to Wear: Avoid a heavy, bulky parka since it'll probably make you too hot and sweaty; then, when you remove it, you may become too cold. Laurie Gullion, a top ski instructor and author of *Nordic Skiing: Steps to Success*, recommends a three-layered system: (1) a wicking layer of long underwear, polypropylene or silk, close to the skin, that moves perspiration away from the body into other layers; (2) an insulating layer in the middle, such as a wool sweater to provide warmth; and (3) a weather-proof layer on the outside to shed wind, rain, or snow.

In addition, you'll want to wear sweat-wicking, insulated socks; depending on the weather and how cold you tend to become, you will probably also want to wear a lightweight hat, gloves, and neck warmer.

To Find Out More:

Start by checking out the "Cross Country Ski Festival Of Fun," which offers free on-snow XC ski lessons for first-timers at ski sites and shops across the United States and Canada. The festival is sponsored by the Cross Country Ski Area Association (CCSAA), a not-for-profit organization that can also help you find XC local ski areas, instruction, and equipment. To find out if there is a host site near you (or for other XC info) contact:

Ski Fest Headquarters
Cross Country Ski Area Association
259 Bolton Road
Winchester, NH 03470
PHONE: 603-239-4341
FAX: 603-239-6387
EMAIL: skifest@xcski.org
WEBSITE: www.xcski.org

Another way to find a qualified XC ski instructor in your area is through this organization:

Professional Ski Instructors of America
A-1 Lincoln Avenue
Albany, NY 12205-4907
PHONE: 518-452-6095

A great website for educational articles, general information and news related to virtually every aspect of cross-country skiing and racing is cross-country ski world at www.xcskiworld.com. It is exclusively an on-line publication.

Finally, the following Nordic skiing magazine can be a great source for up-to-date buyer's guides as well as an easy way to find racing locales and schedules:

Cross Country Skier
P.O. Box 50120
Minneapolis MN
PHONE: 612-377-0312
800-827-0607 subscriptions
WEBSITE: www.crosscountryskier.com

Books to Check Out
Laurie Gullion, *Nordic Skiing: Steps to Success*
(Champaign, Ill.: Human Kinetics, 1993).
This is a great beginner's guide, with all the essentials about equipment, fundamental skills, and techniques.

Paul Parker, *Free-Heel Skiing: Telemark and Parallel Techniques for All Conditions* (Seattle, Wash.: The Mountaineers, 1995).
A good guide for more advanced skiers.

◐ XC Talk:

Binding: The device that holds the toe of the boot securely to the ski.

Herringbone: A way of getting uphill on XC skis, so-called because the tracks left in the snow form a herringbone pattern.

Snowplow: Getting down a hill by moving the tails of the skis outward, while the tips point inward to form an inverted V shape.

CYCLING

Although it's easy to get overwhelmed by the many variations of this sport—and the choices in gear—the truth is you can dust off that old bike in your garage, bring it in for a tune-up, and begin riding for fitness right away. Wear old running or other workout clothes as well as a helmet and design a training schedule as you would when starting out in any other sport: gradually increase your distances, times, and intensity as you build up your leg strength and aerobic capacity. Alternate easy workouts on relatively flat terrain with ones that include some challenging hills.

Of course, if you decide to go further with your cycling, you'll want to learn more—for example, you'll want to master some of the technical skills that allow you to make turns, climb hills, and descend more efficiently. Undoubtedly, too, you'll be faced with bicycling's Biggest Question: What bike should I buy?

How It's Done: There are two main branches of biking:

Road biking—simply, cycling on paved roads: Road races tend to be endurance events, usually 25 miles or more in length, intermixed with a capacity to sprint, since racers often reach speeds of 40 miles per hour or more. For recreational riders, road racing can be a solo endeavor—you race to see how well you perform as an individual. On the competitive level, however, road racing is a team sport—it requires team members to employ an intricate use of tactics to thwart their opponents' progress.

Mountain biking—this is "off-road" biking over unpaved trails, in fields, forests, sand, mud, and anything else that happens to get in the way: The most common type of competition is cross country, races of over 10 miles that traverse terrain that includes hills, twists, and turns. But there are also hill climbing competitions, one-way speed downhill runs, and slalom events.

Other, less common types of biking:

Bicycle motor-cross or BMX racing: The races are conducted on bikes with beefed-up frames and special tires; the bikers wear full protective gear, including motorcycle-like helmets; and the race is conducted on a dirt track that has ramps, mounds for jumping, gravel pits, and sometimes water traps.

Cyclo-cross racing: This is a combination cross-country race and obstacle course. Bikers usually must carry their bikes up loose gravel, slippery ice slopes, or stairways for at least 25 percent of the time. Distances tends to be anywhere from 12 to 20 miles.

Artistic cycling: This kind of racing tends to be more popular in Europe and is basically a type of bicycle gymnastics.

Bicycle polo. This competition is a rough-and-tumble field sport in which the players try to maneuver a ball into their goal while bike-bound, as in regular polo played on horseback.

Key Physical Requirements: Your lungs and legs (especially your calves and quadriceps muscles) get a workout when you bike for fitness. It's not a weight-bearing exercise, so it won't stress your joints.

Some women find riding causes discomfort in their pelvic region—their position on the bike forces their weight onto their pubic bone. If you are riding the right size bike, this problem can usually be corrected by making small adjustments in how you sit on your bike and in the position of your bike's seat in relation to its handlebars. If you adjust your handlebars so that they are slightly lower than your seat, you'll find your weight is automatically distributed more toward the rear of your bike, which takes pressure off your pubic area. Make sure your seat angles downward too, not up. You might also want to investigate buying a bike seat made for women, since these are shaped to support a woman's wider hips and often contain better cushioning.

Equipment: If you are buying a bike, the first decision you need to make is whether you want a mountain bike, a hybrid, or a road bike:

Mountain bikes: These bikes are the biggest sellers right now because they are the most versatile—they can go anywhere although they are slower on the road than road bikes. Mountain bikes have wide, knobby tires and a sturdy, strong frame; you sit upright in the saddle; the handle bars are straight across. Many are amazingly lightweight. If you plan to do a lot of riding on trails or dirt roads, this should be your choice.

Road bikes: These bikes are made to allow for maximum speed and good aerodynamics; they have drop handlebars and require a hunched over position (i.e., you are not in a sitting position). If roads are your venue and speed is your ambition, this is the only choice.

Hybrids: This cross between a mountain and road bike is a great compromise if you aren't sure what type of biking you want to do. If you primarily plan to stay on the roads, but don't want to be excluded from some trail riding, and you prefer to ride sitting upright, this bike is a good choice.

Price will help you narrow down your choices further—decent bikes start at around $200 but can run into the thousands of dollars (many cost more than small cars). Your best place to buy a bike is a bike shop staffed by trained bike mechanics and experienced bikers. They will know how to fit you properly for a bike, they will encourage you to take a bike out on a test ride, they will know how to put your bike together correctly, and they will usually avoid high-pressure selling tactics. Unlike department stores, which plan to sell you a bike then never see you again, a bike store aims to draw you into the fold and have you become a regular customer. They want you to return to them for tune-ups, advice, repairs, upgrades, etc. Bike shops also offer discounts on things like helmets, flat repair kits, water bottle cages, rearview mirrors, car carriers, and other accessories when you buy a bike. (Be forewarned: cycling can quickly become a gear-intensive, expensive sport, but you also do quite well if you need to stick to the bare essentials.) Finally, bike shops are a great place to tap into information about your local biking scene.

What to Wear: The only essential is a helmet; Optional items include biking gloves, which have half-fingers and padded palms; biking shorts, which have built-in cushioning to reduce saddle soreness; biking shoes, which have extra-stiff soles so that you experience less foot pressure and numbness as a result of constant pedaling; and a cycling jersey, which has rear pockets for carrying food, water, maps, or other gear.

To Find Out More

The United States Cycling Federation, the organization responsible for amateur road and track racing in America, and the National Off-Road Bicycle Association (NORBA), which governs the sport of mountain biking, can help you find local, regional, and national biking events as well as clubs: Both organizations function under the umbrella of USA Cycling.

USA Cycling
United States Cycling Federation
National Off-Road Bicycle Association (NORBA)
One Olympic Plaza
Colorado Springs, CO 80909
PHONE: (719) 578-4581
FAX: (719) 578-4628 or (719) 578-4596
E-mail for USA Cycling Federation: uscf@usacycling.org
E-mail for NORBA: norba@usacycling.org
WEBSITE: www.usacycling.org

There are a wide variety of magazines devoted exclusively to cycling; probably the best for beginners is *Bicycling*, since it covers all types and aspects of biking, plus it regularly features articles directed at new cyclists:

Bicycling
33 East Minor Street
Emmaus, PA 18049
PHONE: 610-967-5171
WEBSITE: www.bicyclingmagazine.com

Books to Check Out

James C. McCullagh, *Cycling for Health, Fitness, and Well-Being* (New York: Dell Publishing, 1995).
Written in a conversational style, this is a great beginner's guide—it's filled with commonsense tips (on things like climbing, turning corners, and so on) as well as useful technical information (on what features to look for when buying a bike and which sales pitches to ignore).

Ed Pavelka and the editors of *Bicycling* magazine, *Bicycling Magazine's Complete Book of Road Cycling Skills*. (Emmaus, Penna.: Rodale Books, 1998).
Contains good advice on how to care for your bike, and many specifics on how to boost your efficiency with smooth pedaling and proper form; how to brake without wiping out; how to deal with cycling in a variety of weather conditions.

Dennis Coello, *The New Complete Mountain Biker*
(New York: Lyons and Burford Publishers, 1997).
Besides good sections on mountain biking skills, this book is
strong in its information on how to pack and plan for back
country and wilderness mountain biking tours and camping
trips. It does not contain information about racing.

◐ Bike Talk:

Bonk: A feeling of total depletion during a long race. When
you "bonk" you wonder why you ever wanted to race in the first
place and you struggle with feelings of wanting to quit.

Breakaway: A tactic used in road racing in which a rider or
group of riders surge to the front of the main pack by suddenly
sprinting ahead.

Granny gear: The lowest gear that allows you to spin easily
and is used for extremely steep climbs. Sometimes it's called the
"weenie gear."

Hammer: To pedal all out—full force at top speed; "hammered"
however, means to feel wiped out, completely spent and
exhausted.

GENERAL GYMNASTICS

Although an early start is a must for high-level competitive
gymnastics, women of any age can do what's been dubbed
"general gymnastics," a hybrid form of the sport designed for
recreational gymnasts of all ages and abilities. The governing
body for gymnastic competition in the United States, USA Gymnastics, is actively trying to promote general gymnastics as a
sport "for everyone" and is trying to encourage gyms across
the country to offer instruction in general gymnastics as well.

How It's Done: General gymnastics blends a variety of different elements drawn from traditional gymnastics, dance, aerobics, and calisthenics. A series of classes might include
instruction in headstands, backflips, cartwheels; use of the bal-

ance beam, uneven bars, and vault; use of the hoop, rope, and ribbons in rhythmic gymnastics; rope climbing, trampolining, and all sorts of choreographed dance movements and routines. The logical progression of classes are performances; beyond that, there are national showcase performances, "GymFests," in which you can participate.

Key Physical Requirements: The best gymnasts combine strength (especially upper body strength) with flexibility, coordination, and natural grace and agility. However, many athletes become involved in general gymnastics because, for example, they've become stiff and want to become more flexible.

Equipment: at the very least, you need a gym equipped with mats and horizontal bars. Ideally, the gym should have other traditional gymnastics apparatus as well, such as a balance beam, vault, trampoline, rings, etc.

What to Wear: full body leotard or leggings with a tee-shirt that tucks in, since you may be doing things like flips or headstands. Many athletes prefer to go barefoot, but you can also wear gymnastic slippers or some sort of nonskid sock.

To Find Out More
USA Gymnastics can help you find a gym club that sponsors "general gymnastics" activities.

USA Gymnastics
Attn.: General Gymnastics
Pan American Plaza, Suite 300
201 S. Capitol Avenue
Indianapolis, IN 46225
PHONE: 317-237-5050
FAX: 317-237-5069
E-MAIL: gg@usa-gymnastics.org
WEBSITE: www.usa-gymnastics.org (on the website, there is a search feature "Find a gym club" in which you can type in your city, state, and zip code).

Books to Check Out
Since general gymnastics is something of a hodgepodge of different disciplines, there isn't one tome available (yet) to guide you. In fact, you should be a little leery of standard gymnastics

guides since the "adult version" of gymnastics tends to be less contortionist and progresses at a more moderate pace than the version young children learn.

◖ Gymnastics Lingo:

Arch position: When your body is curved backward.

Rolls: There are many variations on the somersault, including a forward roll, backward roll, straight-leg forward roll, forward straddle roll, and backward straddle roll.

Spotter: A person who gives assurance as well as physical support whenever you are trying a new and/or tricky maneuver, such as a backbend.

IN-LINE SKATING

Many athletes are intrigued by in-line skating because it looks so fluid and fun, but they're also a bit afraid of trying it because they have heard so much about the sport's high rate of injuries. Understandably, they don't want to put their performance in their primary sport at risk by getting injured while in-line skating.

The good news is that if you wear protective gear, in-line skating doesn't appear to be any more dangerous than most sports. According to a study conducted at Tripler Army Medical Center in Hawaii of eighty-one people treated for in-line skating injuries, 90 percent of them were not wearing a complete set of protective gear at the time of injury.

In addition, according to most skating instructors, in-line skating isn't particularly hard to pick up as an adult—especially if you learn by taking a lesson. In fact, if you know how to ice skate, in-line skating should come quite easily to you.

How It's Done: There are all kinds of variations to the sport of in-line skating, including:

- _Outdoor speed skating and competition._ Races can involve short sprints of 200 to 500 meters, 10ks (which most "middle-of-the-pack" skaters can finish in about 25 minutes) or ultramarathons.

- *Skate dancing or artistic skating.* This is very similar, in both movement and appearance, to figure skating and ice dancing.
- *Extreme, stunt, or aggressive skating.* Experts make it look easy, but even the most basic "extreme" maneuvers, such as jumping over obstacles, skating down a flight of stairs, or sliding down the edge of a stair railing, take a tremendous amount of skill and control.
- *Roller hockey.* In the early 1980s, a group of ice hockey players from Minneapolis were looking for a way to train off-season and came up with the original idea for modern in-line skates. Today, the game of roller hockey, which like ice hockey is played with a weighted puck and wooden hockey sticks, has its own distinct set of official rules as well as its own association, The National In-Line Hockey Association. In general, roller hockey is paced faster than ice hockey; it's "gentler" too, since "checking" (body contact) and aggressive behavior are not allowed.

Key Physical Requirements: In-line skating is a lower-impact sport than running; there is less stress placed on your knees, hips, and other joints. But you still need strong legs. If you are a runner or cyclist, in fact, you may find that the stroking motion (the pushing off and to the side with your leg) involved in in-line skating works muscles you normally don't use (primarily the hip and thigh extensor muscles).

In-line skating can also require endurance if you skate to get a workout or to race; daring and an ability to face fear if you aim to try extreme in-line skating stunts; flexibility, especially if you in-line skate dance.

Equipment: If you are not sure what your level of commitment to in-line skating is likely to be, you might consider renting skates for a few sessions before buying. Although rental skates are not likely to be as high a quality as you can buy, they're an economical way for you to get a taste of what the sport involves.

In-line skates start at around $75 and can cost over $400. You probably need to spend between $100 and $200 to get a decent pair of skates for recreational use; if you intend to work out or race on your skates, you may need to spend more. Besides the fit and comfort of the boot, which is of paramount importance, the features you need to pay attention to are as follows:

1. the boot's liner, which should provide good ventilation and cushioning
2. the footbed, which should offer shock absorption features
3. wheel size (the bigger the wheel, the faster the skate)
4. wheel durometer or softness (the harder the wheel, the faster the skate), wheel design (skates made for hockey may have wider wheels), and finally, the quality of your wheels' inner bearings

You can get additional information on how to buy skates from the resources mentioned in the "to find out more" section, below.

What to Wear: full protective gear, which should include a helmet (although there are now helmets made specifically for in-line skating, a Snell safety certified bike helmet provides effective protection too); wrist guards (one for each hand) equipped with plastic braces on the inside of your wrists; knee pads; and elbow guards. The majority of in-line skating injuries are forearm and wrist fractures, followed by ankle, knee and lower leg fractures.

In-skaters tend to wear stretchable biker shorts and close-fitting tops made out of breathable fabric.

To Find Out More

The International Inline Skating Association (INSA) can help you find an instructor, choose gear, as well provide you with information on competition for recreational in-line skating, skate racing, skate dancing, or hockey.

International Inline Skating Association
201 North Front Street
Suite 1306
Wilmington, NC 28401
PHONE: 910-762-7004
FAX: 910-762-9477
WEBSITE: www.iisa.org
E-MAIL: getinline@iisa.org

In addition, an index to virtually every resource available for in-line skating can be found on the World Wide Web at www.skatecity.com/index/

Books to Check Out

Neil Feineman with Team Rollerblade, *Wheel Excitement: The Official Rollerblade® Guide to In-Line Skating* (New York: Hearst Books, 1991).
This is a very well-written introduction to all aspects of in-line skating. The section for beginners is especially strong and filled with useful tips.

Mark Powell and John Svensson, *In-Line Skating* (Champaign, Ill.: Human Kinetics, 1998).
A no-nonsense, solid, information-filled guide, with many photos and illustrations showing skating techniques.

◗ Skate Talk

Black ice: A smooth, recently paved street that is ideal for skating.

Road rash: Scrapes and cuts you get when you fall on unprotected flesh.

Vert skating: "Vert" or vertical skating is a series of aerial tricks, turns, and twists, including flip turns, performed by "extreme" skaters on ramps that curve up to straight walls.

Wall riding: Another "extreme" in-line skate maneuver in which the skater charges the wall at an angle, jumps up, and touches the wall with her inside hand as she uses her leading foot to push herself off and away.

RACQUETBALL

Next to badminton, racquetball is considered one of the simpler racket sports to learn to play. The racket is easy to handle and the ball is very bouncy, which means you have a little leeway in time to get to it before it strikes the floor a second time. Serving is relatively simple, plus there are only three main strokes (forehand, backhand drive, and overhead), none of which is very complicated. The rules are pretty straightforward, too.

Of course, like any sport, the nature of the game changes the more competitively you play it. On a professional level, for example, rallies tend to be spectacularly short and fast moving; on a recreational level, play tends to be more continuous, although still quite fast and energetic.

How It's Played: The game is played on an enclosed court, 40 feet long, 20 feet wide, and 20 feet high. All six surfaces are used in play (in other words, unlike squash, it's okay to hit the ceiling and the upper portions of the walls). The front wall is key since the object of the game is to return each shot to that wall before the ball has bounced on the floor a second time.

You use a short-handled (22 inches in length is the maximum), strung racket; the ball is hollow rubber and bouncy (about the size of a tennis ball but without the fuzz). The first person to get 15 points wins the game; you only score when you are serving. A match is the best two games out of three.

It's possible to play doubles, although it's not as common as in tennis and there are different rules. In addition, many players have strong personal prejudices against racquetball doubles. For example, Victor I. Spear, M.D., in *Sports Illustrated Racquetball* (JP Lippincott Co., 1979), has these strong words to say about racquetball doubles: "I see it as a perversion of a gorgeous sport— finesse transmuted into a brawl. The ultracerebral chess game becomes a chaos of four players seeming to throw the pieces at each other. Both tennis and handball allow for great doubles action without losing the intrinsic soul of the game. Racquetball doubles is not a natural extension of the singles game but a totally different game and, in my view, a poor one."

Key Physical Requirements: The following points are the important requirements to play the game well.

- *Endurance.* Most matches take anywhere from one hour to ninety minutes to play; during most of that time, you are sprinting, pivoting, and diving for the ball. So you need to be able to sustain relatively continuous motion for over an hour. "Fatigue is the assassin of the racquetball player, a foe more dangerous than your opponent," writes Dr. Spear. That's because the more tired you become from lack of proper endurance, the more errors you are likely to make.

- *Forearm and wrist strength.* You generate the power of your swing in racquetball from your forearm and with the snap of your wrist. Authors Charles Brumfield (five times National Champion) and Jeffrey N. Bairstow in *Off the Wall: Championship Racquetball for the Ardent Amateur* suggest doing conventional push-ups to strengthen these muscles as well as doing wrist curls.
- *Agility.* You need to be able to scramble around the court quickly. Warming up before playing a vigorous game, then stretching afterward can help keep you flexible and nimble.

Equipment: Protective goggles are required in most tournaments and recreational facilities, since the speed of the ball (up to 140 mph) can inflict serious damage to your eyes.

Rackets start at around $45 and come in different grip sizes and weights. Balls, which come in specifications set by the United States Racquetball Association, usually cost under $2 to $3 each.

What to wear: Most professional players wear a thin leather glove or half-glove to help them grip the racket better. Loose-fitting, tennis-style attire is usually preferred. Heavy, perspiration-wicking socks are essential to prevent blisters. Workout shoes designed for tennis or other court sports are best.

To Find Out More

Contact the United States Racquetball Association (USRA) or visit their website to find local clubs, instructors, and tournament dates.

United States Raquetball Association
1685 West Uintah Street
Colorado Springs, CO, 80904
PHONE: 719-635-5396
FAX: 719-635-0685
WEBSITE: www.racquetball.org or www.usra.org

Book to Check Out

Stan Kittleson, *Racquetball: Steps to Success* (Champaign, Ill.: Human Kinetics, 1996).

As with all the books in the Steps to Success series, this is a copiously illustrated workbook that delineates virtually every detail of how to play the game. There is not a lot of narrative (i.e., there is no chatty talk about the nature and history of the game); instead the emphasis is on exercises and drills.

◆ Racquetball Lingo:

Hinders: Similar to a foul ball in other sports, hinders come in two varieties. Avoidable hinders, which result in a loss of a rally by the offender, are those that a player causes by not moving out of the way of another player or deliberately pushing an opponent. Deadball hinders, which don't result in any penalties, are caused unintentionally. For example, if a ballpasses through the legs of a player and there is no fair chance of returning it, a deadball hinder is called and the rally is replayed.

Shooter: Also called a gunner or killer, the term refers to a player who uses a high number of kill shots.

Z-ball: A defensive shot in which the ball travels in three directions, off the front wall into the side wall, then diagonally into the back court where it zings and jumps with a lot of sidespin off the second side wall. Executed correctly, it can be almost impossible to return.

ROWING

In the past few years there's been a small boom in recreational rowing among adult women of all ages and abilities (in other words, many of these women are well over age twenty-one and never rowed in college).

In its essence, the sport of rowing is about "pulling a perfect stroke"—having your oar bite the water at just the proper depth so it creates maximum power and minimal drag. In crew (team rowing), you not only aim for a perfect stroke, you aim for perfect synchronization, too, since you need to time your movements perfectly with the rowing cadence of the other rowers. By all accounts, rowing takes intense concentration. But when everything "clicks," rowing should feel natural, fluid, and comfortable.

How It's Done: In this sport a boat is called a shell, which is an apt term considering that the hull on the boats is only about ⅛ to ¼ inch thick to make it as light as possible (some shells weigh as little as 14 pounds). Shells, in general, are long and narrow. Racing shells are as narrow as possible while recreational ones can be rather wide. The seats in a shell are mounted on wheels that are mounted on runners: they slide so that you can row in tandem while extending your legs and then bending your knees. In a shell, you face backward in order to go forward.

In crew or sweep rowing, every rower has one oar, which she uses two hands to power. Crews can consist of two, four, or eight people. Sometimes, boats are manned with a coxswain, a person who faces the rowers (and thus looks out in the direction the boat is headed) and gives steering directions.

In sculling, a rower has two oars, one hand on each. Generally, sculls are single, one-person boats. In competition, it's usually one scull against another, a one-on-one contest. Less common are double and four-person sculls.

If you crave friendship and camaraderie, sweep rowing or crew tends to foster it, since it involves some of the most intense, finely tuned teamwork of any sport. In contrast, if what you really want is time alone and/or don't want to deal with the pressure that comes with having to perform as part of team, you might prefer sculling since it is such a solitary activity.

Key Physical Requirements: You need endurance capacity since a half hour of hard rowing is roughly equivalent to running 5 miles, according to author D. C. Churback in *The Book of Rowing* (The Overlook Press, 1988). There's no doubt that rowing works out your whole body, although it particularly requires strong arm, shoulder, back, and abdominal muscles.

Expect your hands to become blistered and callused—it's an inevitable consequence of pulling an oar regularly. As for gloves, most coaches don't recommend them because they dull your ability to feel and respond to the oar. Plus, developing tough calluses does eventually become an asset for a rower, since they allow you to row for long periods without pain.

◓ Rowing's Winter Alternative: Indoor Regattas

The primary off-season training for virtually all serious rowers is to use the Concept II rowing ergometer (a flywheel rowing machine that is a fixture in most health clubs as well as rowing clubs). There are even "indoor" or "erg" regattas—competitions in which hundreds of rowers compete on gym equipment. The most famous of these competitions is the World Indoor Rowing Championships, also known as the CRASH-B sprints, which is usually held in Cambridge/Boston, Massachusetts, in mid-February and boasts over 1,200 participants. The usual "distance" (as measured on an electronic monitor) is 2,000 meters. There are erg regattas all over the country; a complete listing of indoor regattas is available from Concept II:

Concept II
R.R. 1, Box 1100
Morrisville, VT 05661-9727
PHONE: 800-245-5676
WEBSITE: www.concept2.com
E-MAIL: rowing@concept2.com

Equipment: Your boathouse should provide virtually everything you need, including oars. Single sculls usually can be rented, too.

What to Wear: Having a change of clothes is the first rule of rowing, since there is always the chance that your boat will capsize. The other rule is to avoid clothing that dangles down or is too loose, since it can get caught in and jam the seat mechanism. Most rowers opt for clothes that are fairly tight fitting so as to avoid this problem. In the heat of summer, you might wear cycling shorts, a close-fitted tee-shirt, and water shoes. In cooler weather, you'll want to wear breathable layers that provide warmth, can be easily removed if you become too hot and aren't too bulky. Rowers tend to get dirty (dealing with the grease on the oars, the mud on the shore, and so on), so older, even ripped or tattered clothing, is generally part of the unofficial uniform.

Most rowers wear caps and/or sunglasses to keep the glare out of their eyes.

To Find Out More

A good place to start looking for information is U.S. Rowing, the National Governing Body for the sport (it's responsible for the selection, training, and management of the U.S. Rowing National Team that represents the United States in the Olympics and other competitions). U.S. Rowing publishes *U.S. Rowing,* the only magazine devoted exclusively to rowing, maintains a Resource Library of over six hundred articles on rowing, and provides many services for recreational rowers of all ages. It can help you find a rowing organization near you as well as help you locate regional races and regattas.

> U.S. Rowing Association
> Pan American Plaza, Suite 400
> 201 South Capitol Avenue
> Indianapolis, IN 46225
> A toll-free member services number: 800-314-4ROW
> PHONE: 317-237-5656
> FAX: 317-237-5646
> E-MAIL: usrowing@aol.com
> WEBSITE: www.usrowing.org

Two useful websites are the Rower's Resource at www.rowers resource.com and Row as One Institute at www.tiac.net/users/rowasone/. Both can link you to clubs, regattas, camps, equipment, and so forth.

Books to Check Out

There are not many books on rowing, and most of the good ones are frequently out of stock. If you can't find these at your local bookseller, your local library may have them.

D. C. Churback, *The Book of Rowing* (Woodstock, N.Y.: The Overlook Press, 1988).
This extremely well-written book does much to capture the spirit of the sport while, at the same time, providing a lot of concrete information and instruction.

Nick Smith, *The Complete Book of Rowing and Sculling from Beginner to Champion* (New York: North South Books, 1989).

> ### ◒ Rowing Lingo
>
> _Crab:_ According to author D. C. Churback in _The Book of Rowing_, a crab "is the biggest mistake a rower can make." It refers to a situation in which the blade of the oar slices downward, goes out of control, and gets "stuck" in the water. A crab can severely slow a boat down or even cause it to capsize.
>
> _Feathering:_ The act of rotating or turning the blade of the oar. a feathered blade is parallel to the water's surface.
>
> _Rushing:_ Arriving at the catch—the point when the oar first bites into the water—too early. When one rower rushes, the shell's movement gets out of sync.

RUNNING

It could convincingly be argued that running—of all sports—is the easiest to get involved in. All it requires is that you lace up your shoes and head out the door. It can be solitary or social, depending on your mood and circumstances. It can be done at virtually any time of day, so you don't have to be a slave to gym or court schedules. It's accessible for other reasons, too: You can find running clubs in virtually every community across the country. There are road races available in a wide variety of distances (and all but a few welcome the participation of recreational runners). And there's a mountain of good information—in the form of books, magazines, newsletters, and websites—that makes starting a running program (or revising your present routine) extremely easy.

How It's Done: Running can be ritualistic and nothing else: Your involvement in the sport might not go beyond running once or twice a week, by yourself, a certain distance and route each time. Many runners find this monotonous approach to running is just what the doctor ordered at times—it keeps them fit and helps clear their minds when they are experiencing a lot of stress or engagement in other areas of their lives.

The step up to racing can be made at any time. Thanks to the popularity of the sport, at most local and large-scale races there are large numbers of first-timers—entrants who have never raced at all or who have never raced the distance before. Included among the competition opportunities available for recreational runners are (1) road races, which vary in length from one mile to 5 k (3.1miles) to 10 k to marathons (26.2 miles); (2) trail competitions, which are held off-road, usually in woodsy terrain on dirt paths; and (3) less commonly, track events, which generally involve sprinting for shorter distances.

Key Physical Requirements: Although elite runners tend to be lean and sometimes quite long-legged, you don't need to possess any particular body type to be good at the sport. If you have ever observed a marathon, you'll have noted that runners come in all heights, weights, and ages. *Runners World* magazine even runs a monthly column titled "The Penguin Chronicles," which details the experiences of an avid runner (John Bingham) who also happens to be quite slow and stout.

Equipment: Virtually none. Many serious runners use a heart rate monitor to evaluate the progress of their training. For information, the *Runner's World* website (www.runnersworld.com) has some past articles posted on the pros and cons of heart rate monitors; the book *Serious Training for Endurance Athletes* by Rob Sleamaker and Ray Browing (Human Kinetics, 1996) contains tips on how to use and select a monitor.

What to Wear: Most important is a pair of running shoes that fit properly. If you need help selecting a running shoe, the American Running and Fitness Association will send you a questionaire to fill out (it asks you about what kind of running you do, the mileage you log in a typical week, requests you trace the outline of your foot, and so on), then matches your responses with the information in the AFRA Running Shoe Database to come up with a list of recommended running shoes for you (the printout includes the cost of all the shoes sold in the United States that might fit your need). For nonmembers, the service costs $10; it's free for members (membership costs $15 and includes a subscription to ARFA's monthly newsletter and maps of local running trails across the country, among other things). To contact ARFA:

American Running and Fitness Association
4405 East-West Highway

Suite 405
Bethesda, MD, 20814
PHONE: 301-913-9517 or 800-776-ARFA
FAX: 301-913-9520
E-MAIL: arfarun@aol.com
WEBSITE: www.arfa.org)

Beyond your all-important shoes, you want good athletic socks and clothes that are lightweight and help manage your perspiration. Simultaneously you don't want your clothes to chafe or constrict your movement. The only hard and fast rule for running garb is to test it out several times to make sure it feels comfortable before you wear it in a race.

To Find Out More

To find a local running club, contact the Road Runners Club of America, a national organization of more than 550 chapter clubs in 46 states with more than 150,000 members.

RRCA National Office
1150 South Washington Street, Suite 250
Alexandria, VA 22314-4493
PHONE: 703-836-0558
E-MAIL: office@rrca.org
WEBSITE: www.rrca.org

To find local trails and trail running events, contact the All American Trail Running Association, which also publishes a quarterly newsletter *Trail Times*:

AATRA
P.O. Box 9175
Colorado Springs, CO 80932
PHONE: 719-570-9795
E-MAIL: trlrunner@aol.com.
WEBSITE: www.trailrunner.com

For information about track events as well as race walking and distance competitions in your area, USA Track and Field will help you find a local member association:

USA Track & Field
One RCA Dome, Suite 140
Indianapolis, IN 46225
PHONE: 317-261-0500
FAX: 317-261-0481
WEBSITE: www.usatf.org

The running magazines are another great source of training advice and up-to-date race information. Two that are easy to find on most newsstands and always contain something of use to a recreational runner are *Runner's World* (which weighs in more heavily with articles specifically geared to beginning and women runners) and *Running Times* (which is slanted a bit more toward the already established, serious runner)

Runner's World
Editorial address: 33 East Minor Street, Emmaus, PA 18098
Subscription address: P.O. Box 7307, Red Oak, IA 51591-0307
PHONE: (for subscription info): 800-666-2828
FAX: 610-967-8883
E-MAIL (for editorial): rwedit@rodalepress.com
E-MAIL (for subscription info): runnerwdm@aol.com
WEBSITE: www.runnersworld.com

Running Times
Editorial address: 213 Danbury Road, Wilton, CT 06897
Subscription address: P.O. Box 50016, Boulder, CO 80322-0016
FAX (for editorial): 203-761-9933
PHONE (for subscription info): 800-816-4735

Books to Check Out
Of the dozens available, these two stand out since they are directed to women runners. Both also include a lot of information about cross-training and nutrition for runners:

Joan Benoit Samuelson and Gloria Averbuch, *Joan Samuelson's Running for Women* (Emmaus, PA.: Rodale Press, 1995).

Gordon Bakoulis Bloch, *How to Train For and Run Your Best Marathon* (New York: Fireside, 1993).

◆ **Runner's Jargon**

Fartlek: A Swedish term for speed play—a type of training in which a runner intersperses intervals of fast running with more moderately paced periods. Its purpose is to make you faster.

Hitting the wall: A feeling of depletion and despair that some runners experience at around mile 20 of a marathon.

Ultramarathon: Races (usually but not always trail events) of distances over 26.2 miles, often 50 to 100 miles long.

SKATING

Gliding on the ice can make you feel unfettered, fluid, and graceful (once you get the hang of it!). In fact, the sense of freedom you can get when skating is similar to what you might experience when riding a bike or cruising down a street on in-line skates.

But skating isn't a single sport, it's divided into three main branches: figure skating, speed skating, and ice hockey.

Figure skating: There are five main disciplines to figure skating:

1. Figures, which consists of forty-one geometrical designs traced on the ice by the skater, all based on the figure eight
2. Freestyle, which consists of jumps, spins, arabesques, footwork, and other movements skated to music over the whole ice surface
3. Pair skating, which is really freestyle done by two people together but includes many daring and difficult lifts and spins
4. Precision skating, a highly technical form of group skating performed by teams of twelve to twenty-four skaters
5. Ice dancing—a type of ballroom dancing on ice

Speed skating: It's just like track racing, except the track is coated with ice and the competitors wear skates. Tracks can be either indoor or outdoor.

Ice hockey: This team sport is growing in popularity among girls and women, who tend to play a cleaner game than men's ice hockey (i.e., there's no "checking" or aggressive body contact allowed). Each team has six players on the ice, three in offensive positions, two in defensive positions, and one goalkeeper. Players use curved hockey sticks to try to land a puck—a hard, round rubber disk—in the opponents' goal.

What's Involved: you need to learn the basic skill of skating. Each branch of skating comes with its own variety of skate, so if you know you want to learn to play ice hockey exclusively, you should probably learn to skate using hockey skates. Otherwise, if you are uncertain about what direction your involvement in the sport will take, figure skates are probably easiest to learn on.

Consider taking lessons if you've never stepped on the ice before and/or if you skated minimally as a child. You'll learn how to step on to the ice without falling, how to get up without slipping, and other important skills much faster than if you try to learn on your own. Many rinks hold adult classes.

Key Physical Requirements: Many people avoid ice skating because of a fear of falling and a belief that they have weak ankles. "This myth of weak ankles has probably been propagated by skaters using poor-quality ice skates. In the absence of a serious medical condition, people don't have weak ankles, they simply have weak ice skates or have not fitted their skates properly," declare Karin Kunzel-Watson and Stephen J. DeArmond in *Ice Skating: Steps to Success* (Human Kinetics, 1996).

But what about falling—is it inevitable? Yes, even the best skaters fall sometimes. Still, falls rarely cause serious injuries, according to Kunzel-Watson and DeArmond: "Several studies have found that the single most significant factor related to injuries is the skater's skill level. Most of those who get hurt have skated less than ten times. Many of these injuries are preventable, as they are often related to unruly behavior, poor ice conditions, 'showing off,' and even alcohol abuse." In addition, the majority of ice skating injuries are to the wrist and hand. If you wear a wrist protector designed for in-line skating as well as thick gloves to guard your hands, you'll cut your risks significantly.

The fitness requirements for skating are similar to running

and in-line skating: you'll need strong legs, a good sense of balance, and a decent base of cardiovascular conditioning. Speed skating is especially aerobically demanding, but figure skating can also be a hard workout, depending on what level you take it to.

Equipment: Rental skates are fine if you aren't sure what kind of skating you want to do or how committed you are to skating regularly. The edges of the blades of rental skates may not be as sharp as those you own and maintain yourself, but are usually adequate. When renting (or buying) skates, make sure they fit snugly. You should be able to move your toes, but the heel shouldn't be loose (i.e., your heel should stay firmly in place in the boot when you bend). Ideally, you should wear sweat-resistant, insulated socks that are thin, not two or three pairs of thick woolen socks. You want to be able to feel the boot's fit through the socks so as to be able to maneuver effectively.

What to Wear: Outfits for figure skating competitions are strictly regulated. Likewise, to reduce wind resistance, competitive speedskaters wear skin suits—close-fitting Lycra suits made to fit the skater like a second skin; in some events, speed skaters wear safety approved helmets, neck guards, shin guards, gloves, and knee pads. Ice hockey players have uniforms; women wear the same basic protective equipment as men, but are encouraged to wear female shoulder/chest pads.

For a skater trying out any of these sports, an outfit consisting of long pants or tights, a long-sleeved shirt, and the required safety gear is sufficient to begin. In fact, the only rule is to dress warmly enough (since even indoor rinks are often quite chilly) while avoiding becoming overheated. Start with thin underclothes made of material with sweat-wicking properties; add layers that you can easily remove if you get overheated. Even if you are skating indoors, you may want to wear a hat, gloves, and a scarf.

To Find Out More

The United States Figure Skating Association (USFSA) is the national governing body for the sport of figure skating in the United States. In conjunction with the U.S. Postal Service, the USFSA promotes the Skate with U.S. program—a basic skills program designed to bring figure skating to the largest possible number of people. To find out more about the USFSA's programs, contact:

United States Figure Skating Association
20 First Street
Colorado Springs, CO 80906
PHONE: 719-635-5200
FAX: 719-635-9548
WEBSITE: www.usfsa.org

For information on speed skating, including where to find local clubs, appropriate tracks, instructors, and gear, contact:

Amateur Speedskating Union (ASU) of the United States
1033 Shady Lane, Glen Ellyn IL 60137
PHONE: 630-790-3230
FAX: 630-790-3235
WEBSITE: www.speedskating.org

You can also get information from the national governing body of Olympic-style speed skating:

U.S. Speedskating
P.O. Box 450639
Westlake, OH 44145
PHONE: 440-899-0128
FAX: 440-899-0109
WEBSITE: www.usspeedskating.org

For information about local women's ice hockey clubs and leagues, contact:

USA Hockey
1775 Bob Johnson Drive
Colorado Springs, CO 80906
PHONE: 719-576-8724
FAX: 719-538-1160
WEBSITE: www.usahockey.com
E-MAIL: usah@usahockey.com

Books to Check Out

Karin Kunzle-Watson and Stephen J. DeArmond, *Ice Skating: Steps to Success* (Champaign, Ill.: Human Kinetics, 1996).
Like most of the books in the Steps to Success series, this book is filled with very clear descriptions and drawings of all the essential skills needed in ice skating. It also has a more chatty narrative than is usual in the series, which some may find welcome.

Although there are many books about ice hockey, few address the game as it is played by women. Given the triumph of the U.S. Women's Hockey Team at the 1998 Winter Olympics in Nagano, Japan, however, it is likely more books will soon become available. In the meantime hockey players should find some helpful hints in this title:

Laura Stamm, *Laura Stamm's Power Skating* (Champaign, Ill.: Human Kinetics, 1990).

The few books on speed skating that are available are not current because they do not give instructions on how to use clap skates—the new skates introduced in the 1998 Winter Olympics in Nagano. If you don't plan to use clap skates, the most complete book on speed skating is aptly titled:

Dianne Holum, *The Complete Handbook of Speed Skating* (Lake Placid, N.Y.: High Peaks Cyclery, 1994).

◖ Skate Talk

Changing on the fly: An ice hockey term that refers to the practice of substituting a player in the middle of play, without stopping play.

Clap skate: A new type of skate that has completely changed the face of long track speed skating, leading to dramatically faster times. With a clap skate, a skater can raise her heel from the blade, which allows for a more powerful, longer push.

Hat trick: Three goals scored by one player in a single ice hockey game.

Mohawk: A figure skating term that means a turn forward to backward (or backward to forward), from one foot to the other.

SKIING

If you didn't learn to ski as a kid, you may be scared to try it as an adult. Yet improved binding and boot designs have contributed to a 48 percent reduction in overall injuries, especially leg and ankle fractures, according to a recent long-term evaluation of the medical records of over eight thousand skiers at two ski resorts in Vermont. In fact, there were fewer than three injuries sustained per every thousand adult skiers.

The one risk that does remain high, especially if you are an aggressive skier who executes lots of jumps and sudden turns, is of "blowing out your knees"—suffering an anterior cruciate ligament (ACL) injury of the knee. While the new boots and bindings protect the ankle and tibia, they also transfer some of the stress to the knee. Still, experts say that the risk of a knee problem is significantly reduced if your ski equipment is properly adjusted and you don't take kamikaze runs down the slopes. Also, the ski industry is actively working on redesigning boots so that they put less stress on knees.

How It's Done: The sport of downhill skiing is all about feeling free, graceful, exhilarated, and unfettered as you start at the top of a mountain then make your way down. But in order to experience the thrill and excitement of actually gliding down a slope, you need to do a fair amount of falling down and getting up as you learn to balance your body weight properly over your skis, keep your skis parallel, carve turns, change directions, and so on.

Self-teaching—or getting a few pointers from a friend—is not a very effective or safe way to learn how to ski. That's why most resorts and ski areas won't even let you on the chair lift until you've had at least one lesson. An even better idea is to sign up for several lessons so that you really get beyond falling and are able to get a taste of how it feels to flow down the mountain. You also greatly reduce your chances of getting injured if you learn from a certified ski instructor.

Beyond the essentials of sliding down the slopes, there are all sorts of variations to the sport of skiing. There is acro-skiing or ballet skiing, which is like figure skating on skis; downhill alpine ski racing—high speed races (elite racers reach speeds up to 80 miles an hour according to the U.S. Olympic Committee) down a mountain in which the winner is whoever clocks the fastest time; aerials, in which the skier is launched from a specially designed jump and goes 50 or more feet above a snowy landing hill, while twisting, turning, and flipping; moguls racing—a race over a wild series of bumps on a ski run; ski jumping, in which the skier skies down a long ramplike jump, then flies through the air for distances greater than the length of a football field before landing; and slalom/giant slalom/super G, in which racers zigzag through gates all the way down the hill. There is also "extreme" or freestyle skiing, which involves daredevil maneuvers similar to those executed in "extreme" snowboarding.

Key Physical Requirements: Skiing demands strong leg muscles as well as muscular strength in your hips, thighs, feet, abdominals, lower back, and buttocks. If you regularly engage in a sport like running, biking, soccer, or a racket sport, you'll have built up much of the leg strength for skiing you need, although you may find your entire hip and pelvic region gets more of a workout than you are used to. Obviously, the greater your muscular strength in your lower body, the better able you'll be to control your movements on your skis and the longer you'll last on the slopes before becoming fatigued and sore.

Equipment: Rent it. Ski equipment is not only expensive, there is an unbelievably baffling array of choices when it comes to ski lengths, shapes, weights, and so forth, not to mention a huge number of new boot styles. You need to find out what kind of skier you are first before you can know what kind of gear might suit you best. Also, you may find the sport is only something you plan to do once or twice a year—in that case, it's far more economical to rent by the day or even week rather than buy skis, boots, bindings, and poles.

Expect the attendant at the rental shop to ask you how well you ski—be honest. The attendant will then match you with a pair of skis, poles, and boots according to your weight, height, and skiing skill. A good and skilled rental shop employee will ask you to walk around in your boots for a few minutes so you can make sure they fit properly (snugly, but not so tight that they are painful). The attendant will also set your bindings (the devices that release your boots from your skis) appropriately—i.e., according to your experience level.

What to Wear: You don't necessarily need a ski outfit, per se. You just need to dress warmly—but not too warmly—as you would for participating in any winter sport. You need a wicking layer next to your skin; an insulating layer (usually of wool or other fleece); then a wind-breaking/moisture-resistant layer for both your upper and lower body. You'll need thin, insulated socks, water-resistant gloves, a scarf or neck warmer, and a hat. Ski goggles are optional, but highly recommended by most instructors.

To Find Out More

Ski magazine is the most up-to-date source on gear. It regularly includes buying guides for boots, skis, and other skiing equipment. You can also get technique tips, ratings of ski instructors and resorts, and health and fitness information that is specific to skiing and skiers. The editorial content of *Ski* is geared to the novice, beginner, and intermediate recreational skier; *Skiing, Ski's* sister magazine, is directed at more serious and more expert skiers.

Ski and *Skiing Magazine*
The Skiing Company
Boulder, CO
SUBSCRIPTIONS: 800-678-0817
WEBSITE: www.skinet.com

○ Ski Lingo

Fall line: A hill's steepest line of descent.

Green Circle: A trail marked by a green circle, which is the symbol for the easiest runs suitable for novices. A blue square denotes a more difficult trail, suitable for intermediate skiers; a black diamond trail is for advanced skiers; two black diamonds signify a trail that is extremely steep and suited only for experts; and a yellow triangle marks an area that is off limits to skiers because of unsafe conditions.

Schuss: Skiing straight down a mountain without making any turns, swerves, or zigzags.

Books to Check Out

Herb Gordon, *Essential Skiing: A Bible for Beginner Skiers* (New York: Lyons and Burford, 1996).
This highly readable guide is truly for beginners—it would be too elementary for anyone who possesses intermediate skiing skills. It also includes information on teaching children to ski, snowboarding, and cross-country.

SNOWBOARDING

It's no longer the exclusive domain of teenage boys wearing ultra-baggy pants and sporting nose rings. Snowboarding has gone mainstream.

In 1997, over 3.7 million people snowboarded more than once, an increase in participation of 32.5 percent from 1996, according to a National Sporting Goods Association Participation Survey. Women's participation has grown tremendously, too—women snowboarders even have their own magazine. What's more, most ski areas now allow snowboarding (whereas almost no resorts allowed boarding fewer than fifteen years ago).

The sport tends to appeal particularly to skiers (many of whom have grown a bit bored with their sport, but still love the slopes), skateboarders (for whom snowboarding is a natural winter alternative), and surfers (snowboarding is, in its essence, surfing on the snow). Athletes coming from these sports (skiing, skateboarding, and surfing) will tend to master snowboarding faster than other athletes partly because they already have the moxie, coordination, and specific muscle strengths needed for it.

There are three main snowboarding riding styles:

1. Free riding, which involves turning, carving, and other techniques that are similar to those used in downhill skiing. Free riding is what most recreational snowboarders do.
2. Free styling, which involves a huge catalog of impressive tricks and maneuvers (not all of which are dangerous, although some are!).
3. Alpine racing, which is exactly what it sounds like, snowboarding at high speeds, often down extreme descents.

For each of these styles, specific types of snowboards are used.

How It's Done: Using a board, you slide over the snow. You don't use poles—your arms are free. Your feet, however, are held fast to your board: Snowboard bindings are designed not to release when you fall, unlike ski bindings for downhill skiing.

What's the learning curve for snowboarding? Once you get the hang of it, you can usually begin to excel quite rapidly. However, getting the hang of it almost always involves a lot of falling down (in fact, how to fall properly is one of the first things you'll learn). In other words, the first day or two is often a tricky and challenging time. For this reason, first-time snowboarders are almost always advised to start by taking a lesson from a qualified ski instructor. A lesson will help you learn much faster and you'll be at less risk for injury too.

Key Physical Requirements: The body parts that snowboarding most stresses are feet, ankles, and calves. Your feet and ankles must be strong in order to control the shifting of your body weight from the front of the board to the back, while your calf muscles are the key to making your board execute turns. You'll need to keep your knees bent much of the time, too, so strong quadriceps muscles (thigh muscles that support the knee) are important as is some upper body strength, since you'll need to push yourself up out of the snow frequently at first, and you'll need to lug your snowboard around.

Equipment: Like skiing, snowboarding is gear intensive and expensive. So rent boards until you know if you like the sport. Also, it doesn't make sense to invest in snowboarding equipment right off the bat since you can't really know what gear is right for you until you've experimented with different boards. Only after you've tried boarding can you know what your riding style is and the kind of board that might best suit you.

Keep in mind that even when renting your equipment, it's extremely important to get a good fit in your boots. Snowboard boots (most recreational snowboarders use ones with a soft shell) shouldn't pinch or be too tight, but they should be snug—a snug fit allows you to use your feet effectively to maneuver the board.

What to Wear: You want your clothes to be (1) roomy, to allow for freedom of movement; (2) water-resistant, since you're bound to fall a lot (which means your jacket should either cover your butt or you should wear water-resistant pants); and (3) warm, but not too warm—that's where the wicking layer, topped by an insulating layer of polypropolene or wool, comes in.

You'll also want to wear close-fitting (not bulky) synthetic sports socks, hat, gloves, and scarf or neck warmer. Essential accessories include ski goggles, wrist guards, and knee pads.

To Find Out More

A local snowboard shop is a logical place to start—employees should be able to answer most questions about the sport, equipment, and where to ride. If you have access to the World Wide Web, SnowSports Industries America's site at www.snowlink.com can help you find a shop near you and/or a list of resorts that offer beginner's lessons and package deals. You can also call the Winter Active Sports Hotline at 703-506-4232 or use Snowlink's fax on demand at: 800-730-3636.

These magazines are also good resources, especially if you are looking for up-to-date information on gear:

Snowboarder
P.O. Box 1028
Dana Point, CA 92629
PHONE: 949-496-5922
FAX: 949-496-7849
WEBSITE: www.snowboardermag.com
E-MAIL: snwbrdrmag@surferpubs.com

Transworld *Snowboarding* or *Snowboard Life*
353 Airport Road
Oceanside, CA 92054
PHONE: 888-TWS-MAGS
WEBSITE: www.twsnow.com
E-MAIL: multmedia@twsnet.com

There is also the first and only women's snowboarding magazine, which tends to be strongest in its profiles of top female snowboarders but a little weak in its coverage of technique and new gear options.

Fresh and Tasty
100 Spring Street
Cambridge, MA 02141
WEBSITE: www.freshandtasty.com

Books to Check Out

Jeff Bennett and Scott Downey, *The Complete Snowboarder* (Camden, Maine: Ragged Mountain Press, 1994).
This book has a breezy, hip, conversational style, many good explanatory line drawings, and solid information on selecting a snowboard, how to get started, and advanced techniques for competition.

Lowell Hart, *The Snowboard Book: A Guide for All Boarders* (New York: W.W. Norton & Company, 1997).
Another good title that you can "grow with"—in other words, it will be useful when you're a beginner, but contains lots of information you'll be able to use as you get to be a better boarder.

Bethany Stevens, *Ultimate Snowboarding* (Chicago: Contemporary Publishing, 1998).
Written by the managing editor of *Fresh and Tasty* magazine, this book contains a lot of history of the sport, interviews with snowboarding personalities, as well as information on how to get started.

◑ Snowboarding Lingo

Bonk: Intentionally knocking something (such as a box that you've jumped or a rail you've ridden on) with your snowboard to make a "bonking" sound.

Crust and crud: Crust is snow that is icy on top, but mushy below; crud is irregular chunks of snow and ice that have been carved up by other skiers or boarders.

Riding fakie: Riding backward, also called "switch-stance."

SNOWSHOEING

Snowshoeing is slowly becoming more popular in this country. According to a survey in 1995 by SnowSports Industries America, a manufacturers' association, 840,000 people snowshoed two or more times per year—up from 444,000 in 1992.

This growing interest can partly be explained by two phenomena:

1. *The discovery of snowshoeing by the running community.* For the past four to five years, national as well as local running magazines have been touting snowshoeing as a way to find "fulfillment in winter training" (that's how one author, Welles Lobb, put it in a quarterly runner's journal *FootNotes*). One of the nation's top snowshoe runners, Tom Sobal of Leadville, Colorado, has often been quoted as saying "Running on snowshoes is the best form of cross-training for runners there is. It's a lot more specific to running than cross-country skiing and much lower impact than regular running."

2. *Improvements in snowshoe design itself, which make the sport less laborious as well as easier to learn.* Today, snowshoes are light-weight, provide good "flotation" (i.e., allow for easy gliding over the snow with little icy buildup), and are activity specific (there are models for walking, for cross-training, racing, and for rugged back country trailblazing). Ten years ago there were only two manufacturers of snowshoes in the United States. Currently, there are at least two dozen.

How It's Done: You walk or run on snowshoes—you don't glide as with skis. You can use poles or go poleless. The chief trick to snowshoeing is getting used to the new "space" your feet take up with shoes (which can measure anywhere from 22 to 32 inches in length and 8 to 10 inches wide). Most people are able to do this with a little practice and trial and error—lessons aren't really necessary. The main reason you might fall face first when snowshoeing is that you inadvertently step on one shoe with the other while in motion; if you fall backward, it's probably because you tried to step backward (you need to make U-turns in snowshoes).

Key Physical Requirements: It really depends on how fast you choose to go. You can walk leisurely on snowshoes or you can pump your arms with your poles and run to get a vigorous, cardiovascularly challenging, whole body–toning workout. Because you can easily choose the pace you want to move at, snowshoeing can be a good way to stair step your way up to greater fitness.

Equipment: Because there is now so much choice in snowshoes, buying them has become more complicated and involves more decisions, such as, do you plan to use the shoes for racing (in which case you'll want a smaller, short shoe) or do you plan to use them primarily for bushwhacking back country (in which case a substantially longer and wider shoe is best). In other words, you need to choose a snowshoe according to the type of shoeing you plan to do. The price range for a pair of snowshoes is anywhere from about $170 to $300.

Ideally, you should rent a pair of snowshoes first and try out the sport to get a feel for what aspects of the shoe model you like. Many ski shops and outdoor equipment stores rent snowshoes, as do many of the resorts and trail areas affiliated with the Cross Country Ski Area Association (CCSAA).

You can also get some pretty reliable and detailed advice from L.L. Bean, which sells snowshoes as well as offers snowshoeing clinics (800-341-4341).

What to Wear: Besides snowshoes, you'll want to wear athletic socks that wick away moisture and lightweight boots or athletic shoes. To keep snow from getting inside your shoes and to help keep your feet warm, you should wear nylon or neoprene boot sleeves or overboots over the top of your shoes.

As for your clothing, start with a base layer of long underwear (top and bottom) made of polypropylene or other synthetic material (as opposed to cotton, which tends to retain sweat). Then you might wear a fleece vest (to allow for free movement of your arms) with a water-resistant windbreaker over it. The idea is to wear layers that are lightweight, breathable, yet warm and easily removed if you overheat. Of course, you'll want gloves, hat, and a neck warmer too.

To Find Out More

This national magazine (the only one for this sport) includes a lot of up-to-date information on equipment, techniques, destinations, etc.:

The Snowshoer Magazine
P.O. Box 458
Washburn, WI 54891
PHONE: 651-523-0666

The Tubbs Snowshoe Company organizes a variety of races and other snowshoe events nationwide; its website is a good all-around source of information on the sport.

Tubbs Snowshoes
52 River Road
Stowe, VT 05672
PHONE: 800-882-2748 or 802-253-7398
FAX: 802-253-9982
WEBSITE: www.tubbssnowshoes.com

Books to Check Out

Sally Edwards and Melissa McKenzie, *Snowshoeing* (Champaign, Ill.: Human Kinetics, 1995).
Edwards (who set the women's record at the 1993 Iditarod 100-Mile Snowshoe Race in Alaska with a time of twenty-four hours, one minute) obviously loves this sport and is quite good at conveying her enthusiasm. If you are contemplating buying a pair of snowshoes, this book provides a lot of solid information and guidance.

⌀ Snowshoe Talk

Crampons: These are "teeth" or spikes along the underside of the snowshoe frame that dig into the snow and give you traction. "Claws" are similar, but shorter in spike length.

Decking: The snowshoe's platform.

Traversing: Taking side steps or moving diagonally across a slope, a pattern of movement that is not recommended in snowshoes.

SOCCER

Nearly 4.6 million adults in the United States played soccer in 1998, according to a 1998 National Soccer Participation Survey, conducted by the Soccer Industry Council of America. Of these players, almost 40 percent were women.

Probably the fastest paced, most aerobically challenging team sport you can play, soccer involves a lot of running, thinking on your feet, and hurling your whole body into the action. In soccer, players use everything from their heads to their feet to their chests to the inside of their thighs to move and control the ball. The only body part you can't employ is your hands; only the goalkeeper can legally handle the ball with both hands.

To enjoy soccer, you need to be comfortable with a fair amount of player-to-player body contact. Although maneuvers like "tackling" in soccer do not involve football-like body crushing (in fact, that kind of contact is illegal) playing soccer inevitably involves bodies touching, crowding, and crashing into one another. A certain amount of aggressiveness and roughness on the field is necessary to play a good and skillful game.

How It's Played: It is often said that the essence of soccer is its simplicity. There are only seventeen rules or laws, all of which are easy to understand. The basic features of the game are that it's played by two teams of eleven players each; games are divided into two forty-five minute halves. Like hockey or football, the object of the game is to get the ball into the opponent's goals. Players move the ball across the field, pass it to one another while dodging opponents, and shoot for goals using a variety of skills. For example, there are at least seven different techniques for kicking the ball with your feet and more than three ways of "heading" it (i.e., using your head to control or direct the ball's flight).

The play in soccer tends to be quite continuous: There are no timeouts as in basketball or football. Coaches and/or team captains can't interrupt the game to discuss strategies. Stoppages are very brief: If a ball goes out of bounds, for example, the game is usually only stopped for the few seconds it takes to get the ball back into play.

Key Physical Requirements: The average soccer player runs 5 miles every game, much of that time at top speed, according to

Deborah Crisfield in *Winning Soccer for Girls* (Facts on File, 1996). "The game, of course, does call for some sprinting, but it's minor compared to the need to run nonstop for forty-five minutes while still maintaining the same level of intensity in terms of ball handling. Because of this, soccer players should be able to run at least 5 miles at a time very comfortably."

Besides endurance training, you also need to develop agility and flexibility in order to juggle and dribble the ball with your various body parts. As in any fast-paced sport, quickness is important.

Equipment: You don't need much to play soccer, but you do need:

- *A field*: Unlike most team sports in which the dimensions of the playing field are strictly determined, a soccer field has only to conform to a few specifications: it must be between 100 and 130 yards long, and the width, which is usually between 50 and 100 yards, must be less than the length.
- *A soccer ball*: The ball is usually made of leather, measures 27 to 28 inches in circumference, weighs 14 to 16 ounces, and has a distinctive geometric pattern on it.
- *Two goal areas*: At each end of the field is a goal consisting of two upright posts 8 feet high and 24 feet apart; in front of this is a 6-yard-by-20-yard area called the goal area; beyond this is another penalty box 44 yards by 18 yards. It's only within this area that the goalie can use her hands; outside of it, she must conform to the rules of the other field players.

What to Wear: Players' uniforms usually consist of shirts, shorts, and calf-high socks in team colors. Shin guards are compulsory. Goalkeepers wear shirts in different colors from teammates, so that the referee can easily distinguish her. Soccer shoes may have studs or cleats across the sole. The rules state that nothing shall be worn that may be dangerous to other players.

To Find Out More

The United States Amateur Soccer Association (USASA), a division of U.S. Soccer, the governing body for Olympic soccer in the United States, is responsible for developing the sport for players over the age of nineteen. To find soccer clubs and leagues in your area, contact your state association, which you can find by calling USASA's headquarters in Bergen, New Jersey, at 800-867-2945. The USASA's website is www.usasa.com.

Soccer America, the leading U.S. soccer magazine, in conjunction with the makers of the candy bar Snickers, maintains a national phone book of over 7,300 listings of soccer organizations, clubs, leagues, contact people, businesses, and companies. You may search the Snickers/Soccer America Yellow Pages database for soccer leagues and clubs across the country (and outside of the United States too) on the Web: www.socceramerica.com.

The United Systems of Independent Soccer Leagues operates a thirty-three-team women's league, the W-League, which is the only national adult soccer league for women. The league, which tends to be filled with current and former college players over age nineteen, is split into two divisions: a fifteen-team W-1, or elite, division and an eighteen-team W-2 division. For information, contact:

> The United Systems of Independent Soccer Leagues
> 14497 North Dale Mabry, Suite 201
> Tampa, FL 33618
> PHONE: 813-963-3909
> FAX: 813-963-3807
> WEBSITE: www.usisl.com

Books to Check Out

Deborah Crisfield, *Winning Soccer for Girls* (New York: Facts on File, 1996).
Even if you don't consider yourself a "girl" anymore, this is a great book—well written, with clear descriptions of all the soccer fundamentals, from "heading" to team tactics.

◆ Soccer Talk

Chip: Short "lofted" pass—i.e., one that sails over the heads of the opponents to reach a teammate.

Dribble: Moving the ball with rapid taps of the foot without passing or shooting.

Throw-in: After a ball has gone out of bounds, a player may use her hands to throw the ball back into play.

SOFTBALL

There are over 260,000 softball teams in the United States registered with the Amateur Softball Association, combining to form a membership of more than 4.5 million. And that doesn't count the untold thousands of women who play in less official, more informal leagues and clubs.

There are two forms of softball—slow pitch and fast pitch. In amateur leagues across the country, slow pitch tends to be predominant. With both, the ball is delivered to a batter with an underhanded motion (unlike baseball, which is pitched overhand). As their different names imply, with slow pitch softball the ball is delivered at a moderately slow speed, while with fast pitch, the ball is allowed to travel as fast as the pitcher can make it go. There are a few other rule differences, too.

But the difference in pitching style is what's key to the different "natures" of slow pitch versus fast pitch softball. Slow pitch ball involves a lot of hitting (and a lot fewer strikeouts) and the strategic emphasis of the game is on hitting, base running, and fielding. Slow pitch enthusiasts often insist that their game is more fun to play (since players are more likely to get a chance to thwack the ball and run the bases) as well as faster paced and more exciting to watch.

In fast-pitch ball, which is what the U.S. Women's Softball team played at the 1996 Summer Olympics in Atlanta, pitching strategy is paramount. Batting strategy is also more complex, since bunting and "chopping" are legal (which they aren't in slow pitch). Fast pitch devotees argue that their game requires faster reflexes, more skill, and a higher level of strategizing.

How It's Played: An official game consists of seven innings. In fast pitch, each team has nine players (with many extras and substitutes for their nine on the sidelines); in slow pitch, there are ten players on a team. This tenth player is the short center fielder and may play as an infielder, outfielder, or rover.

Most of us are familiar with the basic concepts behind a game of softball (such as "three strikes, you're out"), but there are many nuances in the rules that you'll need to learn if you plan to play.

Key Physical Requirements: Most softball movements are sprints. For example, the distance between base paths is 60 feet—as a batter/runner you need to be able to sprint that distance quickly and repeatedly, without it tiring you (since you need to stay strong for an entire game). In addition, you need general upper body (but especially rotator cuff and arm) strength to be able to throw the ball with force and precision as well as bat it with skill and accuracy. Not surprisingly, most serious softball players integrate some weight training and running into their softball-specific drills and practices.

Equipment: The equipment for softball is what you'd expect:

- *A field:* The regulation field size for slow-pitch ball is a radius of 250 feet from home plate; for fast pitch, there needs to be a 200-foot radius.
- *Balls.* Official Olympic softballs must be 12 inches in circumference and weigh between 6¼ and 7 ounces.
- *Bats.* Softball bats may be made of hardwood, metal, plastic, graphite, carbon, magnesium, fiberglass, or other composite materials approved by the Amateur Softball Association. However, bats normally used in softball are of aluminum alloy. Bats can be no longer than 34 inches, must not weigh more than 38 ounces, and must have a 10-inch-long safety grip made of cork, tape, or any composition material other than smooth plastic tape.

What to Wear: You'll want to wear a softball glove when you're playing the field; when batting, you must wear a batting helmet, which you need to keep on as you run the bases.

Most recreational softball players simply wear good supportive athletic shoes that are on the lightweight side, so as to allow for easy sprinting. However, you can wear shoes with metal or soft or hard rubber cleats, although any spikes on the heels or sole must not be longer than ½ inch.

Catchers must wear masks, throat protectors, helmets, body protectors, and shin guards.

If you're playing in an official league, you'll probably have a specific uniform, as well as rules dictating what kind of ball cap, headbands, and jewelry you may—and may not—wear.

To Find Out More

For more information on how to get started playing softball in your area, your best source is the Amateur Softball Association (ASA), which provides competition for over 4.5 million players each season. The ASA's competition schedule includes some sixty divisions of play in slow pitch, fast pitch, and modified pitch softball. To find your local ASA representative, contact the national office:

Amateur Softball Association
2801 N.E. 50th Street
Oklahoma City, OK 73111-7203
PHONE: 405-424-5266
FAX: 405-424-3855
WEBSITE: www.softball.org
E-MAIL: info@softball.org

Books to Check Out

Mario Pagnoni and Gerald Robinson, *Softball: Fast and Slow Pitch* (Indianapolis: Masters Press, 1995).
Offers advice on how to select the best equipment as well as how to train for specific positions.

Barry Sammons and Lisa Fernandez, *Fast Pitch Softball: The Windmill Pitcher* (Indianapolis: Masters Press, 1998).
Rather specialized, but great if you want to learn fast-pitch softball pitching mechanics.

◖ Softball Talk

Bag: A base

Designated hitter (DH): In fast pitch, a hitter used as a substitute for any player, provided it is made known prior to the start of the game and her name is indicated on the lineup sheet. The DH must remain in the same position in the batting order for the entire game and may not enter the game on defense.

Pivot foot: In fast pitch, the pivot foot is the pitcher's foot that must remain in contact with the pitcher's plate until the other foot, which takes a small step toward home plate right before the ball is released, has touched the ground. In slow pitch, it is the foot that the pitcher must keep in consistent contact with the pitcher's plate until the ball is released.

SQUASH

The appeal of this game is that it can be fast, furious, and very challenging, both aerobically and mentally. And even though it can be an intense one-on-one game, there is a strong element of built-in sportsmanship to it, since it is against the rules to muscle in on your opponent's freedom of movement and/or obstruct her ability to make a shot of her choice.

Still, squash is considered one of the harder racket sports to learn and to master. This largely has to do with the nature of three essentials of the game: the ball, the racket, and the playing court.

The ball is low-bouncing; it's not as springy and it's smaller than the ones used in tennis or racquetball, which makes it harder to hit.

A squash racket is long-handled (27 inches long), so it doesn't feel like an extension of your hand, and it has a smaller hitting surface (8½ inches by 8) than a tennis racket, for example. So again, it's harder to strike a ball with it.

Finally, squash is played in a small, enclosed court, a four-walled room 32 by 21 feet wide. There are illegal zones on each wall, which makes playing in such a restricted, tight court particularly challenging. Plus there are strict rules of "close contact" that indicate how a player must move around the court so as to allow her opponent a fair chance to make a shot without being blocked. These rules also help ensure the safety of the players. "They are designed to deal with the problems arising from the fact that both players are in the same limited space, moving at high speed and swinging rackets," notes Dick Hawkey in *Play the Game: Squash* (Blandford, 1994).

How It's Played: Both players face the front wall. The object of the game is to get the ball to hit this front wall (instead of crossing a net as in tennis, for example) in such a way that your opponent can't return it. The two tricky aspects of the game are that the ball can rebound off any of the side walls or back wall on its way to and from the front wall, and there are lines on all four walls marking the boundary limits of the play area.

To remain in play, a ball must be struck before it has bounced twice on the floor and you can only hit it once (you can't "double-hit" a ball during a volley). Throughout the game, it is up to you to move in such a way as to not block your opponent's shots. In the United States, the winner is the one who scores 9 points first, with only the server scoring. However, in international competitions, the game is usually played to 15 points and both server and receiver can score. Most matches consist of the best of three to five games.

Key Physical Requirements: As you might guess, endurance, strong legs, and flexibility are the qualifications for squash.

- Endurance, since you need to move quickly and constantly while the ball is in play (the average game lasts 45 to 60 minutes). Of course, the endurance capacity you need will depend a great deal on how aggressively you play.
- Leg strength and speed, since you need to make sudden starts and stops and fast changes of direction.
- Flexibility, especially in your upper body, because you often need to twist and stretch to reach a ball.

Equipment: Rackets start at around $50. Look for the most comfortable grip and a lighter weight variety. Experts warn beginners against spending too much on a first racket, since there is a good chance you'll damage it by hitting the wall or floor with it while you're learning the game. Balls start at about $3.

What to Wear: Protective eyegear, since a ricocheting ball can cause serious damage if it hits your eye.

Like most racket sports, white or soft pastels are worn for competition, but anything loose and comfortable with sweat-wicking properties is fine. You should wear shoes designed for court sports—i.e., ones that provide good gripping for sudden stops and turns but also a lot of shock absorption to cushion your jumps. As in the other racket games, blisters are often a problem, but you can frequently prevent their formation by wearing padded, sweat-resistant sports socks.

To Find Out More

The U.S. Squash Racquets Association (USSRA) can help you locate squash clubs, tournaments, and instructors in your area. Their address is as follows:

U.S. Squash Racquets Association
P.O. Box 1216

Bala-Cynwyd, PA 19004-1216
PHONE: 610-667-4006
FAX: 610-667-6539
E-MAIL: 75471.2207@compuserv.com

The USRA also maintains a website filled with useful information, plus it hosts a talk forum in which you can ask questions and make queries for information. The website address is www.us-squash.org

Books to Check Out

The majority of newer books on squash are directed to seasoned players; they don't contain enough clear basics for a beginner. And, unfortunately, many of the tried and true books on learning to play squash are out of print or their publishers are out of stock. But you might try your local library or used bookseller for either of these titles—each provides easy-to-follow instructions and explanations for first-time players:

Dick Hawkey, *Play the Game: Squash* (London: Blandford, 1994).

Heather McKay, *Heather McKay's Complete Book of Squash* (New York: Ballantine Books, 1979).

◔ Squash Lingo

Nick: A ball that rolls out because it has hit the point where the floor meets the side or back wall, thus making it impossible to retrieve (and usually resulting in a point for the striker).

Philadelphia boast: A trick shot hit from the center of the court that first hits the front wall high on the opposite side, then the side wall, and then comes back out with reverse spin.

Telltale (sometimes called a tin): A 17-inch-high rectangle of sheet metal at the bottom of the front wall that gives off a ringing sound when struck by the ball. If the ball hits the telltale, a fault is called.

SURFING

Surfer girl used to mean a babe in a thong bikini who sat on the sand waiting for her man to finish riding the waves. No longer. More and more women are breaking into what was once the exclusive domain of men. In fact, female surfers now have their own schools, their own surf shops, and their own magazines, as well as their own competitions.

How It's Done: The whole idea of surfing is to slide down the front of a wave, usually as you are standing on a board. In order to do this you need to learn how to balance and hold your body while on a moving surfboard. Learning to surf is similar—although a lot more difficult!—to learning to ride a bike. In both cases, one of the main feats facing you is to master perching and balancing yourself on a "device" while in motion. Also, as is true on a bike, the faster a surfboard is going, the easier it is to balance.

But unlike a cyclist, a surfer must navigate on terrain that is ever-changing: like fingerprints, no two waves are alike. So another chief element of surfing is learning to understand and "read" waves. Some waves are "unsurfable" and so, for her own safety, a surfer must acquire a certain amount of basic knowledge about wave formations, tides, currents, and wind conditions. In other words, surfing does not start at the moment you catch a wave—it starts on the beach when you are sizing up the state of surf.

If you are a beginner, most experts advise you consider taking lessons, or at the very least, start out with a friend who is not only experienced but is patient and prudent. If you attend a school, don't be surprised if a lot of your instruction is on dry sands. The best schools have you practice maneuvers and proper surfing positions first on terra firma, then in the shallow shore-break whitewater, only then gradually moving you out into the swells.

Key Physical Requirements: Upper-body strength. A large part of surfing is paddling out—often against fierce resistance—to catch waves; you also need to be able to comfortably lug your surfboard (which may weigh more than 25 pounds) around.

Needless to say, you also need to be a strong, alert swimmer who is confident (but not too cocky!) about ocean swimming. Wipeouts, in which you get knocked from your board and tumbled in the surf, are inevitable, for both beginners and experienced surfers.

Finally, you need to have good endurance as a swimmer, since if you lose your board in the crest of a wave, your board may end up on the beach while you are faced with a long swim in.

Equipment: Rent a board if you're a beginner—that way you can find out, via trial and error, what you like best in a board in terms of style, weight, stability, and so on. (There are many different types of boards: longboards, which are approximately 9 feet long; shortboards, about 6 feet long; as well as bodyboards, which are smaller, soft boards used lying down.)

What to Wear: You may need a wet suit if you're surfing in cool waters; if the water's warm, check to see if your bathing suit offers protection from bruising when paddling out. Some women wear "board shorts" and body shirts to protect their upper torsos. In addition, applying waterproof sunscreen at least 30 minutes before you hit the beach is an absolute must; make sure to reapply every hour or two.

To Find Out More

There are two new surf magazines for women. Both offer advice specifically for women, including guides on where to find good clinics and instruction schools, how to find stores that stock wet suits, boards, and other surfing gear suited for women, and so on. Both magazines have print as well as on-line versions:

Wahine Magazine
5520 East Second Street, Suite K
Long Beach, CA 90803
PHONE: 562-434-9444
E-MAIL: wahinemag@aol.com
WEBSITE: www.wahinemagazine.com

SurferGirl Magazine
P.O. Box 3618
Half Moon Bay, CA 94019
PHONE: 650-726-5795

FAX: 650-726-3299
E-MAIL: wahine@surfergrrl.com
WEBSITE: www.surfergrrl.com (yes, it's grrl not girl!)

You might also want to look into Waterwomen, an international organization, formed in 1996, for women of all ages and ability levels in surfing, bodyboarding, and other ocean sports. The main objectives of Waterwomen are to foster a supportive environment for competition at all levels, from amateur to professional, and to educate and train women in ocean sports. You can contact the organization at:

Waterwomen, Inc.
P.O. Box 293
Cardiff by the Sea, CA 92007
PHONE: 760-603-0029

In addition, you can get information from the International Surfing Association (ISA), which is the world governing authority for surfing and bodyboarding. Every other year the ISA holds the World Surfing Games. It also organizes the ISA World Pro-Junior Championship (tour of events around the world) and sanctions a large number of competitions worldwide.

ISA Headquarters
5580 La Jolla Boulevard, Suite 145

◒ Surf Talk

Snaps: Rebounding the surfboard off the breaking part of the waves and into the face of the wave. Sometimes called off-the-tops or off-the-lip.

Turn turtle: A maneuver in which you hold your board, then roll under it so it's on top in order to let a big wave get past you.

Tube ride: A tube is the hollow, concave portion of a wave; a tube ride is when the surfer is inside this pocket. If you are viewing the surfer, you won't be able to see her until she suddenly catapults from a barrel of cascading water. To the surfer inside the wave, it's like being inside a tunnel of water.

La Jolla, CA 92037
PHONE: 619-551-5292
FAX: 619-551-5290
E-MAIL: surf@isasurf.org
WEBSITE: www.isasurf.org

Book to Check Out

To many, surfing isn't just a sport but a way of life. So it should come as no surprise that the number of books written on the subject is mind-boggling. But if you're looking for a basic, uncomplicated, conversationally written, how-to guide, expressly directed at people who have never so much as picked up a surfboard in their lives, the following title is an excellent choice:

James MacLaren, *Learn to Surf* (New York: The Lyons Press, 1997).

SWIMMING

Swimming activities fall into these main categories:

Simple lap swimming. Just as some runners do the same route and distance three times a week, with no variations, some swimmers simply like to take to the pool and swim back and forth, nonstop, for a set amount of time or distance. They like the monotony and the even rhythm of their routine and aren't terribly interested in breaking from it.

If, however, you ever get bored by this routine or feel an itch to improve, you should try "interval training"—a method of training in which you swim hard for a short while, rest, then swim hard again. The books mentioned in the Books to Check Out section all contain good explanations of interval training and map out drills you can follow.

Competitive swimming. There are many opportunities for swimmers of all abilities and ages, no matter what their favorite stroke, to compete. In order to compete you need to learn the rules of competition, since it's easy to be disqualified. For example, if you fail to touch a pool wall properly when making a turn, you can be eliminated from the race.

Open water and distance swimming. Triathletes and endurance swimmers often race in oceans, bays, lakes, and rivers, which is a whole lot different from clocking laps in a pool, since you have to deal with currents, wind, and sometimes things like jellyfish and sharks. The definitive guide to this sport is *Open Water Swimming* by Penny Lee Dean, a world-record holder in thirteen events, including crossing the English Channel (Human Kinetics, 1998).

Water fitness. This activity now ranks as one of the fastest growing exercise categories in the United States, with more than 9 million participants, according to *American Fitness* magazine. Surprisingly, you don't have to know how to swim to do an aquatic workout, which usually involves standing in the water as you jog, use weights, do stretches, and perform a variety of steps and jumps. Many athletes take to water fitness as a way to get a good cardiovascular workout while recovering from injuries; runners recovering from any kind of foot or ankle injury can keep their leg muscles in shape with aqua jogging or deep-water running.

Diving: This is a spectacular sport, not unlike a form of gymnastics in the air that requires skill, precision, and a certain amount of daring.

Synchronized swimming. Usually done in groups of up to sixteen swimmers, this is a form of ballet or choreographed dance performed in the water. Swimmers precisely coordinate their movements and body positions to perform group stunts as well as to make floating formations. One of the key skills in synchronized swimming is learning the nine types of "sculling"—a way of using your hands to propel your body in the water (or keep it stationary).

How It's Done: Swimming is all about learning how to polish your strokes so your body moves through the water faster and more efficiently (and more gracefully, as is the case with diving and synchronized swimming).

Key Physical Requirements: Different swim strokes tax different sets of muscles, but as a general rule, you'll get an excellent upper body workout from the arm work demanded of swimming. If you kick correctly, your entire leg gets worked out too, but without any jarring of your joints. In addition, even though you don't notice you're sweating in a pool, you can get a good cardiovascular workout from swimming if you do laps, interval training, or vigorous water fitness routines.

Equipment: You might want to use a kickboard, a small, buoyant, (usually blue), Styrofoam rectangle. You hold it with your arms to keep your upper body afloat while you focus on your kicking technique and power. In reverse, as a way to focus on your arm strokes while keeping your lower body afloat, you might want to use a pull buoy—buoyant cylinders of Styrofoam that you hold between your legs.

What to Wear: Swimsuits are now made in a variety of quick-drying fabrics that don't sag, stretch, and/or become heavy in the water. Goggles protect your eyes from the burning, irritating effects of chlorine—the more expensive choices ($10 to $20) tend to be worth the price since they fit around your eye socket more tightly than the cheaper brands, and they hold up when you use them repeatedly.

You'll want to wear a latex or Lycra swim cap, too—it helps protect your hair from the effects of chlorine, cuts down on the water entering your ears, assists in keeping your goggles secure, and helps cut down on water resistance that might be caused by your free-flowing hair.

To Find Out More

A good place to find swimming instructors, classes, and groups is through your local YMCA, YWCA, or any other fitness center that has a pool. Sometimes sports shops that sell swimming gear can be helpful, too. In addition, United States Swimming or United States Masters Swimming can help you locate a local swim team and can provide you with information about synchronized swimming:

U.S. Swimming
One Olympic Plaza
Colorado Springs, CO 80909-5770
PHONE: 719-578-4578

FAX: 719-578-4669
WEBSITE: www.usswim.org

The United States Water Fitness Association (USWFA) is a nonprofit educational organization that promotes the benefits of water exercise worldwide. It can help you locate a certified water fitness instructor and class in your area.

United States Water Fitness Association
P.O. Box 3279
Boynton Beach, FL 33424
PHONE: 561-732-9908
FAX: 561-732-0950
E-MAIL: uswfa@emi.net
WEBSITE: www.emi.net/uswfa/public_html/

The best source of information about diving programs, lessons, and competitions, for both beginning, novice divers, and masters divers is U.S. Diving.

U.S. Diving
Pan American Plaza
201 South Capitol Avenue, Suite 430
Indianapolis, IN 46225
PHONE: 317-237-5252
FAX: 317-237-5257
E-MAIL: usdiving@aol.com
WEBSITE: www.usdiving.org

A good all-around source of information on swimming techniques and workouts, *Fitness Swimmer* magazine also regularly contains gear guides (such as, "Best New Goggles") and health care articles (such as "How Swimming Can Improve Asthma Symptoms").

Fitness Swimmer
P.O. Box 7420
Red Oak, IA 51591-2420
PHONE: 800-846-0086

Books to Check Out

Jane Katz and Nancy P. Bruning, *Swimming for Total Fitness: A Progressive Aerobic Program* (New York: Main Street Books, 1993).
Good book for true beginners. Offers a progressive program for those who want to learn to swim, as well as for swimmers at every level. Katz explains how to swim in detail and offers drills to improve stroke techniques, tips on improving starts and turns, and a series of progressive workouts designed to increase strength and stamina.

Terry Laughlin and John Delves, *Total Immersion : The Revolutionary Way to Swim Better, Faster, and Easier* (New York: Simon & Schuster, 1996).
Authored by masters swimmer and coach Terry Laughlin, who holds "Total Immersion" workshops across the United States, this book focuses on simple, step-by-step drills that are designed to teach you to stroke through the water faster and more efficiently. The book deals only with the freestyle stroke.

Steve Tarpinian, *The Essential Swimmer* (New York: Lyons and Burford, 1996).
From the basics to advanced techniques, the focus here is on teaching you to identify flaws in your stroke, kick, body position, and breathing; the book then provides detailed drills and instructions on correcting.

◑ Swimmer Speak

False start: Just as it sounds, it's when a swimmer leaves the starting block before the race is officially begun. But unlike track events, where runners often fly from their blocks prematurely several times before the gun goes off, in swimming one false start results in an automatic disqualification from the race.

Splits: Your intermediate time in a race (say halfway). A negative split is when you go faster in the second half of the race than you did in the first half.

Turnover: The number of times you execute a stroke cycle in a given distance or time during a race.

Steve Tarpinian and Brian J. Awbrey, M.D., *Water Workouts : A Guide to Fitness, Training, and Performance Enhancement in the Water* (New York: Lyons and Burford Publishers, 1997).
This book goes beyond lap swimming and includes tough workout prescriptions for aqua aerobics, deep-water running, water strength training, and sport-specific training.

TENNIS

When played well, it looks easy. As a concept, it seems simple too. After all, the general idea of tennis, just as in games like badminton and volleyball, is to hit the ball into your opponent's court in such a way that she is unable to return it to your court or that she returns it so weakly that you can surely "put it away" with your next shot.

In actuality, tennis is quite a complicated game. The strokes, the footwork, and even (or especially!) the scoring are not easy to master. "In fact, tennis is so difficult that we would call it the Everest of the racket sports—it poses the highest challenges and offers the most frustration of any of the major racket sports," write Herbert S. FitzGibbon II and Jeffrey N. Bairstow in *The Complete Racquet Sports Player* (Simon & Schuster, 1979).

But the satisfactions of tennis are as abundant as the challenges, note authors FitzGibbon and Bairstow: "Played outdoors on a bright, sparkling summer's day with breezes rippling the nearby trees, tennis has a feeling of openness, of freedom that is rarely matched by any other sport, whether individual or team. And even if you don't make it to the top, there is an innate pleasure in trying, just as the mountain climber will enjoy a 50-foot rock face even though she knows that Everest is out of her reach. There are enough small pleasures in a game of tennis to make it more than worthwhile."

How It's Played: It is played on a court 78 feet long and 36 feet wide divided by a tautly strung net 3 feet 6 inches high at the posts but only 3 feet high at the center. Singles is played on a narrower court (27 feet wide), usually marked off with white lines. Courts may be made of asphalt, clay, or grass or they can be indoors.

The server delivers the ball from behind the baseline. Two tries are permitted for each service. The served ball must bounce in the proper service court, but after the serve, a player can return balls before they bounce. After a successful serve the ball is hit back and forth until one player or side fails to return the ball successfully.

At the end of the first game, the server becomes the receiver and vice versa. Players alternate thus throughout the match.

Tennis has its own unique and arcane scoring system, unlike that of any other sport (but at least the system is the same for singles and doubles).

A contest or match in tennis is based on three units of scoring: points, games, and sets. A player must win at least 4 points to win a game, at least 6 games to win a set, and at least 2 sets to win a match. In other words, the minimum number of points in a match is 48.

That's easy enough, except that in tennis each point won by a player is called by its own name, not by the cumulative number of points that have been won. If you have no points, your score is called love; if you have 1 point, your score is 15; if you have 2 points, your score is 30; if you have 3 points, your score is 40; and if you win 4 points, you win the game. To win a game, you must not only have won 4 points, you must be at least 2 points ahead of your opponent; to win a set, you must be 2 games ahead.

Key Physical Requirements: Matches last anywhere from one to two hours. In general, tennis is probably less aerobic than other racket sports, but it really depends on the style of tennis game you play. Also, the more quickly you can get around the court, the stronger your arm when it comes to driving a ball across the net, and the more stamina you have, the better player you'll be.

Equipment: tennis balls, which are fabric-covered, fuzzy, hollow, have good bounce and measure between 2½ and 2⅝ inches in diameter and weigh between 2 and 2 1/16 ounces. Yellow and white balls are used in competition, but many players prefer iridescent green ones for practice, since they can be easier to find.

The maximum racket length is 32 inches; the maximum width is 12.5 inches; as with most racket sports, finding a racket that is comfortable to grip and is of a comfortable weight is paramount. Tennis rackets are all over the map in price, but start at around $50.

What to Wear: Players usually wear lightweight clothing, traditionally white or light-colored, and athletic shoes specifically designed for tennis (NOT the flimsy canvas sneakers many of us still refer to as "tennis shoes"). Thick, sweat-repellent socks that give extra cushioning to absorb shocks can help prevent blisters.

To Find Out More

As the national governing body for tennis, the United States Tennis Association (USTA), offers a wide array of information and opportunities. If you just want to try the game to see if you like it, the USTA will arrange for you to have a free lesson in your area. You can then sign up for nine hours of additional lessons at low cost.

If you decide to become a member of USTA (membership costs $25 a year), your USTA membership card lets you play in adult and/or senior tennis leagues in your area. There are also a wide range of USTA-sanctioned tournaments, available only to members, for all ages and ability levels. USTA contact information:

USTA
70 West Red Oak Lane
White Plains, NY 10604
PHONE: 914-696-7000
FAX: 914-696-7167
WEBSITE: www.usta.com

Books to Check Out

There are literally hundreds of books on tennis and there seems to be a steady stream of new additions. Here are two really basic guides that are addressed to players who are picking up a racket for the first time:

Mike Shaw, Ed., *How to Play Tennis : A Step-By-Step Guide* (Cincinnati: Seven Hills Book Distributors, 1993).

Jim Brown, *Tennis : Steps to Success (Steps to Success Activity)* (Champaign, Ill:, Human Kinetics, 1995).

◐ Tennis Talk

Love: The term used in scoring to mean zero or no points served.

Mixed doubles: A type of competition in which a man and woman play as partners against another doubles team composed of a man and woman.

Seeding: A process by which the best entrants in a tournament are placed in the draw so that they will not meet each other in the early rounds of a tournament. Seedings are based on rankings and upon recent tournament performance.

Upset: When a seeded player is defeated by an unseeded one.

TRIATHLON

Although there are an estimated 200,000 plus active triathletes in the United States, there would probably be even more participants except for the common misconception that a triathlon *necessarily* follows the format of the famous—and famously grueling—Ironman, which consists of a 2.4-mile swim, a 112-mile bike ride, and a full 26.2 marathon.

In reality, the majority of triathlons are much, much shorter. The Olympic distance, for instance, is a 1.5k swim, a 40k bike, and a 10k run. A series of women-only triathlons (the Danskin Women's Triathlon Series) held throughout the spring and summer in different cities across the country, is composed of a .75k swim (about a ⅓ mile) a 20k bike (12 miles), and a 5k run (3.1 miles). What's more, most triathlons allow for relay competition. That means you could team up with two friends and parcel out the swim, bike, and run segments of the race among yourselves, so that each of you only races in one sport.

How It's Done: You compete in three different events—a swim, a bike, and a run—consecutively (and almost always in that order). You literally come out of the water after your swim and jump onto your bike, then when the cycle portion of your race is completed, you jump off and hit the pavement running. The clock starts when you jump into the water and only stops when you run across the finish line. That means any time you spend running from the water to your bike or changing your footgear or clothes is calculated in your overall performance time.

The basic rules of the swim are few—any stroke is acceptable, although most athletes use the crawl because it is fastest. You need to stay within the designated swim area (which is usually marked by buoys) during the race. Some triathlons are held at local YMCAs—in those you do laps in a pool, then run outside to jump on your bike.

Most bike racing rules apply to the triathlon. Drafting, in which you gain an aerodynamic advantage by riding close to another cyclist, is forbidden. Each cyclist is supposed to have a safety zone of 2 meters by 7 meters—no rider is allowed to violate and enter this zone except for passing, which needs to be done within fifteen seconds. You are not allowed to walk your bike (although in less competitive, local triathlons, this rule is unlikely to be applied).

Running rules are like most races—no headsets, no baby strollers, and so on. You can break your stride and walk if you need to.

Key Physical Requirements: Although it depends on the distances you choose to race, the triathlon is essentially an endurance sport. You need to be strong and fit in three different sports. One of the biggest challenges is learning how to cope with the fatigue that carries over from one event to another, as well as the cumulative fatigue of the event. But, at the same time, you don't necessarily need to train six hours a day to do triathlons. You can do quite well on less training. In fact, few triathletes train in all three events every day. Instead, they alternate workouts, only combining two sports each time. Then, once a week or every other week, they might combine all three sports in one workout. Whatever training plan you adopt, however, you need to set up a workout schedule that's tailored to the specific event you plan to enter.

Equipment: If your main objective is to compete with yourself and see if and/or how well you can finish, your equipment needs don't have to be terribly complicated. Essentially, for the swim, you'll need a swimsuit, a bathing cap, goggles; for the bike, you'll need a road bike and a helmet; for the run, a good pair of shoes, shorts, and a shirt. Of course, the more competitive you aim to be, the more complicated and expensive equipment choices become. From pedal and shoe systems designed specifically to cut down on bike-to-run transition times to bikes that cost more than many cars, an elite triathlete can easily spend thousands of dollars equipping herself.

What to Wear: Basically, what you wear will depend a lot on the weather conditions you are racing in as well as how competitive you hope to be. Competitive, elite triathletes usually do not change out of their bathing suits for the entire race. But many recreational triathletes find they are more than willing to sacrifice a minute or two in their overall finish times in order to change into something comfortable during a transition. For example, many recreational athletes will wear a wet suit if the waters are cool and/or will switch out of their bathing suit and put on something dry and warm for the bike portion. It pays to remember that if you become too chilled and uncomfortable, you may lose more time and your performance may suffer more than if you took a minute or two to change.

You will usually have your race number printed in a grease pencil on your upper arms, a race number also needs to be attached to your bike, and you'll need to wear your number pinned to a shirt or shorts during the run.

Swimming caps and cycling helmets are usually compulsory. Sometimes the sponsors of the triathlon will provide swim caps. Your helmet must be approved by an official testing authority, such as ANSI or SNELL and must be securely fastened from the time you remove your bicycle from the rack at the start of the cycle, until after you have placed your bike on the rack at the finish of the cycle.

To Find Out More

USA Triathlon, the national governing body for the sport, sanctions over 500 events each year, and also publishes a national magazine, *Triathlon Times*. Membership costs $25 a year.

USA Triathlon
P.O. Box 15850
3595 East Fountain Boulevard F-1
Colorado Springs, CO 80910
PHONE: 719-597-9090
FAX: 719-597-2121

E-MAIL:USATriathlon@usatriathlon.org
WEBSITE:www.usatriathlon.org

For information about the Danskin Women's Triathlon Series (which helps benefit the Susan G. Komen Breast Cancer Foundation):

Danskin Women's Triathlon Series
749 South Lemay A3-221
Fort Collins, CO 80524-3251
PHONE: 800-452-9526
FAX: 970-221-4196

Books to Check Out

Glenn Town, Ph.D., and Todd Kearney, M.S., *Swim, Bike, Run* (Champaign, Ill.: Human Kinetics, 1993).

Steven Jonas, *The Essential Triathlete* (New York: Lyons and Burford, 1996).

John Mora, *Triathlon 101* (Champaign, Ill.: Human Kinetics, 1999).

Each of these books covers most of the bases, and do it well. Especially if you have never trained or competed in a triathlon before, you'll find most of your questions are answered, from how to select the right equipment to what to wear on race day.

There are also two magazines dedicated to the sport:

Triathlete
1415 Third Street, Suite 303
Santa Monica, CA 90401
PHONE: 800-441-1666

⚠️ **Triathlon Lingo**

Duathlon: A run-bike-run event that tends to be particularly appealing to athletes who have trouble with the swim portion of triathlons. The standard duathlon comprises a 5k run (3.1 miles), followed by a 30k bike (18.6 miles), followed by another 5k run.

Self-seed: To place yourself appropriately in the pack of starting swimmers. If you are a slower swimmer, for example, it's important you move to the back, not only so that you don't slow down the others but so that you don't get trampled, kicked, and crowded in your swimming space as the faster swimmers overtake you.

Transitions: The switch from one portion of the event, such as swimming, to another, such as biking. Triathletes will often practice transitions so they lose as little time as possible doing things like switching from biking to running shoes.

VOLLEYBALL

It's an American invention, dreamed up in 1895 by William G. Morgan, an instructor at the Young Men's Christian Association (YMCA) in Holyoke, Massachusetts. And just like its country of origin, volleyball is a melting pot of different elements. It blends aspects of basketball, baseball, tennis, and handball to become a new game that is relatively uncomplicated and extremely versatile. For example, volleyball can be played indoors or outdoors, on grass, in sand, or on a wooden gym floor; it can be played with teams of six players (the number used for indoor competition) anywhere on down to teams of two players (the number used for beach volleyball); and it lends itself well to mixed co-ed teams.

How It's Played: The object of the game is for each team to send the ball regularly over the net to ground it on the opponent's court and to prevent the ball from being grounded on its own court. A team is allowed to hit the ball three times to return it to the opponent's court. A player is not allowed to hit the ball twice consecutively, except when attempting a block. The rally continues until the ball touches the ground/floor, goes out of bounds, or a team commits a fault.

When played indoors with six-person teams, players are positioned on the court in two rows of three. The three players in the front row are called left front, center front, and right front while the players in the back row are called (not surprisingly!) left back, center back, and right back. These playing positions rotate one position clockwise whenever the receiving team wins a rally.

As a rule, beach volleyball is played with two players on a team.

Only the serving team may score a point. The serve switches sides whenever the serving team fails to return the ball to the opponent's court. A team wins a game by scoring 15 points with a 2-point advantage and wins the match by winning the best of three or five games.

Key Physical Requirements: Unlike most other team sports, you use your whole upper torso and both of your arms, including your forearm, when playing volleyball. Your arms are in constant motion, extending and swinging as your hands and fists are punching, slamming, and slapping.

In order to return the ball explosively, you need to be able to leap or jump for it quickly and powerfully. So your legs need to be strong yet with a lot of spring action in them. Not surprisingly, many elite players do jump training based on plyometrics (an intensive training regimen in which jumps, hops, leaps, dives, and rhythmic movements are exaggerated as intensely and rapidly as possible so as to increase speed and strength of ballistic, sudden moves). Strong arms and shoulders are essential for reaching and returning the ball, plus your lower back must be both limber and strong to sustain the impact of diving maneuvers.

You need an ability to sprint, so as to get to the ball quickly, and you need good endurance capacity; volleyball matches can last anywhere from an hour to three hours.

As a rule, beach volleyball is more demanding aerobically since there are only two players to cover the entire court.

Equipment: In its official form, volleyball is played on a rectangular court, approximately 59 feet long and 29 feet wide. For women, a net 7 feet, 4.125 inches high is suspended across the court. The ball, which is made of soft leather, weighs approximately 8½ ounces.

What to Wear: For indoor volleyball, your clothes should ideally protect you from scrapes and burns you can get when you dive for the ball on the gym floor. Long-sleeve shirts or jerseys and lightweight long leggings provide a good sliding surface and skin protection. However, many athletes don't like having their arms and legs constricted by this longer garb. Whatever you choose, if you are playing on a hard gym floor, you should wear knee pads to cushion your falls. Some athletes also wear elbow protectors.

Many athletic shoe manufacturers now have shoes designed specifically for indoor volleyball—look for good ankle support and cushioning for jumping, landing, twisting, lateral movements, and diving.

For beach and grass volleyball, you'll need a visor, sunglasses, and plenty of sunscreen. The game is usually played barefoot in a bathing suit or in loose-fitting lightweight shorts, preferably with a slit in the side to allow for complete freedom of movement, and a breathable, moisture-managing shirt. You want your clothes to fit you loosely enough so that sand can flow through—you don't want sand to stick to your skin and irritate it.

To Find Out More

USA Volleyball sponsors adult programs and indoor competition at several levels in all areas of the country. To find out about adult programs in your area, contact:

USA Volleyball
3595 East Fountain Boulevard, Suite I-2
Colorado Springs, CO 80910-1740
PHONE: 719-228-6800
FAX: 719-228-6899
WEBSITE: www.volleyball.org/usav

Books to Check Out

Barbara L. Viera and Bonnie Jill Ferguson, *Volleyball: Steps to Success* (Champaign. Ill.:, Human Kinetics, 1996).
Provides a thorough, detailed explanation, with illustrations, of how to master the basic skills of indoor volleyball.

Karch Kiraly with editor Jon Hastings, *Karch Kiraly's Championship Volleyball* (New York, Fireside Books, 1996).
This book has a good chapter on the dynamics of beach volley-

ball, although the whole book may be a bit advanced for the very beginning player.

◯ Volleyball Lingo

Dink: A gentle, soft shot or push of the ball around or over the opposing team's blockers.

Pancake: A one-hand floor defensive technique where the hand is extended and slid along the floor palm down while the player dives or extension rolls, so that the ball bounces off the back of the hand.

Spike: It's like the slam dunk in basketball—dramatic and decisive. The player jumps up, then smashes the ball with such force into the opposing team's court that it's difficult, if not impossible, to return.

Stuff: A solid block that is deflected back to the attacking team's floor and puts an end to the volley.

WALKING

Perhaps the most surprising thing about walking is that there is so much to say about it. You would think "put one foot in front of the other" would just about sum it up. But there's been an explosion of information about walking over the past ten or fifteen years partly because walking is now considered an aerobic sport. Not only is there a U.S. National Racewalking Team, but you can compete in racewalks throughout the country, you can buy shoes specially designed for walking, sign up for tours targeted at fitness walkers, and even subscribe to a magazine devoted entirely to the subject of walking.

How It's Done: When you walk to get a workout, your pacing should be purposeful—you need to go beyond strolling at a leisurely pace if you want to strengthen and build your cardiovascular system. As a rule, it's a good idea to vary your workouts, walking long on some days (to build endurance) and going faster on others (to build speed). Focus on taking quick strides, bending your arms at the elbow, and letting your arms pump as you propel forward. You want to roll smoothly from heel to toe, and you'll want to pay attention to posture: Stand tall, hold your head high. Avoid looking down at the ground the entire time and/or slouching your back.

The competitive sport of racewalking has some specific rules regarding walking technique: There is the straight knee rule, which says that your advancing leg must be straightened (i.e., not bent at the knee) from the moment of first contact with the ground until in the vertical position. Essentially, this rule helps distinguish racewalking from running, since when you run your knee is flexed when it makes contact with the ground. There is also the contact rule, which says that one limb of the walker must always maintain contact with the ground—again, this rule helps make a distinction between walking and running, and helps ensure that racewalkers don't "cheat" by breaking into a runner's stride.

Key Physical Requirements: The great thing about walking is that almost everyone can safely embark on a program of exercise walking, regardless of their fitness level or age. And unlike most sports, walking isn't likely to make beginners feel uncoordinated or inept. Regular aerobic walking will build a healthy heart, burn calories, firm and strengthen your calves, thighs, ankles, feet, hips, and buttocks. The strong arm swing that is an element of a balanced, proper stride also will help tone your shoulders, upper back, chest, and arm muscles.

Equipment: The one essential is a good pair of shoes, with first-rate shock absorbency in the heel—the point of impact is concentrated in your heel when you walk. Make sure you have ample toe room so you can solidly roll forward and then off your toes.

What to Wear: You can wear street clothes, but specific workout clothing that can breathe and wicks away sweat is better. You'll also want clothing that's warm enough (but not too warm) in the winter and cool enough in the summer. Most garb designed for runners also works well for walkers.

To Find Out More

Walking Magazine, which is published every other month, features articles about walking gear, walking adventures, walking plans during pregnancy, how to get started, taking your training to new levels, etc.

Walking
45 Broomfield Street
Boston, MA 02108
PHONE: 617-574-0076
SUBSCRIPTIONS: 800-829-5585
FAX: 617-338-7433
WEBSITE: www.walkingmag.com

www.racewalk.com is a website sponsored by U.S. Track & Field, which is the governing body for the sport of racewalking. It includes very good, detailed information on the biomechanics of proper racewalking technique as well as information on how to get involved in competition.

An organization devoted to promoting the development of racewalking throughout the United States and Canada, the North American Racewalking Foundation, specifically matches inquirers with racewalkers and racewalking clubs throughout the country, provides information on shoes, on racewalking technique and training, and on racewalking books and videos as well as publishing a newsletter, the *U.S. Racewalking Journal.* For information, contact:

North American Racewalking Foundation
P.O. Box 50312
Pasadena, CA 91115-0312
PHONE: 626-441-5459
FAX: 626-799-5106
E-MAIL: NARWF@aol.com

Books to Check Out

Therese Iknoian, *Walking Fast* (Champaign, Ill.: Human Kinetics, 1998).
Maps out strenuous walking workouts that will challenge athletes who are already in good shape from playing other sports. If you doubt that walking can be a serious aerobic activity, this book will change your mind.

Mark Fenton and Seth Bauer, *The 90-Day Fitness Walking Program* (New York: Perigee, 1995).
If you are in good aerobic condition already, this book will be too elemental for you, since it starts from the assumption that you are an absolute beginner who doesn't exercise. Written by editors of

> ### ◐ Walk Talk
>
> *Excessive hip drop:* This condition occurs when you rotate your hips too much. Good racewalking form emphasizes hip rotation without much vertical movement of the hip joint and without much lateral, side-to-side swing.
>
> *PaceWalking:* A term once used to describe fast walking for fitness, coined in the late 1980s by Steven Jonas, M.D., a professor of preventive medicine at the School of Medicine of the State University of New York at Stony Brook.

Walking magazine, it presents a day-by-day, progressive walking program and discusses things like how to choose the right shoes, warm up properly, and employ weights while walking.

WINDSURFING

There are a lot of misconceptions about this sport. For example:

- You don't necessarily have to possess superior upper body strength to try it. Light board sailing—in which you use a big board with a small sail in wind under 10 mph—is no more demanding than walking, according to author Ken Winner in *Windsurfing* (Human Kinetics, 1995).
- You don't need a lot of sailor know-how or technical knowledge. Unlike windsurfing's sister sport, sailing, for example, you don't really need to know how to tie a nautical knot in order to windsurf.
- You don't need strong winds. You can windsurf in the lightest breeze. Most professional-level windsurfing is done in high winds (about 20 mph), but most recreational windsurfing is done in less than 10 mph winds.

Of course, windsurfing can be more strenuous if you want it to be. Wave sailing, for example, involves a lot of aerial jumping and turning and requires tremendous strength, endurance, as well as a "thrill-seeking" mentality.

How It's Done: There are five basic beginner skills you'll need to learn in order to set sail; by most estimates, you should be able to pick them up with as little as two to six hours of qualified instruction.

1. Standing on board: You need to learn how to balance your weight on the board.
2. Uphauling the sail: You need to learn how to pull the sail from the water so you can get underway.
3. Powering the sail: Setting the sail at the right angle so you get power is one of the hardest things to figure out.
4. Steering: Maneuvering the board to go where you want it is the next tricky thing you'll need to learn.
5. Mastering the tack and jibe: These are techniques for turning around (and getting you back to where you started).

In addition, windsurfers need to become familiar with the basic water etiquette that prevails in their area. You need to learn, for example, if you have the right of way when encountering a power boat or vice versa.

Key Physical Requirements: Serious windsurfing requires more lower body strength—i.e., good legs—than would seem apparent from watching from shore. Hill running or walking, in particular, builds the quadriceps muscles in your thighs that need to be strong for more aggressive windsurfing. Good strong abdominal and arm muscles also become increasingly more important as you become more experienced and adventurous in the sport. The equation is simple: the stronger the winds you venture out in and the bigger the size sail you use, the more you'll need your body strength to counter the force of the wind and control the sail.

Equipment: There are two types of windsurfers: longboards and shortboards. Longboards, an all-purpose board that can be used in a wide range of wind and water conditions, are recommended for beginners (although professionals and racers use them too). Shortboards are designed for speed and higher winds. The sails and board of a windsurfer need to be matched to the wind conditions you plan to sail in as well as your weight and height. Although you can often pick up a good, basic set for a few hundred dollars (or less if you buy second hand), it probably doesn't make sense to buy a board until you try out the sport several times and get a feel for what type of equipment best suits you.

What to Wear: In ideal summer conditions, you'll just need a bathing suit and sunscreen. However, in some waters, wearing a life jacket is necessary (if the water is calm and you are a competent swimmer, your board can usually suffice as an emergency buoyancy device).

If the beach bottom is rough—i.e. contains twigs, shells, or other debris, you might want to wear water shoes. If the air and/or water temperature is cool, you'll want to wear, at the very least, a short lycra body suit made of thin neoprene. In colder weather a wetsuit is essential to preventing hypothermia (a condition in which your body's core temperature falls and which can result in unconsciousness). A good snug fit is key for waterproofing, especially at the wrist, neck, and ankles. A wetsuit is often part of the package when you rent a board.

To Find Out More

Discover Sailing was established by the National Sailing Industry Association (NISA) to encourage windsurfing (as well as sailing) nationwide; often the program can link you up with no-cost introductory lessons through community centers and sailing schools near your home. The toll free number is 800-535-SAIL. You can visit their website at www.discoversailing.com.

You can also get information about where to find windsurfing lessons, schools, and camps as well as equipment from these two sources:

United States Windsurfing Association
P.O. Box 978
Hood River, OR 97031
PHONE: 541-386-8708
FAX: 541-386-2108
E-MAIL: USWA@aol.com

◐ Windsurfer Speak

Kneesurfer: A windsurfer in which the base is inflatable—i.e., not hard like a surfboard.

Rig: It's what you call the sail when it is assembled with boom, mast, and mast base.

Waterstart: A maneuver in which you use the sail to pull you out of the water (instead of you having to pull the sail out).

American Windsurfing Industries Association
1099 Snowden Road
White Salmon, WA 98672
PHONE: 800-963-7873; 509-493-9463
FAX: 509-493-9464
WEBSITE: www.awia.org
E-MAIL: awia@gorge.net

Books to Check Out

Ken Winner, *Windsurfing* (Champaign, Ill.:Human Kinetics, 1995).
This is a solid beginner's guide; includes some nice information on windsurfing games, tricks, and races.

Algis Steponaitis, *The American Sailing Association's Let's Go Windsurfing* (New York: Hearst Marine Books, 1994).
Includes more than one hundred illustrations, diagrams, and black-and-white photos to help illustrate rig-handling techniques, wind theory, and gear.

SPORT SHORTS

Archery

The skills of archery—using a bow and arrow to hit a target—are used in a variety of different practices. The most common form is target archery, which involves standing behind a line that is a designated distance from the target (a circle with multicolored concentric circles within it). You then try to shoot your arrows as close to the innermost circle (since that has the most points) as you can. In field archery, you shoot at various inanimate objects at different distances while walking in the fields or woods. In ski-archery, you cross-country ski a course making a number of designated shooting stops: the winner is determined by combining the fastest skiing time with the most accurate arrow shots.

Resources

National Archery Association
One Olympic Plaza

Colorado Springs, CO 80909
PHONE: 719-578-4576
FAX: 719-632-4733
WEBSITE: www.usarchery.org

This is the governing body for the sport; via membership, you can get connected with local clubs, instructors, competitions, and so on.

National Field Archery Association
31407 Outer I-10
Redlands, CA 92373
PHONE: 909-794-2133 or 800-811-2331
FAX: 909-794-8512

Besides helping you make connections to "shooter's schools" and field archery events, this organization publishes *Archery* magazine, which is filled with articles on shooting techniques, the latest equipment, etc.

Bobsledding

For this sport, you are part of a team of either two or four that drives a special sled down a track that has various technical challenges, such as curves and tricky descents, built into it. Besides driving and braking skill, you need to be able to sprint powerfully and push the sled aggressively to get it as quickly as possible onto the track. The two-man sled weighs 860 pounds, while the four-man sled has a maximum weight of 1,388 pounds according to the United States Olympic Committee.

Resources

U.S. Bobsled & Skeleton Federation (USBSF)
P.O. Box 828
421 Old Military Road
Lake Placid, NY 12946-0828
WEBSITE: www.usabobsled.org
E-MAIL: info@usabobsled.org

The national governing body for the sport of bobsledding, the USBSF holds training programs for the sport. If you want to try the sport for the fun of it, you can pay for a ride at the Olympic Training Center in Lake Placid, New York—there are also a few recreational tracks at ski resorts across the country.

Bodybuilding

The weight room is the heart and soul of this sport in which weight training is an end unto itself (i.e., athletes aren't trying to get strong for other sports). Athletes strive to have superior muscle definition over their entire body; muscle appearance is a vital aspect of bodybuilding competition.

Resources

National Amateur Bodybuilders Association U.S.A.
P.O. Box 531
Bronx, NY 10469
PHONE: 718-882-6413
FAX: 718-882-6847
WEBSITE: www.nabba.com

Promotes competitions for amateurs of all ages, heights, and weights. Also sponsors Ms. Figure contests, which are similar to traditional bodybuilding contests but with an emphasis on a more feminine look.

Amateur Bodybuilding Association
1307 West Sixth Street
Corona, CA 91720
PHONE: 909-734-3900
FAX: 909-735-6219
WEBSITE: www.getbig.com

The ABA is dedicated to "natural" bodybuilding—that is, without the use of steroids or other drugs. It hosts competitions as well as publishes *Natural Fitness & Muscle Magazine*.

Boxing

It's still a male-dominated sport, but the opportunities for interested women to get involved are growing. Keep in mind, boxing is not the same as classes in boxaerobics (gym workouts that employ shadow boxing maneuvers and punching of heavy bags). In boxing, you fight a real opponent, which means there is the real chance you'll get a black eye or blow to your belly.

Resources
If you have access to the Internet, a great site specifically for women boxers, with links to most major boxing organizations, is www.femboxer.com

U.S.A. Boxing (Women's Division)
One Olympic Plaza
Colorado Springs, CO 80909-5776
PHONE: 719-578-4506
FAX: 719-632-3426
WEBSITE: www.usaboxing.org

Caving

Not for the claustrophobic since it involves exploring dark, often damp, cold, slippery tunnels, caving is an adventure sport that tends to attract people interested in archeology, crystals, conservation, and even bats.

National Speleological Society
Cave Avenue
Huntsville, AL 35810
PHONE: 205-758-2328
WEBSITE: www.caves.org

The society can help you find a local caving club; it also publishes a newsletter and other literature on caving.

Golf

This game of finesse and subtlety is attracting more and more women, many of whom are using the sport as an important social setting to conduct business. The first rule of learning to play is *not* to make your first attempt at hitting a golf ball while playing on a golf course—a move that virtually every seasoned player will tell you is only bound to lead to high frustration. Instead, begin golf at a driving range with a series of lessons from a professional. A pro can teach you the proper grip, stance, and alignment, and the mechanics of the swing to prevent you from falling into bad habits. Be careful about getting instructions from friends and/or your husband—just because someone can play golf doesn't mean he or she knows how to teach it.

Resources

Ladies Professional Golf Association (LPGA)
100 International Golf Drive
Daytona Beach, FL 32124-1092
PHONE: 904-274-6200
FAX: 904-274-1099
WEBSITE: www.lpga.com

The LPGA hosts one-day instruction clinics for beginners across the country; it can also help you find a certified teaching professional in your area.

Lacrosse

The uniqueness of this fast-moving field sport, which is descended from a game played by Native Americans, lies in its use of the crosse—a webbed basket on a stick. You must learn to catch, throw, run backward and forward while using both your hands to hold and maneuver your lacrosse stick, which is used to field a hard rubber ball. "Lax heads" must have strong running legs (since an official game has two periods of 25 minutes, with virtually no timeouts) and good flexibility (to twist and dodge for the ball while holding the crosse).

Resources

U.S. Lacrosse
113 University Parkway
Baltimore, MD 21210
PHONE: 401-235-6882
FAX: 410-366-6735
E-MAIL: info@lacrosse.org
WEBSITE: www.lacrosse.org

This organization can help you find leagues in your area.

An online magazine source for camps, equipment reviews, playing tips, and so forth is www.e-lacrosse.com

Martial Arts

Karate, t'ai chi chuan, kung fu, aikido, judo, qigong, kendo, jujitsu—these are just a few of the martial arts that are well known and widely practiced in this country. Although each martial art has its own distinct traditions, methods of training, and underpinning philosophy, there is one commonality among almost all of them: They all blend and combine a system of self-defense and a technique of mental discipline with a regimen of physical conditioning. As a rule, there are very few physical prerequisites for beginners when it comes to studying any of the individual martial art forms. However, as you become more expert, many of the martial arts become quite physically demanding, both in terms of your overall strength and fitness level and in terms of your ability to fight and spar.

So how do you find the practice that is best suited to you? Unfortunately, there is no easy answer to that question. Even if you think, for example, it's karate you want to study, there are huge variations in the way different schools and instructors practice karate in this country. So rather than dwell on the issue of what martial art might be best for you, it's probably better to get practical and focus on what disciplines are taught in your area. Then, visit the schools or instructors and observe (or take) a class. "Clicking" with a school or instructor is paramount, since most people who become committed to practicing a martial art also form a strong allegiance with their instructor(s) or school.

Resources

Jennifer Lawler, *Martial Arts for Women: A Practical Guide* (Wethersfield, Conn.: Turtle Press, 1998).

This book focuses on many issues that women, in particular, face when they become involved in a martial art. Subjects covered including sparring against taller partners, adjusting to contact, dressing for class, training during pregnancy, dealing with sexist attitudes, choosing the right school, and figuring the cost. The publisher of this book specializes in martial arts and its website—www.turtlepress.com—is a good place to get information about the different martial arts.

Nicklaus Suino, *Arts of Strength, Arts of Serenity: Martial Arts Training for Mental, Physical, and Spiritual Health* (Trumbull, Conn.: Weatherhill, 1996).

Offers a clear, focused discussion and descriptions of many different styles of martial arts with good advice on what to look for in a martial arts school, in the instructor, and the attitude of the students.

Orienteering

This sport combines the physical skills of trail running with navigational skills—i.e., the ability to read a compass and a topographical map. In an "O" competition, "o-nuts" line up at the starting line, with maps and compass in hand, then attempt to find their way through an outdoor course (often unmarked wilderness, although orienteering events have even been held in places like malls, and there are ski orienteering events as well) as fast as possible, stopping at various checkpoints to prove they have reached an area. The winner is the person who arrives at the finish the fastest and who makes the fewest navigational errors.

Resources

This organization will help connect you to everything you need—from a local club to magazines to international competitions to outfitters who specialize in orienteering clothes and compasses.

United States Orienteering Federation
P.O. Box 1444
Forest Park, GA 30298
PHONE: 404-363-2110
WEBSITE: www.orienteering.org

Rock Climbing

There are two types of climbing:

1. *Sport climbing*: A form of climbing that involves little risk and does not demand a huge commitment in terms of learning time. It's done on an artificial wall in a sports center or in manageable outdoor terrain. Usually you wear safety ropes that prevent hard falls. A variation on sport climbing is bouldering—a sport in which you scramble up small hills of rocks using just your hands and feet (you don't wear ropes).
2. *Adventure climbing:* A high-risk endeavor that may be done on the sides of steep mountains, cliffs, snowy terrain, frozen waterfalls, and ice. It's a sport that can be deadly. As such, it demands you acquire a great deal of skill and technical knowledge before you set out.

For both versions of the sport, you need strong fingers (since you use your hands to grip rock and/or rope) and strong muscles in your forearms (since they support the tendons in your hands). You also need to be good at "pull-ups" (i.e., have strong chest, shoulder, and upper arm muscles) since you use your upper body to hoist yourself up.

Resources
A huge book filled with detailed information on all variations of climbing is *Mountaineering: The Freedom of the Hills* published by The Mountaineers (1001 S.W. Klickitat Way, Seattle, WA 98134). Another good book is *Rock Climb!* by John Long (Chockstone Press, P.O. Box 3505, Evergreen, Colo. 80437). In addition, these magazines can provide up-to-date information on gear as well as lots of specific "how-to" advice:

Climbing Magazine
P.O. Box 339
Carbondale, CO 81623
PHONE: 970-963-9449

Rock & Ice Magazine
P.O. Box 3595
Boulder, CO 80303
PHONE: 303-499-8410

Rugby

Rugby has over 6000 active female players in the U.S., 88 percent of whom are between eighteen and forty-nine, according to U.S.A. Rugby, the national governing body for the sport. There are also about 1,200 rugby clubs in this country. So what is it? It's a combination of football (tackling is part of the sport, the ball is similar in shape and feel, but you don't wear a helmet and other protective gear) and soccer (since play involves a lot of continuous running and ball fielding). It's played on a field called a pitch, which is longer and wider than a football field. Each side has fifteen players, and the aim of the game is to get the ball beyond the opponents' goal line. Like football, you need to be willing to be aggressive and not fearful of full body contact; like soccer, you'll need good endurance, strength, and speed to keep up with the game's fast pace.

Resource

USA Rugby
3595 East Fountain Boulevard, Suite M2
Colorado Springs, CO 80910
PHONE: 719-637-1022
E-MAIL: info@usarugby.org
WEBSITE: www.usarugby.org

Sailing

Learning to sail, whether your ambition is to sail a one person dingy (a small open boat) or participate on a boat with a cabin and a crew, involves learning a whole new language. Sailor talk isn't just cool slang. Phrases like "hard alee" and "jibe ho" refer to specific actions that you need to understand and respond to appropriately: the "leech," "luff," and "halyards" are parts of a sail that you need to know how to distinguish.

Being an occasional recreational sailor doesn't require any special physical conditioning, other than being reasonably fit and healthy and possessing an ability to swim. However, if you choose to sailboat race, physical endurance and strength become increasingly important because they enable you to react quickly to changes in the wind as well as stay on the water for long periods of time without becoming fatigued.

Resources

Discover Sailing was established by NSIA, the National Sailing Industry Association, to expose thousands of nonsailors nationwide to the sport annually. The program will often allow you to try sailing in no-cost situations through community centers and sailing schools near your home. Call the toll-free number: 800-535-SAIL or visit their website: www.discoversailing.com

A good source of information about sailing schools, instruction, books, and manuals is the following:

American Sailing Association
13922 Marquesas Way
Marina del Rey, CA 90292
PHONE: 310-822-7171
FAX: 310-822-4741
WEBSITE: www.american-sailing.com
E-MAIL: info@american-sailing.com

A primary source for finding information on the Internet about the entire sailing industry, the SailNet site has links to sailing schools and information on developing sailing skills: www.sailnet.com

Ultimate Frisbee

According to the Ultimate Frisbee Players Association, the game is played competitively by over 25,000 amateur athletes in over 35 countries—not to mention countless casual players. It's a team sport played with a Frisbee on a field. It's hands-off, no body contact involved. You can't run with the Frisbee in your hand. Ideally, there are two teams of seven players each; the object of the game is for a team to pass the disk from player to player, all the way up the field, and catch the disk in the end zone, which scores a point. Like soccer, the game tends to be continuous so you should expect to do a lot of running and flying for the disk.

Resource

Ultimate Frisbee Players Association
3595 East Fountain Boulevard, Suite J2
Colorado Springs, CO, 80910
PHONE: 800-872-4384 or 719-591-1168
FAX: 719-591-2461
E-MAIL: upa_hq@upa.org
WEBSITE: www.upa.org

The UPA can help you find pickup games, tournaments, and other events near you.

Yoga

Almost all forms of yoga—and there are dozens of them—will help increase your flexibility. Beyond that, some styles of yoga, such as kundalini, emphasize breathing, chanting, and meditation, while others, such as ashtanga, are aerobic, power-ful, and muscular. In many ways, there is something for every-one in yoga—the trick is finding the style and instructor that suit you.

Resources

A great article to track down (at your local library—or check to see if it is still posted on Self's website www.phys.com) is "Yoga: The Ultimate Guide," which was published in the July 1998 issue of *Self* magazine—it really helps sort through the differences of all the different varieties of yoga.

An informative guide, with careful, detailed explanations of yoga's core stretching positions is

Mara Carrico, *Yoga Journal's Yoga Basics: The Essential Beginner's Guide to Yoga for a Lifetime of Health and Fitness* (New York: Henry Holt & Co., 1997).

Afterword

I would love to hear from you. What kinds of health and diet challenges have you faced as an athlete? What kinds of solutions have you discovered? Have your experiences been similar to those of the athletes I interviewed, or do you have a different perspective that wasn't mentioned? Have you delved into any new sports, and what did it feel like to be a "beginner" again? I am very interested in hearing any feedback, criticisms, or anecdotes you would like to share. You can E-mail me at: jgraham1@clarityconnect.com. Or write me at: Janis Graham, author of *The Athletic Woman's Sourcebook*, Avon Books, 1350 Avenue of the Americas, New York, NY 10019.

Of course, my hope is that you found this book to be helpful and informative. If you did, a lot of the credit goes to all of the experts and athletes who so generously gave of their time and who so willingly shared their knowledge and experience with me. I was honored to have the opportunity to speak with so many interesting, informed, and talented people. I owe them all a huge thank you. I especially owe thanks to Lisa R. Callahan, M.D., who painstakingly took the time to review the entire manuscript.

I would also like to thank my editor, Lyssa Keusch, who understood the concept of this book from the very beginning and who has been encouraging, pleasant, and insightful throughout. As always, my husband Bob and my two children, Addie and Kaspar, deserve special thanks for being so supportive of my writing as well as my running, swimming, and biking. Finally, I would like to say thank you to my exercise companions Steve, Catherine, and Claudia, who patiently listened to my chatter about this book during many workouts.

References

PART ONE: YOUR ACTIVE HEALTH
Chapter 1: Your Menstrual Cycle

Agostini, R., ed. *Medical and Orthopedic Issues of Active and Athletic Women*. Philadelphia, Penna.: Hanley and Belfus, 1994.

Bennell, K. L., Malcolm, S. A., et al. "Risk Factors for Stress Fractures in Female Track and Field Athletes: A Retrospective Analysis," *Clin J Sport Med* 1995; 5 (4): 229–35.

Broocks, A., Pirke, K. M., et al. "Cyclic Ovarian Function in Recreational Athletes," *J Appl Physiol* 1990; 68 (5): 2083–86.

Bullen, B. A., Skrinar, G. S., et al. "Induction of Menstrual Disorders by Strenuous Exercise in Untrained Women," *New England Journal of Medicine (NEJM)* 312 (1985): 1349–53.

Collaborative Group on Hormonal Factors in Breast Cancer. "Breast Cancer and Hormonal Contraceptives: Further Results," *Contraception* 1996; 54 (3 Suppl): 1S–106S.

Costa, D. M., and Guthrie, S. R., eds. *Women and Sport: Interdisciplinary Perspectives*. Champaign, Ill.: Human Kinetics, 1994.

De Souza, M. J.; and Metzger, D.A. "Reproductive Dysfunction in Amenorrheic Athletes and Anorexic Patients: A Review," *Med Sci Sports Exerc* 1991; 23 (9): 995–1007.

———, Maguire, M. S., et al. Effects of Menstrual Phase and Amenorrhea on Exercise Performance in Runners, *Med Sci Sports Exerc* 1990; 22(5): 575–80.

Drinkwater, B. L. "Exercise and Bones: Lessons Learned from Female Athletes," *Am J Sports Med* 1996; 24 (6): S-33–35.

Fort, I., De Brezzo, R., et al. "Activity Level and Menstrual Cycle Function," *Melpomene J* 1993; 12 (2): 18–20.

Harel, Z., Biro, F. M., et al. "Supplementation with Omega-3 Polyunsaturated Fatty Acids in the Management of Dysmenorrhea in Adolescents," *Am J Obstet Gyncecol* 1996; 174 (4): 1335–38.

Lebrun, C. M., McKenzie C., et al. "Effects of Menstrual Cycle Phase on Athletic Performance," *Med Sci Sports Exerc* 1995; 27 (3): 437–44.

Loucks, A. B. "Effects of Exercise Training on the Menstrual Cycle: Existence and Mechanisms," *Med Sci Sports Exerc* 1990; 22 (3): 275–80.

Loucks, A. B., Vaitukaitis, J., et al. "The Reproductive System and Exercise in Women," *Med Sci Sports Exerc* 1992; 24 (6 Suppl); S288–93.

Monahan, T. "Treating Athletic Amenorrhea: A Matter of Instinct," *Phys Sportsmed* 1987; 15 (7): 184–87.

Nattiv, A., and Armsey, T. D., "Stress Injury to Bone in the Female Athlete," *Clin Sports Med* 1997; 16 (2): 197–224.

Nygaard, I. "Efficacy of Pelvic Floor Muscle Exercises in Women with Stress, Urge, and Mixed Urinary Incontinence," *Am J Obstet Gynecol* 174 (1996): 120–25.

Olson, B. R., Forman, M. R., et al. "Relation Between Sodium Balance and Menstrual Cycle Symptoms in Normal Women," *Ann Int Med* 125 (1996): 564–67.

Pasquale, S. A., and Cadoff, J. *The Birth Control Book.* New York: Ballantine Books, 1996.

Pearl, A. J, editor. *The Athletic Female.* Champaign, Ill.: Human Kinetics, 1993.

Prior, J. C., Vigna, Y., et al. "Conditioning Exercise Decreases Premenstrual Symptoms: A Prospective, Controlled Six-Month Trial," *Fertil Steril* 47 (1987): 402–408.

Shangold, M., Rebar, R. W., et al. "Evaluation and Management of Menstrual Dysfunction in Athletes." *Journal of the American Medical Association (JAMA)* 263 (1990): 1665–69.

Warren, M. P., "Amenorrrhea in Endurance Runners," *J Clin Edocrinol Metab* 1992: 75 (6): 1393–97.

Chapter 2: Your Diet

Armstrong, L. E., Costill, D. L., et al. "Influence of Diuretic-Induced Dehydration on Competitive Running Performance," *Med Sci Sports Exerc* 1985; 17 (4): 456–61.

Beals, K. A., and Manore, M. M. "The Prevalence and Consequences of Subclinical Eating Disorders in Female Athletes," *Int J Sport Nut* 4 (1994): 175–95.

Below, P. R., Mora-Rodriguez, R., et al. "Fluid and Carbohydrate Ingestion Independently Improve Performance During One Hour of Intense Exercise," *Med Sci Sports Exerc* 1995; 27 (2): 200–210.

Clark, N. "Caffeine: A User's Guide." *Phys Sportsmed* Online 1997; 25 (11):

Clark, N. *Nancy Clark's Sports Nutrition Guidebook*. Champaign, Ill.: Human Kinetics, 1990.

Coggan, A., Hopkins, W., et al. "Dietary Fat and Physical Activity: Fueling the Controversy," *Science Exchange Roundtable Articles #25* (1996) 7. Gatorade Sports Science Institute website.

Convertino, V. A., Armstrong, L.E., et al. "Exercise and Fluid Replacement: The American College of Sports Medicine Position Stand," *Med Sci Sports Exerc* 1996; 28 (1): i–viii.

Dueck, C. A., Manore, M.M., et al. "Role of Energy Balance in Athletic Menstrual Dysfunction," *Int. J. Sport Nut* 6 (1996): 165–90.

———, and Matt, K. S., "Treatment of Athletic Amenorrhea with a Diet and Training Intervention Program," *Int J Sports Nut* 6 (1996): 24–40.

Febbraio, M. A., Murton P., et al. "Effect of CHO Ingestion on Exercise Metabolism and Performance in Different Ambient Temperatures," *Med Sci Sports Exerc* 1996; 28 (11): 1380–87.

Graham, T. E., and Spriet, L. L., "Caffeine and Exercise Performance," *Science Exchange Articles #60* 9 (1996) Gatorade Sports Science Institute website.

———. "Metabolic, Catecholamine, and Exercise Performance Responses to Various Doses of Caffeine," *J Appl Physiol* 1995; 78 (3): 867–874.

Grandjean, A. C. "Diets of Elite Athletes: Has the Discipline of Sports Nutrition Made an Impact?" *J Nutr* 1997; 127 (Suppl): S874–877.

Ivy, J. L., Katz, A. L., et al. "Muscle Glycogen Synthesis after Exercise: Effect of Time of Carbohydrate Ingestion," *J Appl Physiol* 1988; 64 (4):1480–85.

Kleiner, S. M. "The Role of Meat in an Athlete's Diet: Its Effect on Key Macro-and Micro Nutrients," *Sports Science Exchange #58* 8 (1995) Gatorade Sports Science Institute website.

Maughan, R. J., "Gastric Emptying During Exercise," *Sports Science Exchange #46* 6 (1993). Gatorade Sports Science Institute website.

———, Leiper, J. B., et al. "Rehydration and Recovery after Exercise," *Sports Science Exchange #62* 9 (1996). Gatorade Sports Science Institute website.

Mellion, M. B. ed. *The Team Physician's Handbook*. Philadelphia: Hanley and Belfus, 1997.

Messina, V., and Messina, M. *The Vegetarian Way*. New York: Crown Trade, 1996.

Millard-Stafford, M., Rosskopf, L. B., et al. "Water Versus Carbohydrate-Electrolyte Ingestion Before and During a 15-km Run in the Heat," *Int J Sports Nut* 7 (1997): 26–38.

Nattiv, A. "The Female Athlete Triad," *Phys Sportsmed* Online 1994; 22 (1).

———, Agostini, R., et al. "The Female Athlete Triad," *Clin Sports Med* 1994; 13 (2): 405–18.

Nicholas, C. W., Green, P. A., et al. "Carbohydrate Intake and Recovery of Intermittent Running Capacity," *Int J Sport Nut* 7 (1997): 251–60.

Pedersen, A. B., Bartholomew, M. J., et al. "Menstrual Differences Due to Vegetarian and Nonvegetarian Diets," *Am J Clin Nut* 53 (1991): 879–85.

Pendergast, D. R., Horvath, P. J., "The Role of Dietary Fat on Performance, Metabolism and Health," *Am J Sports Med* 1996; 24 (6 Suppl): S53–58.

Rajaram, S., Weaver, C. M., et al. "Effects of Long-Term Moderate Exercise on Iron Status in Young Women," *Med Sci Sports Exerc* 1995; 27 (8): 1105–1110.

Ryan, A. J., Chang, R., et al. "Gastrointestinal Permeability Following Aspirin Intake and Prolonged Running," *Med Sci Sports Exerc* 1996; 28 (6): 698–705.

Schwenk, T. L., "Psychoactive Drugs and Athletic Performance,". *Phys Sportsmed* Online. 1997; 25 (1).

Snow, R. C., Schneider, J. L., et al. "High Dietary Fiber and Low Saturated Fat Intake among Oligomenorrheic Undergraduates," *Fertil Steril* 54 (1990): 632–37.

Sundgot-Borgen, J. "Risk and Trigger Factors for the Development of Eating Disorders in Female Elite Athletes," *Med Sci Sports Exerc* 1994; 26 (4): 414–19.

Swain, R. A. "Exercise-Induced Diarrhea: When to Wonder," *Med Sci Sports Exerc* 1994; 26 (5): 523–26.

Tsintzas, O., Williams, C., et al. "Influence of Carbohydrate Supplementation Early in Exercise on Endurance Running Capacity," *Med Sci Sports Exerc* 1996; 28 (11): 1373–79.

Williams, M. H. *The Ergogenics Edge*. Champaign, Ill.: Human Kinetics, 1998.

Williams, N. I., and Young J. C. "Strenuous Exercise with Caloric Restriction: Effect on Luteinizing Hormone Secretion," *Med Sci Sports Exerc* 1995; 27 (10): 1390–98.

Wolinsky I. *Nutrition in Exercise and Sport*. Boca Raton, Fla.: CRC Press, 1998.

Yeager, K. K., Agostini, R., et al. "The Female Athlete Triad:

Disordered Eating, Amenorrhea, Osteoporosis," *Med Sci Sports Exerc* 1993; 25 (7): 775–77.

Zarkadas, P. C., Carter, J. B. "Taper Increases Performance and Aerobic Power in Triathletes," *Med Sci Sport Exerc* 1994; 26 (Suppl): abstract 194.

Chapter 3:   Your Skin, Hair, Feet . . .

Arendt, E. A. "Common Musculoskeletal Injuries in Women," *Phys Sportsmed* Online. 1996; 24 (7).

Basler, R. S. W, Basler, D. L, et al. "Cutaneous Injuries in Women Athletes," *Derm Nurs* 1998; 10 (1): 9–18.

Beck, J. L. "The Female Athlete's Knee," *Clin Sports Med* 1985; 4 (2); 345–66.

Frey, C. "Helping the Athletic Woman Find a Shoe That Fits," *J Musculoskel Med* 1998; 15 (3): 35–45.

Frey, C., Thompson, F., et al. "Update on Women's Footwear," *Foot & Ankl J* 1995; 16 (61): 328–31.

———. "American Orthopaedic Foot and Ankle Society Women's Shoe Survey," *Foot & Ankl J* 1993; 14 (2): 78–81.

Gehlsen, G., and Stoner, L. J. "The Female Breast in Sports and Exercise," *Med Sport Sci* 24 (1987) 13–22.

Huston, L. J. and Wojtys, E. M. "Neuromuscular Performance Characteristics in Elite Female Athletes," *Am J Sports Med* 1996; 24(4): 427–36.

Lawson, L., and Lorentzen, D. "Selected Sports Bras: Comparisons of Comfort and Support," *Clothing and Textiles Res J.* 1990 8 (4): 55–60.

Leshaw, S.M. "Itching in Active Patients: Causes and Cures," *Phys Sportsmed* Online 1998; 26 (1).

Mahler, D. A. "Exercise-Induced Asthma," *Med Sci Sports Exerc* 1993 25 (5): 554–61.

Martin D. R. "Athletic Shoes: Finding a Good Match," *Phys Sportsmed* Online. 1997; 25 (9).

———. "How to Steer Patients Toward the Right Sport Shoe," *Phys Sportsmed* Online 1997; 25 (9).

Matheson, G. O., Clement D. B., et al. "Stress Fractures in Athletes: A Study of 320 Cases," *Am J Sports Med* 15(1987): 46–58.

Maves, K. K., and Weiler, J. M. "Running and Wheezing: The Athlete with Asthma," *Pharm Times.* June 1993: 31–39.

Moeller, J. L., and Lamb, M. M. "Anterior Cruciate Ligament Injuries in Female Athletes: Why Are Women More Susceptible?," *Phys Sportsmed* online 1997; 25 (4).

Mujika, I., Busso, T., et al. "Modeled Responses to Training and

Taper in Competitive Swimmers," *Med Sci Sports Exerc* 1996; 28 (2): 251–58.

Novick, N. L. *You Can Do Something About Your Allergies.* New York: Macmillan, 1994.

Pharis, D. B., Teller, C., et al. "Cutaneous Manifestations of Sports Participation," *JAm Acad Derm* 1997; 36 (3): 448–59.

Potera, C. "Help Patients Get Serious About Sunscreens," *Phys Sportsmed* Online 1997; 25(5).

Ramsey, M. L. "Avoiding and Treating Blisters," *Phys Sportsmed* Online 1997; 25 (12).

Ramsey, M. L. "Pitted Keratolysis: A Common Infection of Active Feet," *Phys Sportsmed* Online 1996; 24 (10).

———. "Skin Care for Active People." *Phys Sportsmed* Online 1997; 25 (3).

Savin, R. C., and Donofrio, L. M. "Aggressive Acne Treatment: As Simple as One, Two, Three?" *Phys Sportsmed* Online 1996; 24 (24).

Stamford, B. "Sports Bras and Briefs: Choosing Good Athletic Support," *Phys Sportsmed* Online 1996; 24 (12).

Chapter 4:   Your Mind and Emotions

Burfoot, A. "The Brain Connection," *Runner's World* 1994; 29(8): 70.

Curtis, J. D. *The Mindset for Winning,* La Crosse, Wisc: Coulee Press, 1991.

Evans, L., and Hardy, L. "Sport Injury and Grief Responses: A Review," *J Sport & Exerc Psych* 17 (1995): 227–45.

Gould, D., and Udry, E. "Psychological Skills for Enhancing Performance: Arousal Regulation Strategies," *Med Sci Sports Exerc* 1994; 26 (4): 478–85.

Hooper, S. L., Mackinnon, L. T., et al. "Markers for Monitoring Overtraining and Recovery," *Med Sci Sports Exerc* 1995; 27 (1): 106–12.

Kyllo, B.L. and Landers, D. M., "Goal Setting in Sport and Exercise: A Research Synthesis to Resolve the Controversy," *J Sport & Exerc Psych* 17 (1995): 117–37.

Lehmann, M., Foster, C., et al. "Overtraining in Endurance Athletes: A Brief Review," *Med Sci Sports Exerc* 1993; 25 (7): 854–863.

Mechikoff, R. A. *Sport Psychology for Women.* New York: Harper & Row, 1987.

Mondin, G. W., Morgan, W. P., et al. "Psychological Consequences of Exercise Deprivation in Habitual Exercisers," *Med Sci Sports Exerc* 1996; 28 (9): 1199–1203.

Morgan, W. P., "Mind Games: The Psychology of Sport," *Perspectives in Exercise Science and Sports Medicine* 10 (1997): 1–62.

————. "Psychological Components of Effort Sense," *Med Sci Sports Exerc* 1994; 26 (9): 1071–77.

Murphy, S. M., "Imagery Interventions in Sport," *Med Sci Sports Exerc* 1994; 26 (4): 486–94.

Raglin, J. S., Koceja, D. M, et al. "Mood, Neuromuscular Function, and Performance During Training in Female Swimmers," *Med Sci Sports Exerc* 1996; 28 (3): 372–77.

Singer, R. N., Murphey, M., et al. *Handbook of Research on Sport Psychology.* New York: Macmillan, 1993.

Syer, J., and Connolly, C. *Sporting Body, Sporting Mind.* New York: Cambridge University Press, 1984.

Thaston, L. "Physiological and Psychological Effects of Short-term Exercise Addiction on Habitual Runners," *J Sport Psychol* 4 (1982): 73–80.

Turner, P. E., and Raglin, J. S. "Variability in Precompetition Anxiety and Performance in College Track and Field Athletes," *Med Sci Sports Exerc* 1996; 28 (3): 378–385.

Van Raalte, J. L., Brewer, B. W., et al. "The Relationship Between Observable Self-Talk and Competitive Junior Tennis Players' Match Performances," *J Sport & Exerc Psych* 16 (1994): 400–415.

Vealy, R. S. "Current Status and Prominent Issues in Sport Psychology Interventions," *Med Sci Sports Exerc* 1994; 26 (4): 495–502.

Weinberg, R. S. "Goal Setting and Performance in Sport and Exercise Settings: A Synthesis and Critique," *Med Sci Sports Exerc* 1994; 26 (4): 469–77.

Wischnia, B. "Comeback at Comrades," *Runner's World* 1994; 29 (8): 76.

Chapter 5: Your Pregnancy

American Academy of Pediatrics. "Breastfeeding and the Use of Human Milk," *Pediatrics* 1997; 100 (6): 1035–39.

Araugo, D. "Expecting Questions About Exercise and Pregnancy?," *Phys Sportsmed* Online 1997; 25 (4).

Artal, R., Wiswell, R., et al. "Pulmonary Response to Exercise in Pregnancy," *Am J Obstet Gynecol* 154 (1986): 378–83.

Camporesi, E. M. "Diving and Pregnancy," *Semin Perinat* 1996; 20 (4): 292–302.

Carey, G. B., Quinn, T. J., et al. "Breast Milk Composition after Exercise of Different Intensities," *J Hum Lact* 1997; 13 (2): 115–20.

Clapp, J. F. "Morphometric and Neurodevelopmental Outcome at Age Five Years of the Offspring of Women Who Continued to Exercise Regularly Throughout Pregnancy," *J Pediatr* 129 (1996): 856–63.

————"Pregnancy Outcome: Physical Activities Inside Versus Outside the Workplace," *Semin Perinat* 1996; 20 (1): 70–76.

————"The Changing Thermal Response to Endurance Exercise During Pregnancy," *Am J Obstet Gynecol* 165 (1991): 1684-9.

————"The Course of Labor after Endurance Exercise During Pregnancy," *A J Obstet Gynecol* 163 (1990): 1799–805.

————and Capeless, E. "The Changing Glycemic Response to Exercise During Pregnancy," *Am J Obstet Gynecol* 165 (1991): 1678–83.

————. "The VO2max of Recreational Athletes Before and After Exercise," *Med Sci Sports Exerc* 1991; 23 (10):1128–33.

————and Little, K. D. "Effect of Recreational Exercise on Pregnancy Weight Gain and Subcutaneous Fat Deposition," *Med Sci Sports Exerc.* 1995; 27 (2): 170–77.

————and Rizk, K. H. "Effect of Recreational Exercise on Midtrimester Placental Growth," *Am J Obstet Gynecol* 167 (1992): 1518–21.

————, Rokey, R, et al. "Exercise in Pregnancy," *Med Sci Sports Exerc* 1992; 24 (6 suppl): S294–300.

————, Simonian, S, et al. "The One-Year Morphometric and Neurodevelopmental Outcome of the Offspring of Women Who Continued to Exercise Regularly Throughout Pregnancy," *Am J Obstet Gynecol* 178 (1998): 594–9.

Dewey, K. G. "Effects of Maternal Caloric Restriction and Exercise During Lactation," *J Nut* 1998; 128 (2 Suppl): S386–89.

————, Lovelady, C. A., et al. "A Randomized Study of the Effects of Aerobic Exercise by Lactating Women on Breast-Milk Volume and Composition," *N Eng J Med* 330 (1994): 449–53.

Hale, R.W., and Milne, L. "The Elite Athlete and Exercise in Pregnancy," *Semin Perinat* 1996; 20(4): 277–84.

Hatch, M. C., Shu X., et al. "Maternal Exercise During Pregnancy, Physical Fitness, and Fetal Growth," *Am J Epidemiol* 137 (1993): 1105–1114.

Horns, P. N., Ratcliffe, L. P., et al. "Pregnancy Outcomes Among Active and Sedentary Primiparous Women," *J Obstet Gynecol Neonatal Nurs* 1996; 25 (1): 49–54.

Hotoum, N., Clapp, J. F., et al. "Effects of Maternal Exercise on Fetal Activity in Late Gestation," *J Matern Fetal Med* 1997; 6 (3): 134–39.

Huch, R. "Physical Activity at Altitude in Pregnancy," *Semin Perinat* 1996; 20 (4): 303–14.

Jones, R. L., Botti, J. J., et al. "Thermoregulation During Aerobic Exercise in Pregnancy," *Obstet Gynecol* 65 (1985): 340–45.

Kardel, K. R., and Kase, T. "Training in Pregnant Women: Effects on Fetal Development and Birth," *Am J Obstet Gynecol* 178 (1998): 280–86.

Katx, J. *Water Fitness During Your Pregnancy*. Champaign, Ill.: Human Kinetics, 1995.

Katz, V. L. "Water Exercise in Pregnancy," *Semin Perinat* 1996; 20 (4): 285–91.

Koltyn, K. F., and Schultes, S. S. "Psychological Effects of an Aerobic Exercise Session and a Rest Session Following Pregnancy," *J Sports Med Phys Fitness* 1997; 37 (4): 287–91.

Lokey, E. A., Tran, Z. V., et al. "Effects of Physical Exercise on Pregnancy Outcomes : A Meta-Analytic Review," *Med Sci Sports Exerc* 1991; 23(11): 1234–39.

Lovelady, C. A, Lonnerdal, B., et al. "Lactation Performance of Exercising Women," *Am J Clin Nutr* 52 (1990): 103–109.

———, Nommsen-Rivers, L. A., et al. "Effects of Exercise on Plasma Lipids and Metabolism of Lactating Women," *Med Sci Sports Exerc* 1995; 27 (1): 22–28.

McMurray, R. G., Hackney, A. C., et al. "Metabolic and Hormonal Responses to Low-Impact Aerobic Dance During Pregnancy," *Med Sci Sports Exerc* 1996; 28 (1): 41–46.

———, Mottola, M. F., et al. "Recent Advances in Understanding Maternal and Fetal Responses to Exercise," *Med Sci Sports Exerc* 1993; 25 (12): 1305–21.

Mottola, M. F. "The Use of Animal Models in Exercise and Pregnancy Research," *Semin Perinat* 1996; 20 (4): 222–31.

Penttinen J., and Erkkola R. "Pregnancy in Endurance Athletes," *Scand J Med Sci Sports* 1997; 7 (4): 226–28.

Ohtake, P. J. and Wolfe, L. A. "Physical Conditioning Attenuates Respiratory Responses to Steady-State Exercise in Late Gestation," *Med Sci Sports Exerc* 1998 30 (1):17–27.

Pivarnik, J. M. "Cardiovascular Responses to Aerobic Exercise During Pregnancy and Postpartum," *Semin Perintal* 1996; 20(4): 242–49.

———. "Potential Effects of Maternal Physical Activity on Birth Weight: Brief Review," *Med Sci Sports Exerc* 1998; 30 (3): 400–406.

———, Ayres, N. A, et al. "Effects of Maternal Aerobic Fitness on Cardiorespiratory Responses to Exercise," *Med Sci Sports Exerc* 1993; 25 (9): 993–98.

Soultanakis H.N., Artal R., et al. "Prolonged Exercise in Pregnancy: Glucose, Homeostasis, Ventilatory and Cardiovascular Responses," *Semin Perinat.* 1996; 20 (4): 315-27.

Sternfeld, B. "Physical Activity and Pregnancy Outcome," *Sports Med* 1997; 23 (1): 33–47.

Sternfeld, B., Quesenberry, C. P., et al. "Exercise During Pregnancy and Pregnancy Outcome," *Med Sci Sports Exerc* 1995; 27 (5): 634–40.

Veille, J., Hohimer, A. R., et al. "The Effect of Exercise on Uterine

Activity in the Last Eight Weeks of Pregnancy," *Am J Obstet Gynecol* 151 1985: 727–30.

Wolfe, L. A., Walker, R. M. C., et al. "Effects of Pregnancy and Chronic Exercise on Respiratory Responses to Graded Exercise," *J Appl Physiol* 1994; 76 (5): 1928–36.

Chapter 6: What to Expect as You Age

Blair, S. N., Kampert, J. B., et al. "Influences of Cardiorespiratory Fitness and Other Precursors on Cardiovascular Disease and All-Cause Mortality in Men and Women," *JAMA* 1996; 276 (3): 205–10.

Davy, K. P., Evans, S. L., et al. "Adiposity and Regional Body Fat Distribution in Physically Active Young and Middle-Aged Women," *Int J Obes Relat Metab Disord* 1996; 20 (8): 777–83.

DiPietro, L. "The Epidemiology of Physical Activity and Physical Function in Older People," *Med Sci Sports Exerc* 1996; 28 (5): 596–600.

Dook, J. E., James C., et al. "Exercise and Bone Mineral Density in Mature Female Athletes," *Med Sci Sports Exerc* 1997; 29 (3):291-96.

Douglas, P. S., Clarkson, T. B., et al. "Exercise and Atherosclerotic Heart Disease in Women," *Med Sci Sports Exerc* 1992; 24 (6 suppl): S266–76.

Douglas, P. S., and O'Toole, M. "Aging and Physical Activity Determine Cardiac Structure and Function in the Older Athlete," *J Appl Physiol* 1992; 72 (5): 1969-73.

Eastall, R. "Treatment of Postmenopausal Osteoporosis," *NEJM* 1998; 338 (11): 736–46.

Erickson, S. M., and Sevier, T. L. "Osteoporosis in Active Women: Prevention, Diagnosis and Treatment," *Phys Sportsmed* Online 1997; 25 (11).

Frisch, R. E., Wyshak G., et al. "Lower Prevalence of Diabetes in Female Former College Athletes Compared with Nonathletes," Diabetes 1986; 35 (10): 1101–1105.

———. "Lower Lifetime Occurrence of Breast Cancer and Cancers of the Reproductive System Among Former College Athletes," *Am J Clin Nutr* 45 (1987): 328–35.

Gutin B., and Kasper, M. J. "Can Vigorous Exercise Play a Role in Osteoporosis Prevention? A Review," *Osteoporos Int* 1992; 2 (2): 55–69.

Hammar, M., Berg G., et al. "Does Physical Exercise Influence the Frequency of Postmenopausal Hot Flushes?," *Acta Obstet Gynecol Scand* 69 (1990): 409–412.

Hargarten, K. M. "Menopause: How Exercise Mitigates Symptoms," *Phys Sportsmed* Online 1994; 48.

Jackson, A. S., Wier, L. T., et al. "Changes in Aerobic Power of Women, Ages 20–64 Yr.," *Med Sci Sports Exerc* 1996; 228 (7): 884–91.

Kohrt, W. M., Malley, M. T., et al. "Effects of Gender, Age, and Fitness Level on Response of VO2 max to Training in 60–71-yr-olds," *J Appl Physiol* 1991; 71 (5): 2004-2011.

Kramer, M. M., and Wells, C. L. "Does Physical Activity Reduce Risk of Estrogen-Dependent Cancer in Women?," *Med Sci Sports Exerc* 1996; 28(3): 322–34.

Kushi, L. H., Fee, R. M., et al. "Physical activity and mortality in postmenopausal women," *JAMA* 1997; 277 (16): 1287–92.

Landau, C., Cyr, M. G., and Moulton, A. W. *The Complete Book of Menopause*. New York: Perigee Books, 1995.

Love, S. *Dr. Susan Love's Hormone Book*. New York: Random House, 1997.

Martinez, M. E., Giovannuci E., et al. "Lesiure-Time Physical Activity, Body Size, and Colon Cancer in Women," *J Natl Cancer Inst* 1997; 89 (13): 948–55.

Morganti, C. M., Nelson, M. E., et al. "Strength Improvements with 1 yr of Progressive Resistance Training in Older Women," *Med Sci Sports Exerc* 1995; 27 (6): 906–912.

Nelson, M. E., Fiatarone, M. A., et al. "Effects of High-Intensity Strength Training on Multiple-Risk Factors for Osteoporotic Fractures," *JAMA* 1994; 272 (24): 1909–1914.

Ryan, A. S., Nicklas, B. J., et al. "A Cross-Sectional Study on Body Composition and Energy Expenditure in Women Athletes During Aging," *Am J Physiol* 271 (1996): 916–21.

Seiler, K. S., Spirduso, W. W., et al. "Gender Differences in Rowing Performance and Power with Aging," *Med Sci Sports Exerc* 1998; 30(1): 121–27.

Siscovick, D. S., Fried L., et al. "Exercise Intensity and Subclinical Cardiovascular Disease in the Elderly," *Am J Epidemiol* 1997; 145 (11): 977–86.

Tanaka, H., and Seals, D. R. "Age and Gender Interactions in Physiological Functional Capacity: Insight from Swimming Performance," *J Appl Physiol* 1997; 82 (3): 846–51.

Tang, M. X., Jacobs, D., et al. "Effect of Oestrogen During Menopause on Risk and Age at Onset of Alzheimer's Disease," *Lancet* 1996; 348 (9025): 429–32.

Thune, I., Brenn, T., et al. "Physical Activity and the Risk of Breast Cancer," *NEJM* 1977; 336(18): 1269–75.

Willett, W. C., Manson, J. E., et al. "Weight, Weight Change, and Coronary Heart Disease in Women," *JAMA* 1995; 273(6): 461–65.

Wood, P. D. "Exercise and Lipids," *Am J Sports Med* 1996; 24 (6 Suppl): S59–60.

Yamanouchi, K., Nakajima, H., et al. "Effects of Daily Physical Activity on Insulin Action in the Elderly," *J Appl Physiol* 1992; 73 (6): 2241–45.

Part Two: Your Sports Resource

Craib, M. W., Mitchell, V. A., et al. "The Association Between Flexibility and Running Economy in Sub-Elite Male Distance Runners," *Med Sci Sports Exerc* 1996; 28 (6): 737–43.

Flynn, M. G., Carroll, K. K., et al. "Cross Training: Indices of Training Stress and Performance," *Med Sci Sports Exerc* 1998; 30 (2): 294–300.

Hickson, R. C., et al. "Potential for Strength and Endurance Training to Amplify Endurance Performance," *J Appl Physiol* 1988 Nov; 65 (5): 2285–90.

Lindsay, F. H., Hawley, J. A., et al. "Improved Athletic Performance in Highly Trained Cyclists After Interval Training," *Med Sci Sports Exerc* 1996; 28 (11): 1427–34.

Marcinik E. J., Potts J., et al. "Effects of Strength Training on Lactate Threshold and Endurance Performance," *Med Sci Sports Exerc* 1991; 23 (6): 739–43.

McFarland, E. G., and Wasik M. "Injuries in Female Collegiate Swimmers Due to Swimming and Cross Training," *Clin J Sport Med* 1996; 6(3): 178–82.

Potera, C. "Cross-Training Can Lead to Injuries," *Phys Sportsmed* Online 1997; 25 (9).

Index

Page numbers in italics indicate sidebars.